Bladder Cancer

Editor

JOAQUIM BELLMUNT

HEMATOLOGY/ONCOLOGY CLINICS OF NORTH AMERICA

www.hemonc.theclinics.com

Consulting Editors
GEORGE P. CANELLOS
H. FRANKLIN BUNN

April 2015 • Volume 29 • Number 2

ELSEVIER

1600 John F. Kennedy Boulevard • Suite 1800 • Philadelphia, Pennsylvania, 19103-2899

http://www.theclinics.com

HEMATOLOGY/ONCOLOGY CLINICS OF NORTH AMERICA Volume 29, Number 2
April 2015 ISSN 0889-8588, ISBN 13: 978-0-323-35976-4

Editor: Jessica McCool
Developmental Editor: Stephanie Wissler

Hematology/Oncology Clinics (ISSN 0889-8588) is published bimonthly by Elsevier Inc., 360 Park Avenue South, New York, NY 10010-1710. Months of issue are February, April, June, August, October, and December. Business and Editorial Offices: 1600 John F. Kennedy Blvd., Ste. 1800, Philadelphia, PA 19103—2899. Customer Service Office: 3251 Riverport Lane, Maryland Heights, MO 63043. Periodicals postage paid at New York, NY and at additional mailing offices. Subscription prices are $385.00 per year (domestic individuals), $633.00 per year (domestic institutions), $190.00 per year (domestic students/residents), $440.00 per year (Canadian individuals), $783.00 per year (Canadian institutions) $520.00 per year (international individuals), $783.00 per year (international institutions), and $255.00 per year (international and Canadian students/residents). International air speed delivery is included in all *Clinics* subscription prices. All prices are subject to change without notice. **POSTMASTER:** Send address changes to *Hematology/Oncology Clinics of North America*, Elsevier Health Sciences Division, Subscription Customer Service, 3251 Riverport Lane, Maryland Heights, MO 63043. Customer Service (orders, claims, online, change of address): Elsevier Health Sciences Division, Subscription Customer Service, 3251 Riverport Lane, Maryland Heights, MO 63043. Tel: 1-800-654-2452 (U.S. and Canada); 314-447-8871 (outside U.S. and Canada). Fax: 314-447-8029. E-mail: journalscustomerservice-usa@elsevier.com (for print support); journalsonlinesupport-usa@elsevier.com (for online support).

Reprints. For copies of 100 or more, of articles in this publication, please contact the Commercial Reprints Department, Elsevier Inc., 360 Park Avenue South, New York, New York 10010-1710; Tel.: 212-633-3874, Fax: 212-633-3820, E-mail: reprints@elsevier.com.

Hematology/Oncology Clinics of North America is covered in *MEDLINE/PubMed (Index Medicus), EMBASE/ Excerpta Medica, and BIOSIS.*

Contributors

CONSULTING EDITORS

GEORGE P. CANELLOS, MD
William Rosenberg Professor of Medicine, Department of Medical Oncology, Dana-Farber Cancer Institute, Boston, Massachusetts

H. FRANKLIN BUNN, MD
Professor of Medicine, Division of Hematology, Brigham and Women's Hospital, Harvard Medical School, Boston, Massachusetts

EDITOR

JOAQUIM BELLMUNT, MD, PhD
Director, Bladder Cancer Center, Dana-Farber Cancer Institute, Dana-Farber/Brigham and Women's Cancer Center; Associate Professor, Harvard Medical School, Boston, Massachusetts

AUTHORS

WASSIM ABIDA, MD, PhD
Fellow, Genitourinary Oncology Service, Department of Medicine, Memorial Sloan Kettering Cancer, New York, New York

TOM J.H. ARENDS, MD
Department of Urology, RadboudUMC, Nijmegen, The Netherlands

HARM C. ARENTSEN, MD, PhD
Department of Urology, RadboudUMC, Nijmegen, The Netherlands

DEAN F. BAJORIN, MD
Attending, Genitourinary Oncology Service, Department of Medicine, Memorial Sloan Kettering Cancer, New York, New York

JOAQUIM BELLMUNT, MD, PhD
Director, Bladder Cancer Center, Dana-Farber Cancer Institute, Dana-Farber/Brigham and Women's Cancer Center; Associate Professor, Harvard Medical School, Boston, Massachusetts

RICHARD CATHOMAS, MD
Division of Oncology/Hematology, Kantonsspital Graubünden, Chur, Switzerland

STEVEN L. CHANG, MD, MS
Department of Urology, Bladder Cancer Center, Dana-Farber/Brigham and Women's Cancer Center; Assistant Professor of Surgery, Division of Urology, Center for Surgery and Public Health, Brigham and Women's Hospital, Harvard Medical School, Boston, Massachusetts

WOONYOUNG CHOI, PhD
Departments of Urology and Cancer Biology, U.T. M.D. Anderson Cancer Center, Houston, Texas

TONI K. CHOUEIRI, MD
Dana Farber Cancer Institute, Boston, Massachusetts

BOGDAN CZERNIAK, MD, PhD
Department of Pathology, U.T. M.D. Anderson Cancer Center, Houston, Texas

MARIA DE SANTIS, MD
Ludwig Boltzmann Institute for Applied Cancer Research (LBI-ACR VIEnna) - LBCTO, 3rd Medical Department, Centre for Oncology and Haematology, Kaiser Franz Josef Hospital, Vienna, Austria

COLIN P.N. DINNEY, MD
Department of Urology, U.T. M.D. Anderson Cancer Center, Houston, Texas

JASON A. EFSTATHIOU, MD, DPhil
Associate Professor, Department of Radiation Oncology, Massachusetts General Hospital, Harvard Medical School, Boston, Massachusetts

ANDRÉ P. FAY, MD
Bladder Cancer Center, Dana-Farber/Brigham and Women' s Cancer Center, Harvard Medical School, Boston, Massachusetts

MATTHEW D. GALSKY, MD
Associate Professor of Medicine, Director of Genitourinary Medical Oncology, The Tisch Cancer Institute, Icahn School of Medicine at Mount Sinai, New York, New York

LAUREN C. HARSHMAN, MD
Lank Center for Genitourinary Oncology, Dana-Farber Cancer Institute, Harvard Medical School, Boston, Massachusetts

ASHESH B. JANI, MD, MSEE
Professor, Department of Radiation Oncology, Emory University, Atlanta, Georgia

BENJAMIN S. JONES, MD
University of Alabama at Birmingham (UAB) Comprehensive Cancer Center, Birmingham, Alabama

ASHISH M. KAMAT, MD, MBBS, FACS
The University of Texas MD Anderson Cancer Center, Houston, Texas

ADAM S. KIBEL, MD
Professor, Division of Urology, Brigham and Women's Hospital, Harvard Medical School, Boston, Massachusetts

DAVID J. KWIATKOWSKI, MD, PhD
Professor of Medicine, Senior Physician, Department of Medicine, Brigham and Women's Hospital, Harvard Medical School, Boston, Massachusetts

JEFFREY J. LEOW, MBBS, MPH
Department of Urology, Bladder Cancer Center, Dana-Farber/Brigham and Women's Cancer Center; Division of Urology, Center for Surgery and Public Health, Brigham and Women's Hospital, Harvard Medical School, Boston, Massachusetts; Department of Urology, Tan Tock Seng Hospital, Singapore

SETH P. LERNER, MD
Professor, Beth and Dave Swalm Chair in Urologic Oncology, Scott Department of Urology; Director of Urologic Oncology; Director of the Multidisciplinary Bladder Cancer Program; Faculty Group Practice Medical Director, Baylor College of Medicine Medical Center, Houston, Texas

ILARIA LUCCA, MD
Department of Urology, Comprehensive Cancer Center, Medical University of Vienna, Vienna General Hospital, Vienna, Austria; Department of Urology, Centre Hospitalier Universitaire Vaudois, Lausanne, Switzerland

NÚRIA MALATS, MD, PhD, MPH
Genetic and Molecular Epidemiology Group, Spanish National Cancer Research Centre (CNIO), Madrid, Spain

WILLIAM MARTIN-DOYLE, MD, MPH
Resident Physician, Department of Medicine, Brigham and Women's Hospital, Harvard Medical School, Boston, Massachusetts

DAVID J. McCONKEY, PhD
Professor and Director of Urologic Research, Departments of Urology and Cancer Biology, U.T. M.D. Anderson Cancer Center, Houston, Texas

STEPHANIE A. MULLANE, BS
Bladder Cancer Center, Dana-Farber/Brigham and Women's Cancer Center, Harvard Medical School, Boston, Massachusetts

SUJATA NARAYANAN, MD
Department of Medicine, Stanford University School of Medicine, Stanford, California

ANDREA OCHOA, BS
Departments of Urology and Cancer Biology, U.T. M.D. Anderson Cancer Center, Houston, Texas

ANNA ORSOLA, MD, PhD
Bladder Cancer Center, Dana Farber Cancer Institute, Harvard Medical School, Boston, Massachusetts

JOAN PALOU, MD, PhD
Urology Department, Fundacio Puigvert, Barcelona, Spain

MARK A. PRESTON, MD, MPH
Instructor in Surgery, Harvard Medical School; Division of Urology, Brigham and Women's Hospital, Boston, Massachusetts

FRANCISCO X. REAL, MD, PhD
Epithelial Carcinogenesis Group, Spanish National Cancer Research Centre (CNIO), Madrid, Spain; Department of Experimental and Health Sciences, Universitat Pompeu Fabra, Barcelona, Spain

JONATHAN E. ROSENBERG, MD
Associate Attending, Genitourinary Oncology Service, Department of Medicine, Memorial Sloan Kettering Cancer Center, New York, New York

SHAHROKH F. SHARIAT, MD
Professor and Chairman, Department of Urology, Comprehensive Cancer Center, Medical University of Vienna, Vienna General Hospital, Vienna, Austria; Adjunct Professor, Department of Urology, University of Texas Southwestern Medical Center, Dallas, Texas; Adjunct Professor of Urology and Medical Oncology, Department of Urology, Weill Cornell Medical College, New York-Presbyterian Hospital, Cornell University, New York, New York

WILLIAM U. SHIPLEY, MD, FACR
Professor, Department of Radiation Oncology, Massachusetts General Hospital, Harvard Medical School, Boston, Massachusetts

ARLENE SIEFKER-RADTKE, MD
Department of Genitourinary Medical Oncology, U.T. M.D. Anderson Cancer Center, Houston, Texas

EDUARDO SOLSONA, MD, PhD
Urology Department, Instituto Valenciano de Oncologia, Calle del Profesor Beltrán Bàguena, València, Spain

GURU SONPAVDE, MD
University of Alabama at Birmingham (UAB) Comprehensive Cancer Center, Birmingham, Alabama

SANDY SRINIVAS, MD
Department of Medicine, Stanford University School of Medicine, Stanford, California

CORA N. STERNBERG, MD
Chief, Department of Medical Oncology, San Camillo Forlanini Hospital, Rome, Italy

MAXINE SUN, PhD
Cancer Prognostics and Health Outcomes Unit, University of Montreal Health Center, Montreal, Canada

QUOC-DIEN TRINH, MD
Division of Urologic Surgery, Center for Surgery and Public Health, Brigham and Women's Hospital, Harvard Medical School, Boston, Massachusetts

YME WEIJERS, MD
Department of Urology, RadboudUMC, Nijmegen, The Netherlands

DANIEL WILLIS, MD, FACS
The University of Texas MD Anderson Cancer Center, Houston, Texas

J. ALFRED WITJES, MD, PhD
Department of Urology, RadboudUMC, Nijmegen, The Netherlands

Contents

Bladder cancer incidence is higher in old men, shows geographic variation, and is mostly an environmental disease. Cigarette smoking, occupational exposures, water arsenic, *Schistosoma haematobium* infestation, and some medications are the best established risk factors. Low-penetrance genetic factors also contribute to its origin, some through interaction with environmental factors. Bladder cancer has high prevalence and a low mortality, being largely a chronic disease. Data on environmental and genetic factors involved in the disease outcome are inconclusive.

Classic as well as more recent large-scale genomic analyses have uncovered multiple genes and pathways important for bladder cancer development. Genes involved in cell-cycle control, chromatin regulation, and receptor tyrosine and PI3 kinase-mammalian target of rapamycin signaling pathways are commonly mutated in muscle-invasive bladder cancer. Expression-based analyses have identified distinct types of bladder cancer that are similar to subsets of breast cancer, and have prognostic and therapeutic significance. These observations are leading to novel therapeutic approaches in bladder cancer, providing optimism for therapeutic progress.

Bladder cancer (BCa) is a heterogeneous disease with a variable natural history. Most patients (70%) present with superficial tumors (stages Ta, T1, or carcinoma in situ). However, 3 out of 10 patients present with muscle-invasive disease (T2–4) with a high risk of death from distant metastases. Moreover, roughly between 50% and 70% of superficial tumors do recur, and approximately 10% to 20% of them progress to muscle-invasive disease. However, BCa has a relatively low ratio of mortality versus incidence of new cases. In consequence, there is the danger of overdiagnosis and overtreatment.

While UTUC is relatively uncommon, it has an aggressive natural history and poor prognosis, which has not substantially improved over the past two decades. Nevertheless, continued research has led to the discovery of risk factors improving the prevention and early detection of UTUC. Although RNU remains the standard treatment for localized invasive UTUC, nephron-sparing surgery for selected patients has made considerable progress in the recent years. The stagnation in the prognosis of UTUC over the past two decades highlights the necessity for incorporating multimodal approaches including refinements in systemic chemotherapy and radiotherapy to attain better outcomes for patients with UTUC.

Although cystectomy remains the standard for treatment of muscle-invasive bladder cancer in the United States, there exist potentially curative alternatives for a selected subset of these patients in organ preservation using concurrent chemotherapy with radiation following an aggressive transurethral resection of the tumor. Chemotherapy and radiotherapy in combination, with salvage cystectomy for invasive recurrence, have produced 10-year disease-specific survival rates of 60% to 65% with overall survival similar to that of cystectomy in selected patients. Fine-tuning of the chemoradiotherapy sequencing, timing, and fractionation has been reported in both single-center and cooperative group publications from North America and Europe.

Muscle invasive bladder cancer (MIBC) is an aggressive disease associated with poor survival rates. High rates of relapse, despite radical cystectomy, suggest that administration of systemic therapy in the perioperative period may improve clinical outcomes. Neoadjuvant treatment with cisplatin-based combination regimens is an established standard of care and has improved long-term survival in MIBC. As the use of neoadjuvant chemotherapy steadily increases, clinicians still need to decide about administering adjuvant chemotherapy to patients with high-risk disease. This review examines in detail the latest evidence available for both neoadjuvant and adjuvant chemotherapy, and highlights pertinent studies.

Metastatic urothelial carcinoma is primarily a disease of the elderly, with a median overall survival of approximately 15 months. Cisplatin-based combination chemotherapy is standard first-line treatment for eligible patients, with carboplatin-based regimens used as an alternative for patients considered unfit to receive cisplatin. Prognostic models incorporating clinical risk factors have been validated, and molecular characteristics that predict for treatment response are under investigation. This review summarizes the current status

for breast cancer. Each subtype is enriched with potentially clinically action-able genomic alterations and epigenetic signatures; there are associations between tumor subtype and sensitivity to conventional cisplatin-based chemotherapy. The authors review biological and clinical characteristics of the intrinsic subtypes and describe their implications for the development of conventional and targeted agents. The role that tumor plasticity seems to play in basal and luminal bladder cancer biology and its potential effects on the development of therapeutic resistance is also discussed.

HEMATOLOGY/ONCOLOGY
CLINICS OF NORTH AMERICA

ISSUE OF RELATED INTEREST

Urologic Clinics of North America, May 2014 (Vol. 41, Issue 2)
Early Detection of Prostate Cancer
Stacy Loeb and Matthew R. Cooperberg, *Editors*
Available at: http://www.urologic.theclinics.com/

VISIT THE CLINICS ONLINE!
Access your subscription at:
www.theclinics.com

NOW AVAILABLE FOR YOUR iPhone and iPad

Preface

Bladder Cancer

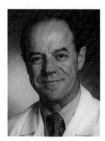

Joaquim Bellmunt, MD, PhD
Editor

After very little advancement in the last two decades, bladder cancer is back in the spotlight with the advent of new immunotherapy approaches and the comprehensive understanding of genetics with the Cancer Genome Atlas Project that provides insights to improve the therapeutic arsenal. Improvements in risk stratification and surgical advances have joined this progress too.

I am privileged and proud to be the editor of the present issue of *Hematology/ Oncology Clinics of North America*, which gathers an outstanding group of contributors from different backgrounds that share passion and commitment for urothelial tumors and that have made possible to put all these recent achievements into perspective.

The entire disease spectrum is covered throughout the different articles. Detailed and updated epidemiology/molecular epidemiology (see Real and Malats) and molecular biology (see Martin-Doyle and Kwiatkowski) for bladder cancer set the basis for a better diagnosis and staging (see Sun and Trinh). For non-muscle-invasive bladder cancer, newer data from individual patient data and meta-analysis set new cutoffs for progression that will eventually move into detailed nomograms that will help select patients for prompt cystectomy (see Weijers, Arentsen, Arends, and Witjes as well as Orsola, Palou, and Solsona). The role of molecular markers and the relevance and customized management for nonurothelial bladder cancer and rare variant histologies (see Willis and Kamat) are addressed from an expert approach.

To follow, we get into two major surgical articles written in extremely comprehensive language and filled with up-to-date novelties. For the new trends in the surgical management of invasive bladder cancer, Preston, Lerner, and Kibel have put together and updated data on the development of robotic-assisted radical cystectomy, the role of extended lymph node dissection, and the evidence supporting the role of Enhanced Recovery After Surgery protocols. All of these approaches are already making a difference in outcomes for the patients undergoing radical cystectomy. The second surgical article provides a comprehensive update on the management of upper urinary tract tumors (see Lucca, Leow, Shariat, and Chang). On the other side of the spectrum

Hematol Oncol Clin N Am 29 (2015) xiii–xiv
http://dx.doi.org/10.1016/j.hoc.2014.12.001
0889-8588/15/$ – see front matter © 2015 Elsevier Inc. All rights reserved.

and as an alternative to surgery in selected patient populations, options and strategies currently available for bladder preservation (see Jani, Efstathiou, and Shipley) are thoroughly described by the best outstanding experts in the field.

Moving along to the management of muscle-invasive disease, nomograms have been developed to predict relapse-free survival more accurately and to help in identifying patients who are the best candidates for neoadjuvant therapy or who might benefit from adjuvant therapy (see Leow, Fay, Mullane, and Bellmunt). The retrospective genomic analysis of the extreme response phenotype (patient obtaining a complete pathologic response [pT0] when receiving neoadjuvant chemotherapy) has made possible the finding of the ERCC2 mutations predicting an exquisite sensitivity to cisplatin-based chemotherapy. The proactive implementation of translational end points in prospective trial design like the Coxen model, together with additional prediction models in both precystectomy and postcystectomy settings, should improve our ability to choose the most efficacious perioperative treatment. The authors present in their article an unbiased and detailed review of the evidence for both neoadjuvant and adjuvant therapy useful for practical clinical application.

Finally, in the metastatic setting, Abida, Bajorin, and Rosenberg summarize the first-line treatment and prognostic factors of metastatic bladder cancer for platinum-eligible patients, depicting the promising future in this setting. For cisplatin-ineligible patients, a comprehensive update of options—recently reported in first line—are presented in the article by Cathomas, Santis, and Galsky. The management of subsequent second-line therapeutic options and a discussion on emerging new therapies are scholarly addressed by Narayanan, Harshman, and Srinivas.

This issue of *Hematology/Oncology Clinics of North America* wraps up with two strong insights into the future of urothelial cancer: the role of recently described targeted therapies in conjunction with the new immunotherapy approaches (Sonpavde, Jones, Bellmunt, Choueiri, and Sternberg) and the new therapeutic opportunities that emerge with the description of the intrinsic subtypes of muscle-invasive bladder cancer based on the analysis of gene expression (McConkey and Dinney).

I hope this work will be enjoyed by many and will help put a twenty-first-century perspective on all the knowledge generated to date.

Joaquim Bellmunt, MD, PhD
Director, Bladder Cancer Center
Dana-Farber Cancer Institute, Dana-Farber/Brigham and Women's Cancer Center
Associate Professor, Harvard Medical School
450 Brookline Ave., Boston, MA 02215, USA

E-mail address:
Joaquim_bellmunt@dfci.harvard.edu

Erratum

In the April 2014 issue (Volume 28, number 2), in the article "The Role of Adenosine Signaling in Sickle Cell Therapeutics," a potential conflict of interest for co-author Joel Linden was inadvertently omitted. Please note that Joel Linden, Ph.D. is an inventor on a patent issued to the University of Virginia, which claims the use of adenosine A2A agonists for the treatment of sickle cell disease; he owns shares in Adenosine Therapeutics LLC, which licensed this patent.

Hematol Oncol Clin N Am 29 (2015) xv
http://dx.doi.org/10.1016/j.hoc.2014.12.002
0889-8588/15/$ – see front matter © 2015 Elsevier Inc. All rights reserved.

hemonc.theclinics.com

Epidemiology of Bladder Cancer

Núria Malats, MD, PhD, MPH[a],*, Francisco X. Real, MD, PhD[b,c]

KEYWORDS

- Bladder cancer • Urothelium • Incidence and prevalence • Smoking
- Occupational risk factors • Arsenic • Genetic susceptibility

KEY POINTS

- Bladder cancer incidence increases with age, is higher in men, and is a major burden to the health systems because of the chronic nature of the most common non–muscle-invasive tumors.
- Cigarette smoking, occupational exposures, arsenic, *Schistosoma haematobium* infection, some medications, and genetic variation are the major risk factors associated with the disease.
- Further evidences are needed to establish the role of disinfection byproducts, fluid intake, urinary tract infections, diabetes, metabolic syndrome, viruses, and medications in bladder cancer.
- *GSTM1*-null and *NAT2* slow acetylator genotypes are associated with modest increase in risk; other low-penetrance genetic susceptibility loci have been identified but are not yet of clinical utility.
- Further work is needed to establish the role of environmental and genetic factors in patient outcome; the effect of smoking cessation strategies should be tested prospectively.

THE BURDEN OF THE DISEASE

Bladder cancer is mainly a disease of aging; its incidence and prevalence increase around the sixth decade and peak in the seventh to eighth decade of life. It is the ninth most common cancer, with 430,000 new cases diagnosed in 2012 worldwide; on average it is 3 to 4 times more common in men than in women. Incidence rates are highest in Europe, the United States, and Egypt (**Fig. 1**).[1,2] Substantial variation exists in the incidence of bladder cancer worldwide, because of differences not only in origin, mainly smoking, but also in registration.[3]

The authors have nothing to disclose.
[a] Genetic and Molecular Epidemiology Group, Spanish National Cancer Research Centre (CNIO), Madrid 28029, Spain; [b] Epithelial Carcinogenesis Group, Spanish National Cancer Research Centre (CNIO), Madrid 28029, Spain; [c] Department of Experimental and Health Sciences, Universitat Pompeu Fabra, Barcelona 08003, Spain
* Corresponding author.
E-mail address: nuria@cnio.es

Hematol Oncol Clin N Am 29 (2015) 177–189
http://dx.doi.org/10.1016/j.hoc.2014.10.001
0889-8588/15/$ – see front matter © 2015 Elsevier Inc. All rights reserved.

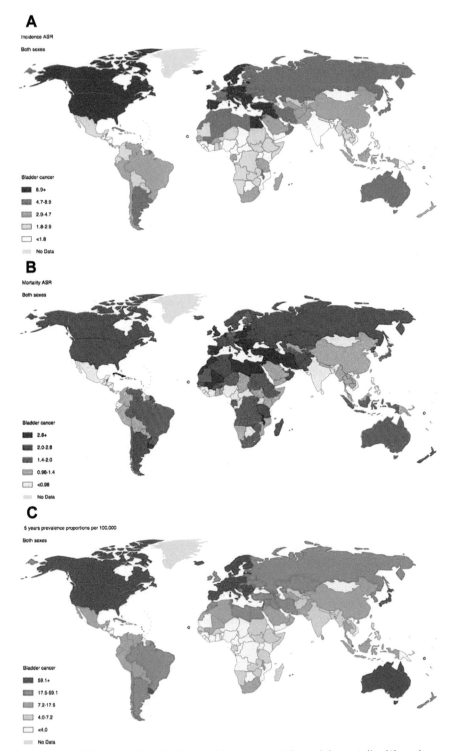

Fig. 1. GLOBOCAN maps of worldwide bladder cancer incidence (*A*), mortality (*B*), and prevalence (*C*) for both sexes. ASR, age-standardized rate. (*From* GLOBOCAN 2012: estimated bladder cancer incidence, mortality and prevalence worldwide in 2012. International Agency for Research on Cancer Web site. Available at: http://globocan.iarc.fr/Pages/Map.aspx. Accessed October 13, 2014.)

The highest mortality rate in men is 8 per 100,000 person-years in Middle East and Northern Africa (see **Fig. 1**).[1] Mortality rates tended to increase in men in most European countries between 1960 and 1990, with a subsequent decline in many countries; no clear pattern of mortality trends could be observed in women.[1] In the United States, incidence and mortality have essentially not changed in the past 25 years, indicating a lack of progress, and bladder cancer is twice as common in white versus African American men (**Box 1**).[4]

In North Africa a predominance of squamous cell carcinomas is seen, mainly from *Schistosoma haematobium* infection.[5] However, urothelial cell carcinoma is the most common form of bladder cancer (urothelial bladder cancer [UBC]) in the Western world, accounting for 95% of all cases. Hence, this review will refer exclusively to this tumor subtype. The incidence of UBC is increasing in developing countries probably as a result of a smoking epidemic.

From a clinical standpoint, UBC is classified as non–muscle-invasive bladder cancer (NMIBC) and muscle-invasive bladder cancer (MIBC), because invasion of the muscle layer is the major determinant for performing a cystectomy. The 5-year relative survival rate for patients with UBC ranges from 97% (stage I) to 22% (stage IV). The 5-year relative survival for all stages combined is higher among men than among women (84% and 75%, respectively). Most patients have a chronic disease that requires continued surveillance and follow-up, and UBC is the most expensive tumor on a per-patient basis and an important economic burden to the health care system.[6]

So far, the major risk factors associated with UBC have not been shown to differentially affect the development of NMIBC versus MIBC.[5] Increasing evidence shows that under the designation "urothelial bladder cancer" multiple molecular entities are included.[7] Therefore, in the next years a new molecular taxonomy with epidemiologic, clinical, and therapeutic implications will likely be established.

An extensive review of the epidemiology of bladder cancer has been published elsewhere.[5] The present article first summarizes the known and suggested risk factors, both genetic and nongenetic, for UBC, and comments on current needs to disentangle the complex etiologic scenario of UBC.

Box 1
Facts about urothelial bladder cancer in the United States

Number of new cases in 2014: 74,690

Incidence: 20.5

Ranking by incidence: 4th (men); 10th (women)

Percentage of new cases: 4.5%

Number of deaths in 2014: 15,580

Mortality: 4.4

Number of living people with urothelial bladder cancer in 2011: 571,518

Lifetime risk of developing urothelial bladder cancer during lifetime: 2.4%

Male to female ratio: approximately 3

THE CAUSES OF THE DISEASE: WHAT IS KNOWN?

Table 1 displays the factors/exposures for which conclusive evidence exists regarding their association with bladder cancer risk.

Table 1
Urothelial bladder cancer

Established Evidence	Suggestive Evidence	Inconclusive Evidence
Age >45	Tobacco inhalation	Pipe and cigar smoking,
Male sex	Low total fluid intake	chewing and snuffing
Cigarette smoking	Low physical activity	tobacco
Occupational exposures	Low consumption of fresh	Alcohol, coffee, tea
to aromatic amines	fruits and vegetables	consumption
and polycyclic	Low plasma levels of vitamin D	Artificial sweeteners
aromatic	Disinfection byproducts	Personal use of hair dyes
hydrocarbons	Diabetes	Energy intake
Water arsenic	Bacterial urinary tract	Meat, fish, milk, and dairy
Medications	infections	products
(phenacetin,	Spinal cord injury and	Other vitamins and
cyclophosphamide,	indwelling catheters	antioxidants
chlornaphazine)	Medications (nonsteroidal	Nitrate in drinking water
Radiation	anti-inflammatory drugs,	Viral infections
Genetic susceptibility	pioglitazone)	Urinary stones
variants (see **Table 2**)	Family history	Urinary acidic pH
	Sulfotransferases (SULT), DNA	Metabolic syndrome
	repair, and cytochrome P450	Ever-parity
	enzymes (CYP) variants	Hormone replacement
		therapy
		Medications (acetaminophen/
		paracetamol, aspirin,
		metformin, isoniazid and
		phenobarbital)

Age

UBC is rare in individuals younger than 40 years. Incidence peaks in the population older than 75 years, and the mean age at diagnosis is approximately 67 years.[1]

Gender

The incidence of UBC is higher in men, at least partly because of their higher tobacco smoking rates. However, both human and animal studies support the notion that gender-related liver metabolism differences and the different effect of androgens and estrogens on bladder carcinogenesis may contribute to gender differences.[8] Importantly, women present with more advanced tumors and have worse survival rates than men.[9]

Smoking

Cigarette smoking accounts for 50% to 65% of UBC cases in men and 20% to 35% in women.[10] The most recent and largest cohort study in the United States shows an increased risk of UBC among current (hazard ratio [HR], 4.06; 95% CI, 3.66–4.50) and former smokers (HR, 2.22; 95% CI, 2.03–2.44) compared with never smokers. This study suggests that the population-attributable risk among women is comparable to that of men.[10] The risk is higher for black tobacco and increases with number of cigarettes smoked daily and number of years of smoking, and with the inhalation of tobacco smoke.[11] Evidence suggests that cessation of smoking reduces the risk of UBC only for blond tobacco.[5]

Occupational Exposures

Occupational exposures have been estimated to account for up to 20% to 27% of bladder cancers; changes in legislation over the past 30 years seem to have led to reduced risks in the Western countries.[12] The risks conferred by occupational exposures range from 1.2 to 1.4.[13] Aromatic amines, to which exposure occurs in the chemical and rubber industries, are major occupational carcinogens. Polycyclic aromatic hydrocarbons (PAHs), used in aluminum production, coal gasification, coal tars, roofing, and carbon black manufacture, are also associated with UBC risk.[14] Several high-quality studies and meta-analyses have shown an excess risk of UBC among dyers in textile industries, painters, varnishers, and hairdressers, although the risk varies over time and place.[5,13] Increased risks have also been reported among truck and bus drivers. The pattern of occupational UBC risk among women is, to some extent, similar to that in men. Despite the banning of some major identified carcinogens, risks have not decreased in certain jobs, such as hairdressers. A substantial concern at the worldwide level is the regulation of exposures among relevant settings in developing countries.[13]

Arsenic

In various geographic areas, studies have consistently shown increased UBC risks associated with exposure to high levels of arsenic in drinking water, and the International Agency for Research on Cancer (IARC) has classified arsenic in drinking water as carcinogenic to humans (bladder, lung, and skin).[15] Recent systematic reviews and meta-analyses have confirmed this relationship; statistically significant increases in risk have been demonstrated for exposures to 50 μg/L or more of arsenic (median odds ratio, 4.2; 95% CI, 2.1–6.3), with less strong evidence for exposures at 10 μg/L.[15]

Medications

The use of phenacetin-containing analgesics has been consistently associated with increased UBC risk in case-control studies. Cyclophosphamide and chlornaphazine also increase the risk of UBC.[5,16] All 3 drugs are considered bladder cancer carcinogens in humans, based on the evaluation of the IARC.

Radiation

Radiation therapy, used in the past for dysfunctional uterine bleeding, and currently for ovarian, cervical, and prostate cancers, is associated with an increase in UBC risk.[5,16] No definite evidence shows an increased UBC risk associated with the use of iodine-131 to treat hyperthyroidism.[17]

Genetic Susceptibility

A cohort study of twins from Sweden, Denmark, and Finland estimated that 31% of the risk of UBC may be explained by heritable factors, although the estimation was not statistically significant.[18] A recent study of the heritability of 12 common sporadic cancers found that UBC showed the smallest inherited component (heritability [h^2_g], 0.01; 95% CI, 0–0.11).[19] Overall, candidate gene studies have yielded inconsistent results regarding the association of genetic variation and UBC risk, an exception being *GSTM1* and *NAT2*. The most reproducible evidence comes from rigorous genome-wide association studies (**Table 2**). The risks associated with tobacco and occupational exposures suggested that variation in genes coding for enzymes involved in the metabolism of urothelial carcinogens, such as aromatic amines and PAHs, might contribute to the individual susceptibility to UBC. Glutathione S-transferases (GST) are

Table 2
Genetic variation associated with bladder cancer susceptibility

Variant	Presumptive Gene	Chromosomal Location	Reference (PMID)
GSTM1-null	GSTM1	1p13.3	García-Closas M, et al (2011)[20] (meta-analysis)
rs1495741	NAT2	8p22	García-Closas M, et al (2011)[20] García-Closas M, et al (2011)[61]
rs17863783	UGT1A	2q37.1	Tang W, et al (2012)[62]
rs7238033	SLC14A1	18q12.3	Garcia-Closas M, et al (2011)[63] Rafnar T, et al (2011)[64]
rs10936599		3q26.2	Figueroa JD, et al (2014)[65]
rs907611		11p15.5	Figueroa JD, et al (2014)[65]
rs62185668	JAG1?	20p12	Rafnar T, et al (2014)[66]
rs9642880	MYC?	8q24.21	Kiemeney LA, et al (2008)[67]
rs710521	TP63	3q28	Kiemeney LA, et al (2008)[67]
rs2736098/rs401681	TERT/CLPTM1L	5p15.33	Rafnar T, et al (2009)[68] Rothman N, et al (2010)[69]
rs2294008	PSCA	8q24.3	Wu X, et al (2009)[70]
rs798766	FGFR3/TACC3	4p16.3	Kiemeney LA, et al (2010)[71]
rs1014971	CBX6/APOBEC3A	22q13.1	Rothman N, et al (2010)[69]
rs8102137	CCNE1	19q12	Rothman N, et al (2010)[69]

?, indicates that it has been proposed that the SNP is associated with the stated gene without conclusive evidence being available.

a large family of enzymes involved in electrophile detoxification by glutathione conjugation to a wide variety of substrates, including PAH epoxides and byproducts of oxidative stress. Gene copy number changes account for GSTM1 variation; approximately 50% of the US Caucasian population is GSTM1-null (ie, lacks the gene and its product). A meta-analysis of 28 case-control studies estimated an odds ratio (OR) of 1.5 (95% CI, 1.3–1.6) for GSTM1-null individuals.[20] N-acetyltransferases (NATs) participate in the bioactivation and detoxification of aromatic amines. NAT2 polymorphisms have been extensively studied as a risk factor of UBC; the lack of 2 functional NAT2 alleles leads to a slow acetylation phenotype that has been consistently, but not universally, associated with an increased risk of UBC.[21] A meta-analysis of 46 case-control studies showed a statistically significant increased risk for UBC among NAT2 slow versus intermediate/rapid acetylators (OR, 1.37; 95% CI, 1.24–1.52) with evidence of geographic heterogeneity.[22] An association of smoking and the NAT2 genetic variants is one of the few examples of consistent gene-environment interactions in the literature.[20] NAT2 has wide genetic variation; genotyping 2 single nucleotide polymorphisms (SNPs) is sufficient to capture this variation (rs1041983 and rs1801280). Beyond GSTM1 and NAT2, a total of 14 independent susceptibility loci have been shown to be significantly associated with UBC risk.[23,24] Several of these lie in regions where functional relationships have been proposed, including rs798766-FGFR3 somatic mutations, rs2294008-PSCA, and rs7238033-SLC14A1, involved in urea transport and urine concentration. All of these associations show modest differences in risk for the variant allele, and therefore currently cannot be used in the clinical setting.[23]

THE CAUSES OF THE DISEASE: WHAT NEEDS TO BE CONFIRMED (OR REFUTED)

Table 1 also lists the factors/exposures for which suggestive or inconclusive evidence exists regarding their association with UBC. This section examines the most important ones in terms of frequency and impact.

Lifestyle Habits

Strong evidence does not show that alcohol, coffee, or tea drinking is associated with an increased risk of UBC. Prior positive reports may have been subject to confounding. Case-control and cohort studies have shown contradictory results on the association of total fluid intake and UBC risk. Insufficient evidence exists on the role of artificial sweeteners as bladder carcinogens in humans.[25–27] Meta-analyses conclude that personal use of hair dyes is not associated with an appreciable risk increase.[28] Recent systematic reviews and meta-analysis of case-control and cohort studies suggest that physical activity is associated with a reduced risk of UBC, with a median OR of 0.85 (95% CI, 0.74–0.98).[29]

Diet

Evidence suggests the consumption of fresh fruits and vegetables has a protective effect against the development of UBC. Elevated risks were identified for diets with a high fat content (relative risk [RR], 1.37; 95% CI, 1.16–1.62); whether energy intake mostly accounts for this increased risk has not been elucidated. Meta-analyses provide no evidence for an association of disease development with the consumption of meat, fish, milk, and dairy products.[5,16] Some evidence suggests that sufficient plasma levels of vitamin D are associated with reduced risk of UBC, possibly associated with selected tumor subtypes.[30] Insufficient evidence exists regarding an association between other vitamins and antioxidants and bladder carcinogenesis.[16] No evidence suggests that dietary or supplementary intake of potassium; sodium; calcium; magnesium; phosphorus; iron; vitamins B_1, B_2, B_6, and B_{12}; niacin; or folic acid affects UBC risk.[31]

Water Contaminants

Contradictory evidence exists regarding the association between nitrate in drinking water and the development of UBC. Several studies have found a positive association between chlorination byproducts in drinking water and UBC.[16,32] A pooled analysis including 6 case-control studies supported these findings. An increased risk of UBC was observed among men exposed to an average of more than 1 µg/L (particles per billion) trihalomethanes (OR, 1.24; 95% CI, 1.09–1.41); no association was observed among women. Investigators have proposed that geographic differences may account for the controversial findings.[33]

Medical Conditions

Evidence regarding the association with cystitis and urinary tract infections is inconclusive, possibly because of difficulties in disease definition and medical diagnosis. Epidemiologic evidence on the role of viruses in UBC is conflicting.[34,35] Tumor genome sequencing has revealed 4% of MIBC expressing cytomegalovirus, human papillomavirus, and BK polyomavirus transcripts.[36] The role of urinary tract stones in UBC risk is controversial. Contradictory evidence exists on the association of an acidic urine pH and bladder cancer risk.[37] As for diabetes, a meta-analysis of 9 case-control studies, 19 cohort studies, and 8 cohort studies of patients with diabetes shows an increased risk of UBC among individuals with diabetes in the case-control studies (median OR, 1.45; 95% CI, 1.13–1.86; $P = .005$) and cohort studies (RR, 1.35;

95% CI, 1.12–1.62; P<.001), but not in the cohort studies of patients with diabetes. The risk of UBC was found to be higher among patients diagnosed within less than 5 years.[38] A systematic review and meta-analysis suggest an association between metabolic syndrome and an increased risk of UBC (median OR, 1.10; P = .013).[39] Spinal cord injury and indwelling catheters are not frequent but may be associated with increased UBC risk.

Menstrual, Reproductive, and Hormonal Factors

Hormonal factors have been proposed as one explanation for the excessive incidence of UBC in women. Several studies, including a meta-analysis, have consistently reported a decreased risk for ever-parous women (OR, ≈0.7–0.8); an increased risk associated with early menopause has also been suggested.[40–42] The studies on contraceptive use and hormone replacement therapy have not been conclusive.[43–45]

Medications

Current evidence does not support an increased risk of UBC among regular users of acetaminophen.[46] Some evidence suggests that regular use of nonaspirin nonsteroidal anti-inflammatory drugs is associated with a reduced risk of UBC (OR, 0.92; 95% CI, 0.81–1.04). The risk reduction was limited to nonsmokers (OR, 0.58; 95% CI, 0.41–0.83; P = .02).[47] In contrast, no evidence suggests an association between risk and regular aspirin use based on a meta-analysis and a pooled analysis of 3 cohort studies. Pioglitazone, a peroxisome proliferator-activated receptor gamma agonist of the thiazolidinedione family used to treat type 2 diabetes mellitus, has been associated with an increased risk of UBC. Both a literature review and a meta-analysis support a slight increase in risk of UBC with use of this agent (median OR, 1.20; 95% CI, 1.07–1.34), with a direct association between risk and treatment duration and cumulative dose.[48,49] Evidence from a systematic review supports the association between metformin use in patients with diabetes and a reduced risk of several cancer types, but not bladder cancer.[50] Evidence is insufficient for several drugs whose use has been considered as a possible risk factor for the development of UBC, including isoniazid and phenobarbital.

Familial History of Bladder Cancer

Familial clustering of UBC is rare. The results of case-control studies have shown a modest increase in risk of UBC among relatives of probands with UBC, but the results are controversial.[16,51] Some evidence suggests that the association is stronger for patients presenting with UBC at an age younger than 45 years.[52] Nevertheless, a role of shared environmental factors cannot be ruled out. Family-based studies also indicate a slightly increased risk of UBC associated with individuals with a family history of cancer, with a higher risk among younger patients and women.[53] Evidence suggests an increase in bladder cancer among patients with Costello syndrome and related germline mutant *RAS* conditions, Lynch syndrome, survivors of hereditary retinoblastoma, and *MUTYH*-associated polyposis.[54–58]

Genetic Variation

Many studies of candidate genes/SNPs were performed during the past 2 decades. Because most of them yielded nonreproducible findings, candidate studies should include built-in replication analyses. Among the genetic pathways that merit additional work are xenobiotic metabolism and DNA repair. Regarding the latter, meta-analyses and pooled analyses have provided some support for a role of variation in *ERCC2*, *NBN*, and *XPC* in UBC susceptibility, with very modest risk increases.[59] Additional genome-wide studies will likely contribute to the identification of novel genetic loci associated with small risk effects.

RISK FACTORS ASSOCIATED WITH URINARY BLADDER CANCER CLINICAL CHARACTERISTICS AND OUTCOME

Because bladder cancer is often a chronic disease, some of the risk factors associated with the development of the initial tumor may also influence outcome. However, little research has been performed in this area, except in regard to smoking. A recent systematic review suggests that, in patients with NMIBC, smoking at diagnosis is associated with increased recurrence after primary treatment, whereas the evidence regarding its association with progression and mortality is weaker.[60] Smoking cessation may influence outcome in patients with NMIBC. More work is needed to determine whether smoking is associated with response to intravesical bacillus Calmette-Guérin. In patients with MIBC, no evidence suggests a major association between smoking and outcome. Overall, the results of available studies are

---

Box 2
Future directions

- Epidemiologic studies predominantly assess risk exposures individually, but subjects are exposed to multiple risk factors concurrently. "Exposome" studies, correcting for correlated risk factors, may help provide a better understanding of bladder cancer development.

- Studies are needed focusing on risk factors (lifestyle and genetic) among subjects lacking any of the established risk factors for the disease ("orphan risk factor subjects").

- Further exploration of the bladder microbiome may provide further insights regarding bladder cancer pathogenesis.

- Why some patients develop an indolent form of the disease and others develop aggressive bladder cancer must be explored. Environmental/lifestyle risk factors have not been found to be selectively associated with one of these disease phenotypes. A few genetic variants seem to be selectively associated with certain phenotypes. Whether the patient's genetic background impinges on the type of bladder cancer that develops must be investigated.

- Using the emerging new bladder cancer taxonomy based on molecular markers, whether the known bladder cancer risk factors selectively associate with molecular subtypes must be determined.

- The combined consideration of multiple genetic susceptibility factors (SNPs, copy-number variation, gross structural rearrangement, mosaicisms) may also help identify common genetic pathways frequently altered in bladder cancer development.

- To further identify factors involved in bladder cancer development, agnostic/omics approaches (epigenomics, metabolomics, massive parallel sequencing) must be applied and integrated with established risk factors.

- Cancer is a dynamic process. Longitudinal studies using urine (and other) biomarkers may shed light on the evolution of the disease. However, improved study designs must be implemented to allow assessment of time-dependent interactions.

- The indolent nature of most non–muscle-invasive bladder cancers is a major health burden. More work is needed to identify the environmental/lifestyle and genetic factors that affect patient outcome.

- In the era of precision medicine, more work is needed on the impact of comorbidities and genetic variation on patient evolution.

inconclusive, with a major flaw being their retrospective nature. These strategies merit further study, but should be tested in the setting of well-designed prospective clinical trials.

SUMMARY

Substantial knowledge exists regarding the causes of bladder cancer, but thus far it has not had a major impact on disease incidence or mortality. Increased awareness about the role of smoking is needed at the population level. Additional suggestions for future directions are listed in **Box 2**.

REFERENCES

1. Ferlay J, Soerjomataram I, Ervik M, et al. GLOBOCAN 2012 v1.0, cancer incidence and mortality worldwide: IARC CancerBase No. 11 [Internet]. Lyon (France): International Agency for Research on Cancer; 2013. Available at: http://globocan.iarc.fr. Accessed October 13, 2014.
2. Bray F, Ren JS, Masuyer E, et al. Estimates of global cancer prevalence for 27 sites in the adult population in 2008. Int J Cancer 2013;132:1133–45.
3. Chavan S, Bray F, Lortet-Tieulent J, et al. International variations in bladder cancer incidence and mortality. Eur Urol 2014;66:59–73.
4. Available at: http://seer.cancer.gov/statfacts/html/urinb.html. Accessed August 4, 2014.
5. Silverman D, Devesa SS, Morore LE, Rothman N. Bladder cancer. In: Schottenfeld D, Fraumeni JF Jr, editors. Cancer epidemiology and prevention. New York: Oxford University Press; 2006. p. 1101–27.
6. Svatek RS, Hollenbeck BK, Holmäng S, et al. The economics of bladder cancer: costs and considerations of caring for this disease. Eur Urol 2014;66(2):253–62.
7. Sjödahl G, Lauss M, Lövgren K, et al. A molecular taxonomy for urothelial carcinoma. Clin Cancer Res 2012;18:3377–86.
8. Zhang Y. Understanding the gender disparity in bladder cancer risk: the impact of sex hormones and liver on bladder susceptibility to carcinogens. J Environ Sci Health C Environ Carcinog Ecotoxicol Rev 2013;31:287–304.
9. Shariat SF, Sfakianos JP, Droller MJ, et al. The effect of age and gender on bladder cancer: a critical review of the literature. BJU Int 2010;105:300–8.
10. Freedman ND, Silverman DT, Hollenbeck AR, et al. Association between smoking and risk of bladder cancer among men and women. JAMA 2011;306:737–45.
11. Samanic C, Kogevinas M, Dosemeci M, et al. Smoking and bladder cancer in Spain: effects of tobacco type, timing, environmental tobacco smoke, and gender. Cancer Epidemiol Biomarkers Prev 2006;15:1348–54.
12. Delclos GL, Lerner SP. Occupational risk factors. Scand J Urol Nephrol Suppl 2008;218:58–63.
13. Reulen RC, Kellen E, Buntinx F, et al. A meta-analysis on the association between bladder cancer and occupation. Scand J Urol Nephrol Suppl 2008;218:64–78.
14. Rota M, Bosetti C, Boccia S, et al. Occupational exposures to polycyclic aromatic hydrocarbons and respiratory and urinary tract cancers: an updated systematic review and a meta-analysis to 2014. Arch Toxicol 2014. [Epub ahead of print].
15. Saint-Jacques N, Parker L, Brown P, et al. Arsenic in drinking water and urinary tract cancers: a systematic review of 30 years of epidemiological evidence. Environ Health 2014;13:44.

16. Murta-Nascimento C, Schmitz-Dräger BJ, Zeegers MP, et al. Epidemiology of urinary bladder cancer: from tumor development to patient's death. World J Urol 2007;25:285–95.

17. Franklyn JA, Maisonneuve P, Sheppard M, et al. Cancer incidence and mortality after radioiodine treatment for hyperthyroidism: a population-based cohort study. Lancet 1999;353:2111–5.

18. Lichtenstein P, Holm NV, Verkasalo PK, et al. Environmental and heritable factors in the causation of cancer–analyses of cohorts of twins from Sweden, Denmark, and Finland. N Engl J Med 2000;343:78–85.

19. Lu Y, Ek WE, Whiteman D, et al. Most common 'sporadic' cancers have a significant germline genetic component. Hum Mol Genet 2014;23(22):6112–8.

20. García-Closas M, Malats N, Silverman D, et al. NAT2 slow acetylation, GSTM1 null genotype, and risk of bladder cancer: results from the Spanish Bladder Cancer Study and meta-analyses. Lancet 2005;366:649–59.

21. Marcus PM, Vineis P, Rothman N. NAT2 slow acetylation and bladder cancer risk: a meta-analysis of 22 case-control studies conducted in the general population. Pharmacogenetics 2000;10:115–22.

22. Moore LE, Baris DR, Figueroa JD, et al. GSTM1 null and NAT2 slow acetylation genotypes, smoking intensity and bladder cancer risk: results from the New England bladder cancer study and NAT2 meta-analysis. Carcinogenesis 2011;32: 182–9.

23. Wang M, Chu H, Lv Q, et al. Cumulative effect of genome-wide association study-identified genetic variants for bladder cancer. Int J Cancer 2014;135(11): 2653–60.

24. McDonagh EM, Boukouvala S, Aklillu E, et al. PharmGKB summary: very important pharmacogene information for N-acetyltransferase 2. Pharmacogenet Genomics 2014;4:409–25.

25. Pelucchi C, La Vecchia C. Alcohol, coffee, and bladder cancer risk: a review of epidemiological studies. Eur J Cancer Prev 2009;18:62–8.

26. Zhou J, Kelsey KT, Giovannucci E, et al. Fluid intake and risk of bladder cancer in the Nurses' Health Studies. Int J Cancer 2014;135:1229–37.

27. Michaud DS, Kogevinas M, Cantor KP, et al. Total fluid and water consumption and the joint effect of exposure to disinfection by-products on risk of bladder cancer. Environ Health Perspect 2007;115:1569–72.

28. Turati F, Pelucchi C, Galeone C, et al. Personal hair dye use and bladder cancer: a meta-analysis. Ann Epidemiol 2014;24:151–9.

29. Keimling M, Behrens G, Schmid D, et al. The association between physical activity and bladder cancer: systematic review and meta-analysis. Br J Cancer 2014; 110:1862–70.

30. Amaral AF, Méndez-Pertuz M, Muñoz A, et al. Plasma 25-hydroxyvitamin D(3) and bladder cancer risk according to tumor stage and FGFR3 status: a mechanism-based epidemiological study. J Natl Cancer Inst 2012;104: 1897–904.

31. Steinmaus CM, Nuñez S, Smith AH. Diet and bladder cancer: a meta-analysis of six dietary variables. Am J Epidemiol 2000;151:693–702.

32. Villanueva CM, Cantor KP, Grimalt JO, et al. Bladder cancer and exposure to water disinfection by-products through ingestion, bathing, showering, and swimming in pools. Am J Epidemiol 2007;165:148–56.

33. Costet N, Villanueva CM, Jaakkola JJ, et al. Water disinfection by-products and bladder cancer: is there a European specificity? A pooled and meta-analysis of European case-control studies. Occup Environ Med 2011;68:379–85.

34. Michaud DS. Chronic inflammation and bladder cancer. Urol Oncol 2007;25: 260–8.
35. Robles C, Viscidi R, Malats N, et al. Bladder cancer and seroreactivity to BK, JC and Merkel cell polyomaviruses: the Spanish bladder cancer study. Int J Cancer 2013;133:587–603.
36. Cancer Genome Atlas Research Network. Comprehensive molecular characterization of urothelial bladder carcinoma. Nature 2014;507:315–22.
37. Alguacil J, Kogevinas M, Silverman D, et al. Urinary pH, cigarette smoking, and bladder cancer risk. Carcinogenesis 2011;32:843–7.
38. Zhu Z, Wang X, Shen Z, et al. Risk of bladder cancer in patients with diabetes mellitus: an updated meta-analysis of 36 observational studies. BMC Cancer 2013;13:310.
39. Esposito K, Chiodini P, Colao A, et al. Metabolic syndrome and risk of cancer: a systematic review and meta-analysis. Diabetes Care 2012;35:2402–11.
40. Dietrich K, Demidenko E, Schned A, et al. Parity, early menopause and the incidence of bladder cancer in women: a case-control study and meta-analysis. Eur J Cancer 2011;47:592–9.
41. Weibull CE, Eloranta S, Altman D, et al. Childbearing and the risk of bladder cancer: a nationwide population-based cohort study. Eur Urol 2013;63:733–8.
42. Hsu I, Vitkus S, Da J, et al. Role of oestrogen receptors in bladder cancer development. Nat Rev Urol 2013;10(6):317–26.
43. Kabat GC, Kim MY, Luo J, et al. Menstrual and reproductive factors and exogenous hormone use and risk of transitional cell bladder cancer in postmenopausal women. Eur J Cancer Prev 2013;22:409–16.
44. Daugherty SE, Lacey JV Jr, Pfeiffer RM, et al. Reproductive factors and menopausal hormone therapy and bladder cancer risk in the NIH-AARP diet and health study. Int J Cancer 2013;133:462–72.
45. Dietrich K, Demidenko E, Schned A, et al. Parity, early menopause and the incidence of bladder cancer in women: a case-control study and meta-analysis. Eur J Cancer 2011;47:592–9.
46. Fortuny J, Kogevinas M, Garcia-Closas M, et al. Use of analgesics and NSAIDs, genetic predisposition and bladder cancer risk in Spain. Cancer Epidem Biomark Prev 2006;15:1696–702.
47. Daugherty SE, Pfeiffer RM, Sigurdson AJ, et al. Nonsteroidal antiinflammatory drugs and bladder cancer: a pooled analysis. Am J Epidemiol 2011;173: 721–30.
48. Bosetti C, Rosato V, Buniato D, et al. Cancer risk for patients using thiazolidinediones for type 2 diabetes: a meta-analysis. Oncologist 2013;18:148–56.
49. Kostapanos MS, Elisaf MS, Mikhailidis DP. Pioglitazone and cancer: angel or demon? Curr Pharm Des 2013;19:4913–29.
50. Franciosi M, Lucisano G, Lapice E, et al. Metformin therapy and risk of cancer in patients with type 2 diabetes: systematic review. PLoS One 2013; 8:e71583.
51. Hemminki K, Bermejo JL, Ji J, et al. Familial bladder cancer and the related genes. Curr Opin Urol 2011;21:386–92.
52. Murta-Nascimento C, Silverman DT, Kogevinas M, et al. Risk of bladder cancer associated with family history of cancer: do low-penetrance polymorphisms account for the increase in risk? Cancer Epidemiol Biomarkers Prev 2007;16: 1595–600.
53. Aben KK, Witjes JA, Schoenberg MP, et al. Familial aggregation of urothelial cell carcinoma. Int J Cancer 2002;98:274–8.

54. Kratz CP, Rapisuwon S, Reed H, et al. Cancer in Noonan, Costello, cardiofacio-cutaneous and LEOPARD syndromes. Am J Med Genet C Semin Med Genet 2011;157C:83–9.
55. Win AK, Lindor NM, Young JP, et al. Risks of primary extracolonic cancers following colorectal cancer in lynch syndrome. J Natl Cancer Inst 2012;104: 1363–72.
56. Skeldon SC, Semotiuk K, Aronson M, et al. Patients with Lynch syndrome mismatch repair gene mutations are at higher risk for not only upper tract urothelial cancer but also bladder cancer. Eur Urol 2013;63:379–85.
57. Marees T, Moll AC, Imhof SM, et al. Risk of second malignancies in survivors of retinoblastoma: more than 40 years of follow-up. J Natl Cancer Inst 2008;100: 1771–9.
58. Vogt S, Jones N, Christian D, et al. Expanded extracolonic tumor spectrum in MU-TYH-associated polyposis. Gastroenterology 2009;137:1976–85.
59. Stern MC, Lin J, Figueroa JD, et al. Polymorphisms in DNA repair genes, smoking, and bladder cancer risk: findings from the international consortium of bladder cancer. Cancer Res 2009;69:6857–64.
60. Crivelli JJ, Xylinas E, Kluth LA, et al. Effect of smoking on outcomes of urothelial carcinoma: a systematic review of the literature. Eur Urol 2014;65:742–54.
61. García-Closas M, Hein DW, Silverman D, et al. A single nucleotide polymorphism tags variation in the arylamine N-acetyltransferase 2 phenotype in populations of European background. Pharmacogenet Genomics 2011;21:231–6.
62. Tang W, Fu YP, Figueroa JD, et al. Mapping of the UGT1A locus identifies an uncommon coding variant that affects mRNA expression and protects from bladder cancer. Hum Mol Genet 2012;21:1918–30.
63. Garcia-Closas M, Ye Y, Rothman N, et al. A genome-wide association study of bladder cancer identifies a new susceptibility locus within SLC14A1, a urea transporter gene on chromosome 18q12.3. Hum Mol Genet 2011;20:4282–9.
64. Rafnar T, Vermeulen SH, Sulem P, et al. European genome-wide association study identifies SLC14A1 as a new urinary bladder cancer susceptibility gene. Hum Mol Genet 2011;20:4268–81.
65. Figueroa JD, Ye Y, Siddiq A, et al. Genome-wide association study identifies multiple loci associated with bladder cancer risk. Hum Mol Genet 2014;23:1387–98.
66. Rafnar T, Sulem P, Thorleifsson G, et al. Genome-wide association study yields variants at 20p12.2 that associate with urinary bladder cancer. Hum Mol Genet 2014;23:5545–57.
67. Kiemeney LA, Thorlacius S, Sulem P, et al. Sequence variant on 8q24 confers susceptibility to urinary bladder cancer. Nat Genet 2008;40:1307–12.
68. Rafnar T, Sulem P, Stacey SN, et al. Sequence variants at the TERT-CLPTM1L locus associate with many cancer types. Nat Genet 2009;41:221–7.
69. Rothman N, Garcia-Closas M, Chatterjee N, et al. A multi-stage genome-wide association study of bladder cancer identifies multiple susceptibility loci. Nat Genet 2010;42:978–84.
70. Wu X, Ye Y, Kiemeney LA, et al. Genetic variation in the prostate stem cell antigen gene PSCA confers susceptibility to urinary bladder cancer. Nat Genet 2009;41: 991–5.
71. Kiemeney LA, Sulem P, Besenbacher S, et al. A sequence variant at 4p16.3 confers susceptibility to urinary bladder cancer. Nat Genet 2010;42:415–9.

Molecular Biology of Bladder Cancer

William Martin-Doyle, MD, MPH, David J. Kwiatkowski, MD, PhD*

KEYWORDS

- Bladder cancer • Urothelial carcinoma • Mutations
- Somatic copy number alterations • Cell cycle • Epigenetics • Molecular subtypes

KEY POINTS

- There is a high rate of both mutations and genomic amplifications and deletions in muscle-invasive bladder cancer.
- *FGFR3* is commonly activated in bladder cancer, through either mutation, gene fusion events, or elevated expression, and is a potential therapeutic target.
- Chromatin regulatory gene mutations, Cell-cycle gene mutations, amplifications (cyclins), and deletions (cyclin-dependent kinase inhibitors) are very common in bladder cancer.
- Viral infection seems to contribute to bladder cancer development in 5% to 10% of cancers.
- The main RNA expression subtypes of bladder cancer are basal and luminal, similar to breast cancer, and confer both prognostic and therapeutic significance.
- The following genes and pathways are frequently affected: the ERBB family (including EGFR, ERBB2, and ERBB3), FGFR3, and the PI3K-mTOR (PI3KCA, PTEN, and TSC1) signaling cascade , many of which are potentially targetable using small molecule kinase inhibitors or antibody therapeutics.

BACKGROUND

Bladder cancer is a leading cause of morbidity and mortality, with nearly 400,000 new cases and 150,000 deaths worldwide.[1] However novel approaches to treatment in the past 2 decades have been sparse. Since 2006, of 126 approvals granted by the US Food and Drug Administration for hematology/oncology medications, none have been for the treatment of bladder cancer,[2] and chemotherapeutic approaches remain rooted in cisplatin-based combinations first introduced 30 years ago. This limited progress has provided major incentive to analyze molecular alterations in bladder cancer in detail in an effort to identify novel treatment approaches.

Bladder cancer genetics and molecular biology have historically provided important general insights into cancer biology, beginning with the discovery of *HRAS* as the first

Department of Medicine, Brigham and Women's Hospital, Harvard Medical School, 75 Francis St, Boston, MA 02115, USA
* Corresponding author. Department of Medicine, Brigham and Women's Hospital, Harvard Medical School, 1 Blackfan Circle, Room 6-213, Boston, MA 02115, USA.
E-mail address: dk@rics.bwh.harvard.edu

Hematol Oncol Clin N Am 29 (2015) 191–203
http://dx.doi.org/10.1016/j.hoc.2014.10.002
0889-8588/15/$ – see front matter © 2015 Elsevier Inc. All rights reserved.

hemonc.theclinics.com

oncogene in a bladder cancer cell line.[3] Since that seminal discovery, multiple genes commonly subject to mutation in bladder cancer have been identified, including *TP53*,[4] *RB1*,[5] *TSC1*,[6] *FGFR3*,[7] and *PIK3CA*.[8,9] Furthermore, comparative genomic hybridization and related techniques were used extensively in bladder cancer, leading to identification of multiple amplified and deleted genes, including *PPARG*, *E2F3*, *EGFR*, *CCND1*, and *MDM2*, which are amplified, and *CDKN2A* and *RB1*, which are commonly deleted.[10–17] These and other molecular alterations involved in bladder cancer have been summarized in previous reviews.[16,18]

Recently, next-generation sequencing has enabled large-scale analyses, mainly focused on muscle-invasive bladder cancer, greatly expanding our understanding of this malignancy.[19–22] The initial next-generation sequencing studies were performed by the Beijing Genomics Institute,[20,21] in studies that focused initially on mutation identification,[20] and then included both mutation analysis and transcriptome studies.[21] More recently, The Cancer Genome Atlas (TCGA) project, funded by the National Cancer Institute, has performed a comprehensive analysis of 131 muscle-invasive bladder cancers, including assessment of mutations, copy number changes, expression profiling by RNA-Seq, micro RNA (miRNA) analysis, CpG methylation analysis, proteomic analysis of about 150 proteins, and integrated analyses of these data sets.

This review summarizes the current understanding of molecular alterations in bladder cancer, and focuses on findings from the TCGA project[19] and the Beijing group.[20,21] We also discuss recent reports providing improved understanding of molecular subtypes of bladder cancer based on expression analyses.

MOLECULAR ALTERATIONS IN BLADDER CANCER

Fig. 1 illustrates the major findings of the TCGA study, showing mutation rates and frequencies, gene deletions and amplifications, and changes in expression for genes of interest.[19]

Mutations in Bladder Cancer: General Findings

The TCGA study identified a relatively high rate of 7.68 mutations per Mb within coding regions, equivalent to 302 exonic mutations per cancer.[19] This mutation rate is exceeded among cancers studied in the TCGA project (now >20) only by lung adenocarcinoma, lung squamous cell carcinoma, and melanoma.[23] The mechanism or cause of this high mutation rate in bladder cancer is not known with certainty. Although smoking is associated with mutation rate and spectrum in lung cancer, this was not seen in bladder cancer,[19] despite the well-known epidemiologic association between cigarette smoking and bladder cancer. On the other hand, 51% of mutations seen in bladder cancer were TCW -> TTW or TGW changes ("TCW mutations" [C > T and C > G mutations] at T-C-A/T [TCW] trinucleotides), a class of mutation likely mediated by one of the DNA cytosine deaminases, in the APOBEC gene family.[24,25] In addition, APOBEC3B was expressed at high levels in all bladder cancers examined, suggesting a major role for APOBEC-mediated mutagenesis in the high mutation rate seen in bladder cancer.[19]

The Beijing group identified a somewhat lower overall mutation rate, but by statistical analyses identified significant levels of mutation in 37 genes. This included many genes identified previously, as well as multiple chromatin remodeling genes, namely, *KDM6A*, *ARID1A*, *CREBBP*, *EP300*, *KMT2A*, *NCOR1*, *CHD6*, and *KMT2C*.[20,21] In the TCGA analysis, 32 genes were identified as sustaining mutations at a significant rate (see **Fig. 1**B). There was considerable overlap between the genes

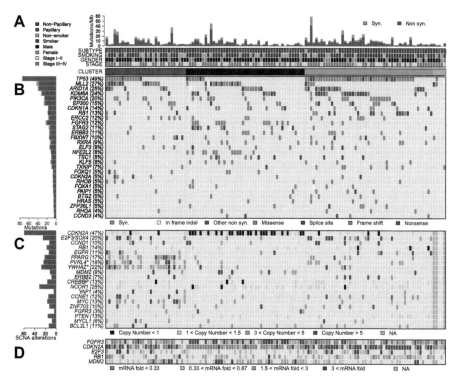

Fig. 1. The genomic landscape of bladder cancer. (*A*) Mutation rate and type, histologic subtype, smoking status, gender, tumor stage, and cluster type. (*B*) Genes with significant levels of mutation and mutation types. (*C*) Deletions and amplifications for genomic regions with statistically significant focal copy number changes. "Copy number" refers to absolute copy number. Note that 2 amplification peaks (*asterisk*) contain several genes, any of which could be the target, as opposed to the single gene listed here. (*D*) RNA expression level for selected genes, expressed as fold change from the median value for all samples. Cancers were grouped into 3 clusters (*red, blue,* and *green*) using consensus non-negative matrix factorization (NMF) clustering. (*From* The Cancer Genome Atlas Research Network. Comprehensive molecular characterization of urothelial bladder carcinoma. Nature 2014;507:316; with permission.)

identified by the Beijing group and those identified in the TCGA analysis, providing significant confirmation, despite the distinctly different populations being studied (Beijing, Chinese; TCGA, mostly American and of European origin). Genes sustaining significant levels of mutation can be organized into several classes.

Somatic copy number alterations in bladder cancer

Somatic copy number alterations (SCNAs) were also common in the TCGA data set, with an average of 204 segmental SCNAs and 22 genomic rearrangements per cancer analyzed.[19] Statistical methods (GISTIC) were used to identify significant recurrent focal SCNAs, and 27 amplified and 30 deleted regions were identified (see **Fig. 1C**). *CDKN2A* was deleted in nearly half of the samples, and other genes that were probable targets of deletion included *KDM6A, RB1, WWOX, PDE4D, FOXQ1, FAM190A, LRP1B,* and *CREBBP*. Many deletions extended over a large genomic region and a single gene target could not be identified. Many genes were focally amplified, including *E2F3/SOX4, CCND1, EGFR, PPARG, MDM2, ERBB2, YAP1, CCNE1, MYC, ZNF703, FGFR3, MYCL1*, and *BCL2L1*. Other chromosomal regions of amplification extended over a large genomic region, containing more than a single gene. This included a region on chromosome 1q22–23.2 containing *PVRL4*, and a region on chromosome 8q22.3 containing *YWHAZ*. Multiple past reports made similar, although more limited, findings.[14,26–28]

Cell-cycle gene aberrations in bladder cancer

Mutation or deletion of cell-cycle genes in cancer has been known for many years, and reported previously in bladder cancer for over 2 decades (for examples[4,17,29,30]). The recent in-depth genomic analyses performed have confirmed and extended our knowledge of cell-cycle gene events in bladder cancer. Reviewing these alterations in the order of frequency, *TP53* (encodes p53) mutations were found in 49% and 24% of bladder cancers by the TCGA and Beijing groups.[19–21] p53 is the "guardian of the genome," and it responds to cellular stress by inducing cell-cycle arrest, apoptosis, senescence, and DNA repair. Its loss leads to bypass of these important effects, enhancing further genome damage, and continued proliferation. *CDKN2A* deletions are also very common in bladder cancer, similar to many other malignancies, with deletions seen in about 50% of samples in both the TCGA and Beijing studies.[19–21] Mutations in *CDKN2A* were also seen in 5% of bladder cancers.[19] *CDKN2A* encodes both p19^ARF and p16^INK4A proteins, which regulate the p53 and RB pathways, respectively. p16^INK4A is a cyclin-dependent kinase (cdk) inhibitor for cdk4 and cdk6, and its loss enhances cell-cycle progression.

RB1 was mutated in 10% and deleted in 15% of TCGA tumors,[19] with similar findings by the Beijing group.[20,21] The RB protein regulates the cell cycle by binding to the E2F transcription factor,[31] and its loss also leads to enhanced cell-cycle progression despite DNA damage or other signals.

A novel finding in the TCGA analysis was inactivation of *CDKN1A* by mutation in 14% and deletion in 6%.[19] Another group reported similar findings simultaneously.[22] *CDKN1A* encodes another cyclin-dependent kinase inhibitor, p21, distinct from p16^INK4A, but its loss similarly pushes the cell toward continued division despite DNA damage or other signals, enhancing cell proliferation and accumulation of additional DNA damage. *CDKN1A* mutation has not been seen at appreciable frequency in any other cancer studied to date by the TCGA.

Three cell-cycle genes were amplified in bladder cancer in these studies: *CCND1* (cyclin D1) in 10% to 21% of bladder cancers, *CCNE1* (cyclin E1) in 12% to 13%, and *MDM2* in 9% to 4% of samples, respectively, in the TCGA and Beijing analyses.[19–21] Both cyclin D1 and cyclin E1 are necessary cofactors for different cdks and hence their overexpression enhances cell proliferation. *MDM2* encodes an E3 ubiquitin–protein ligase, the enzyme that degrades p53 protein; hence, its overexpression lowers p53 levels, thereby inhibiting p53 function. *MDM2* amplification was mutually exclusive of *TP53* mutation for the most part in the TCGA analysis (see **Fig. 1**).[19]

Overall, 1 or more cell-cycle genes were mutated, deleted, or activated by amplification in 93% of the TCGA tumor samples, most often the *TP53* and/or *CDKN2A* genes (see **Fig. 1**).

Kinase signaling: receptor tyrosine kinases and the phosphatidylinositol-3-kinase-mammalian target of rapamycin pathway Given the well-known successes of tyrosine kinase inhibitor therapy for activated kinases in both chronic myelogenous leukemia (driven by BCR-ABL) and lung adenocarcinoma (driven by activating mutations in *EGFR*), there is major interest in the identification of similar activated tyrosine kinases in all types of cancer. Activating mutations in *FGFR3* were first identified in bladder cancer 15 years ago[7]; they are more commonly seen in superficial than in muscle-invasive cancers. *FGFR3* mutations were seen at 11% frequency in the muscle-invasive cancers studied by the TCGA and Beijing groups.[19–21] In addition, 3% of cases had FGFR3 amplification, and another 3% had FGFR3-TACC3 gene fusions.[19] These latter gene fusions have recently been reported by several groups, and shown to be activating.[32,33] Three members of the ERBB family of receptor tyrosine kinases were also altered at significant frequency in bladder cancer.[19] *EGFR* amplification was seen in 11%, *ERBB2* was mutated in 5% and amplified in 7%, and *ERBB3* was mutated in 11% and amplified in 2% of bladder cancers. These events in FGFR3 and ERBB family members are all potentially targetable using either tyrosine kinase inhibitors, or antibody-mediated therapies.[34,35] This potential is underscored by a recent report of the benefit of both erlotinib (EGFR tyrosine kinase inhibitor) and cetuximab (monoclonal antibody against EGFR) in some subsets of muscle-invasive bladder cancers.[36]

Mutations involving genes in the phosphatidylinositol-3-kinase (PI3K)–protein tyrosine phosphatase (PTEN)–AKT–TSC1–TSC2–mammalian target of rapamycin (mTOR) signaling pathway have long been recognized in bladder cancer.[6,8,9] The recent large-scale studies provided further documentation of mutation of both positive and negative regulators in this signaling cascade. *PIK3CA* was mutated in 15% and amplified in 5%, *PTEN* was mutated in 3% and deleted in 13%, *TSC1* was mutated in 8%, and *TSC2* was mutated in 2% in the TCGA analyses, with similar results from the Beijing studies.[19–21] All of these mutations lead to potential therapeutic targets, as highlighted by 2 recent studies showing that bladder cancer patients with *TSC1* and *MTOR* mutations were exceptional responders to treatment with/including everolimus, an mTOR allosteric inhibitor.[37,38]

Other genes and pathways Two genes involved in the response to oxidative stress were found to be mutated in bladder cancer in the TCGA analysis. *NFE2L2* encodes a transcription factor that is induced to mediate the cellular response to oxidative stress, and missense mutations in this gene were identified in 8% of the TCGA samples.[19] Mutations in *NFE2L2* were previously reported in cancer and shown to promote malignancy,[39] although not previously known for bladder cancer. *TXNIP* encodes thioredoxin interacting protein and is also involved in mediating the response to oxidative stress.[40] Mutations were seen in 7% of cancers in the TCGA study.[19]

Mutations in genes involved in lipid metabolism were also identified in the TCGA analysis.[19] *RXRA*, which encodes the retinoid X nuclear receptor alpha,[41] was mutated in 9% of bladder cancers, with 7 of 12 mutations occurring at the same amino acid in the ligand-binding domain. All 7 of these cancers showed increased expression of genes involved in lipid metabolism, consistent downstream effects of RXR activation. *PPARG*, which encodes the peroxisome proliferator-activated receptor gamma (glitazone receptor), was amplified in 17% of bladder cancers.

STAG2 is another relatively novel gene found to be mutated in bladder cancer by several groups at frequencies from 10% to 20%.[19,21,42–44] The STAG2 protein is a subunit of cohesin, a protein complex that regulates the separation of sister chromatids during cell division. Conflicting results were seen in terms of a potential association between *STAG2* mutation and survival in bladder cancer.[21,42–44]

ERCC2 was observed to be mutated in 12% and 7% of bladder cancers in the TCGA and Beijing analyses.[19–21] *ERCC2* is a nucleotide excision repair gene that causes xeroderma pigmentosum.[45] It seems that these mutations may act in a dominant negative fashion, because 15 of 16 were deleterious missense mutations.[19] A recent report described a positive association between *ERCC2* mutation and response to cisplatin-based chemotherapy in bladder cancer, consistent with loss of ERCC2 function leading to an Achilles heel-like sensitivity to cisplatin.[46]

Epigenetics: Chromatin Regulation

The role of epigenetic effects on regulation of gene expression, and their alterations in cancer in general have been studied for many years. However, the potential importance of these events in bladder cancer was advanced considerably by the recent in-depth genomic analyses. Mutations in chromatin regulatory genes in bladder cancer were first identified by the Beijing group, and then confirmed and extended by the TCGA analyses.[19–21] It is known that there are 2 main categories of chromatin modification that influence gene expression. The first is methylation at the C position of CG nucleotide sequences, and other less common modifications to the nucleotide sequence itself. The second is histone modifications, which are generated by chromatin regulatory genes. Chromatin regulatory genes are often referred to as "writers," "erasers," and "readers," based on their function in creating covalent modification of histones (methylation, acetylation), removing such modifications (demethylation, deacetylation), and in binding to such modifications to influence gene transcription. Genes involved in all 3 of these functions are commonly mutated in bladder cancer.

Mutations in *KDM6A*, an "eraser" demethylase acting on histone H3 at lysine 27, are seen in 20% to 25% of bladder cancers.[19–21] *MLL2*, encoding a histone 3 lysine 4 (H3K4) methyltransferase of the trithorax group, is a "writer," and is mutated in 27% of bladder cancers.[19] *ARID1A*, encoding a member of the SWI/SNF family, has helicase and ATPase activity, is a "reader," and is mutated in 25% of bladder cancers.[19] *EP300*, encoding a histone acetylase, is a "writer," which is also a transcription factor, and is mutated in 15% of bladder cancers.[19] Many other chromatin regulatory genes are mutated in more than 10% of bladder cancer samples, including *MLL3, MLL, CREBBP, CHD7* and *SRCAP*.[19] In addition, *CREBBP* and *NCOR1* were deleted in 13% and 25% of bladder cancers, respectively (see **Fig. 1**). Despite the likely importance of these mutations in the chromatin regulation of the genome in bladder cancer cells, there was no association between any of these gene mutations and expression profile or other features in the TCGA analysis.[19]

Viral infection in bladder cancer: cytomegalovirus, BK polyomavirus, and human papillomavirus 16

Exploration of infectious etiologies has long been of interest in bladder cancer: A viral etiology for bladder cancer has been considered for some time, and there is a clear epidemiologic relationship to chronic *Schistosoma* infection. The TCGA analysis identified 7 tumors (6%) with viral DNA sequences and five tumors with viral RNA transcripts.[19] The tumors with viral transcripts were: 3 with cytomegalovirus, 1 with BK polyomavirus, and 1 with human papillomavirus 16. Some of those with viral DNA sequences showed integration of viral DNA into the genome, with 1 instance of integration into *BCL2L1*, an apoptosis regulatory gene, suggesting that insertional mutagenesis might contribute to bladder cancer development in these cases.

Molecular Subtypes of Bladder Cancer

There is considerable heterogeneity in bladder cancer, both in terms of natural history and response to chemotherapy. Many efforts have been made to define molecular subsets of bladder cancer based on mutation profile and/or expression features to attempt to provide prognostic information, as well as guidance in selection of chemotherapy. For example, Takata and colleagues[47] analyzed gene expression profiles of biopsy materials from 27 invasive bladder cancers by microarray to identify 14 "predictive" genes whose expression levels were most correlated with response to methotrexate, vinblastine, doxorubicin, and cisplatin (M-VAC) chemotherapy. Ongoing studies are attempting to validate this expression profile prospectively. In the TCGA analysis, unsupervised clustering by non-negative matrix factorization of mutations and focal SCNAs identified 3 groups (see **Fig. 1A**).[19] Group A (*red*), labeled "focally amplified," was highly enriched in focal SCNAs in several genes, as well as mutations in *MLL2*. Group B (*blue*), labeled "papillary *CDKN2A*-deficient *FGFR3* mutant," was enriched in papillary histology, and the majority had loss of *CDKN2A*, and 1 or more alterations in *FGFR3*. Group C (*green*), labeled "*TP53*/cell-cycle mutant," had *TP53* mutations in nearly all samples, and enrichment for *RB1* mutations, and amplifications of *E2F3* and *CCNE1* (see **Fig. 1**).

The TCGA analysis also used RNA-Seq based expression profiling to identify 4 distinct mRNA expression clusters (**Fig. 2A**).[19] Cluster I ("papillarylike") was enriched in cancers with papillary morphology, *FGFR3* mutations, *FGFR3* copy number gain, elevated *FGFR3* expression, and *FGFR3–TACC3* gene fusions. Cluster II was similar to cluster I in several respects, but did not have an association with papillary morphology or *FGFR3* events. Clusters I and II both expressed high *HER2* (*ERBB2*) levels and had an elevated estrogen receptor beta (*ESR2*) signaling signature, suggesting a relationship to HER2-positive breast cancers. Clusters I and II also had features similar to those of luminal A breast cancer, with high expression of *GATA3* and *FOXA1*. I and II also expressed uroplakins (markers of urothelial differentiation), E-cadherin, and members of the miR-200 family of miRNAs (which target multiple regulators of epithelial–mesenchymal transition), suggesting that these cancers had urothelial differentiation to some extent. In contrast, cluster III ("basal/squamous-like") was similar in some respects to both basal-like breast cancer, and squamous cell cancers of the head and neck and lung with expression of epithelial lineage genes, including several keratin genes. Some also showed some degree of variant squamous histology on pathology review.

Similar but more extensive findings were made simultaneously by 2 other groups.[48,49] Unsupervised clustering using array-based RNA expression data identified 3 robust clusters, termed basal, luminal and p53-like in one of these studies (see **Fig. 2B**).[48] Samples in the basal cluster expressed high levels of keratins 5, 6, and 14, similar to cluster III from the TCGA analysis. This cluster was labeled basal, because the authors recognized that this expression pattern was similar to that of the basal layer of the normal urothelium, which is least differentiated and does not express the usual urothelial marker genes. Several other expression features were common to these 2 independently derived clusters Choi and colleagues also showed that basal bladder cancers had the poorest prognosis, with the shortest disease-specific survival.[19,48] The luminal cluster was similar to clusters I and II identified in the TCGA analysis, with expression of luminal breast cancer markers, as noted. The last cluster, p53-like, was similar to the luminal cluster in terms of luminal breast marker expression, but also had an activated wild-type p53 gene signature. Choi and colleagues did extensive replication analyses to validate their clustering analysis, including reanalysis of a large data set in which similar clusters were identified, though named somewhat differently.[50,51] Pathway analysis led to identification of Stat-3, nuclear factor-κB, Hif-1, and p63 as probable transcriptional drivers of basal gene expression[48]; and correspondingly, peroxisome proliferator activated receptor (PPAR)-γ and the estrogen receptor as drivers of the luminal gene expression pattern. Short hairpin RNA knockdown of p63 in a basal-like bladder cancer cell line, UM-

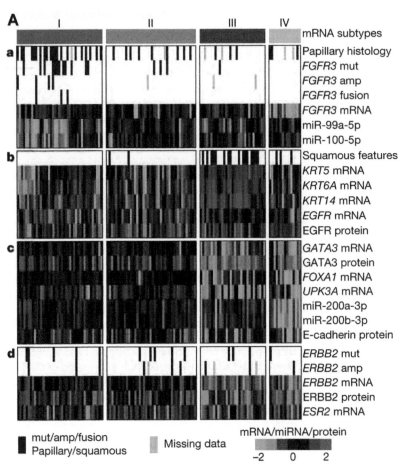

Fig. 2. Molecular subtypes of bladder cancer defined by expression profiling in 3 studies. (*A*) Expression clustering by the TCGA. (*a*), Papillary histology, FGFR3 alterations, FGFR3 expression, and reduced FGFR3-related miRNA expression are enriched in cluster I. (*b*), Expression of epithelial lineage genes and stem/progenitor cytokeratins are generally high in cluster III, some of which show variant squamous histology. (*c*) Luminal breast and urothelial differentiation factors are enriched in clusters I and II. (*d*) ERBB2 mutation and estrogen receptor-beta (ESR2) expression are enriched in clusters I and II. (*B*) Expression clustering and survival by Choi and colleagues (*a*). Array-based RNA expression profiling and hierarchical cluster analysis of a cohort of 73 muscle-invasive bladder cancers. RAS, TP53, RB1, and FGFR3 mutations are indicated below the dendrogram. Black, mutation; white, wild type; gray, data not available. Right, Kaplan-Meier overall survival (*P* = .098) and disease-specific survival (*P* = .028) in the 3 tumor subtypes. (*b*) Expression of basal and luminal markers in the 3 subtypes. The heat maps depict relative expression of basal (*left*) and luminal (*right*) biomarkers. Gene set enrichment analyses (GSEA; data not shown) were used to confirm that basal and luminal markers were enriched in the subtypes. (*C*) Associations between mutations and basal subtypes of bladder cancer by Damrauer and colleagues FGFR3 and TSC1 alterations were significantly enriched in luminal bladder cancer, whereas alterations of the RB1 pathway were enriched in basal-like bladder cancer. TP53 alterations were distributed evenly in the 2 subtypes. (*From* [*A*] The Cancer Genome Atlas Research Network. Comprehensive molecular characterization of urothelial bladder carcinoma. Nature 2014;507:318, with permission; and [*B*] Choi W, Porten S, Kim S, et al. Identification of distinct basal and luminal subtypes of muscle-invasive bladder cancer with different sensitivities to frontline chemotherapy. Cancer Cell 2014;25:153, with permission; and [*C*] Damrauer JS, Hoadley KA, Chism DD, et al. Intrinsic subtypes of high-grade bladder cancer reflect the hallmarks of breast cancer biology. Proc Natl Acad Sci U S A 2014;111:3112, with permission.)

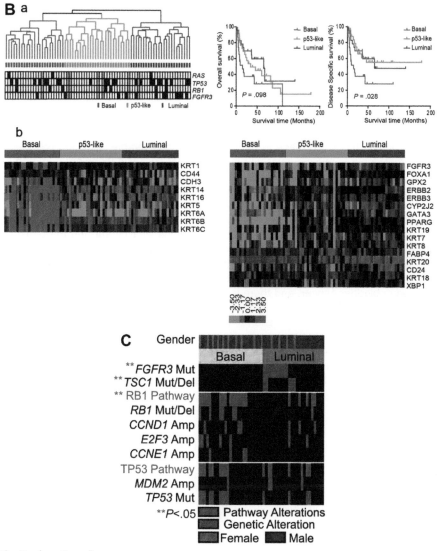

Fig. 2. (continued)

UC14, showed decreased basal gene expression, and increased PPAR-γ pathway expression. Treatment with rosiglitazone, a PPAR-γ activator, also reduced basal gene expression, and enhanced luminal cluster gene expression, providing evidence that p63 and PPAR-γ antagonize each other. Choi and colleagues[48] also noted that patients with bladder cancers in the p53-like expression cluster showed a poor response to cisplatin-based chemotherapy, finding this to be consistent among several different treatment groups they were able to collect. Notably, the p53-like expression cluster, defined by expression of a p53 gene set, did not correlate with mutation of TP53. Gene expression pattern could be assayed using DAZL technology on formalin-fixed, paraffin-embedded samples, enabling wide adoption of this method of bladder cancer expression clustering.[48]

A similar clustering of bladder cancer into basal and luminal subtypes was made independently by the third group, also using multiple data sets.[49] In addition, these investigators found that there was a significant association between mutation and expression subtype. *FGFR3* and *TSC1* mutations were significantly enriched in the luminal subtype, whereas *RB1* pathway alterations including *RB1* mutation/deletion, *CCND1* amplification, *SOX4/E2F3* amplification, and *CCNE1* amplification were significantly enriched in basal-like bladder cancer (see **Fig. 2**C).[49]

SUMMARY

Great progress has been made in deciphering in considerable detail the molecular events that occur in muscle-invasive bladder cancer.[19–22] Mutations are common in multiple signaling pathways in bladder cancer, and typically cancers have several alterations in different pathways that likely all contribute to cancer development. Cell-cycle gene alterations are common in bladder cancer, similar to many other adult malignancies, but therapeutic development in this sphere has not progressed. In contrast, multiple alterations in both receptor tyrosine kinases and the PI3K–mTOR pathway occur commonly in bladder cancer, and there is significant hope that many of these can be targeted effectively with specific kinase inhibitors either in use currently or under development. Chromatin regulatory gene mutations are especially common in bladder cancer, and there is hope for therapeutic development directed at these mutations.

Recent, comprehensive expression profiling studies have been convergent in identifying 2 major types of bladder cancer—basal and luminal—with some significant similarities to the same subtypes in breast cancer.[19,48,49] Moreover, these subtypes have different prognoses and natural histories, and response to conventional chemotherapy. Thus, there is hope that this new understanding will also translate to improved care for the bladder cancer patient.

REFERENCES

1. Jemal A, Bray F, Center MM, et al. Global cancer statistics. CA Cancer J Clin 2011;61:69–90.
2. United States Food and Drug Administration. Hematology/oncology (cancer) approvals & safety notifications. 2014. Available at: http://www.fda.gov/Drugs/InformationOnDrugs/ApprovedDrugs/ucm279174.htm. Accessed August 23, 2014.
3. Parada LF, Tabin CJ, Shih C, et al. Human EJ bladder carcinoma oncogene is homologue of Harvey sarcoma virus ras gene. Nature 1982;297:474–8.
4. Esrig D, Spruck CH, Nichols PW, et al. P53 nuclear-protein accumulation correlates with mutations in the P53 gene, tumor grade, and stage in bladder-cancer. Am J Pathol 1993;143:1389–97.
5. Cote RJ, Dunn MD, Chatterjee SJ, et al. Elevated and absent pRb expression is associated with bladder cancer progression and has cooperative effects with p53. Cancer Res 1998;58:1090–4.
6. Hornigold N, Devlin J, Davies AM, et al. Mutation of the 9q34 gene TSC1 in sporadic bladder cancer. Oncogene 1999;18:2657–61.
7. Cappellen D, De Oliveira C, Ricol D, et al. Frequent activating mutations of FGFR3 in human bladder and cervix carcinomas. Nat Genet 1999;23:18–20.
8. Lopez-Knowles E, Hernandez S, Malats N, et al. PIK3CA mutations are an early genetic alteration associated with FGFR3 mutations in superficial papillary bladder tumors. Cancer Res 2006;66:7401–4.

9. Platt FM, Hurst CD, Taylor CF, et al. Spectrum of phosphatidylinositol 3-kinase pathway gene alterations in bladder cancer. Clin Cancer Res 2009;15:6008–17.
10. Blaveri E, Brewer JL, Roydasgupta R, et al. Bladder cancer stage and outcome by array-based comparative genomic hybridization. Clin Cancer Res 2005;11: 7012–22.
11. Simon R, Burger H, Brinkschmidt C, et al. Chromosomal aberrations associated with invasion in papillary superficial bladder cancer. J Pathol 1998;185:345–51.
12. Richter J, Jiang F, Gorog JP, et al. Marked genetic differences between stage pTa and stage pT1 papillary bladder cancer detected by comparative genomic hybridization. Cancer Res 1997;57:2860–4.
13. Voorter C, Joos S, Bringuier PP, et al. Detection of chromosomal imbalances in transitional cell carcinoma of the bladder by comparative genomic hybridization. Am J Pathol 1995;146:1341–54.
14. Kallioniemi A, Kallioniemi OP, Citro G, et al. Identification of gains and losses of DNA sequences in primary bladder cancer by comparative genomic hybridization. Genes Chromosomes Cancer 1995;12:213–9.
15. Forbes SA, Bindal N, Bamford S, et al. COSMIC: mining complete cancer genomes in the catalogue of somatic mutations in cancer. Nucleic Acids Res 2011;39:D945–50.
16. Goebell PJ, Knowles MA. Bladder cancer or bladder cancers? Genetically distinct malignant conditions of the urothelium. Urol Oncol 2010;28:409–28.
17. Williamson MP, Elder PA, Shaw ME, et al. p16 (CDKN2) is a major deletion target at 9p21 in bladder cancer. Hum Mol Genet 1995;4:1569–77.
18. Knowles MA. Molecular pathogenesis of bladder cancer. Int J Clin Oncol 2008; 13:287–97.
19. The Cancer Genome Atlas Research Network. Comprehensive molecular characterization of urothelial bladder carcinoma. Nature 2014;507:315–22.
20. Gui Y, Guo G, Huang Y, et al. Frequent mutations of chromatin remodeling genes in transitional cell carcinoma of the bladder. Nat Genet 2011;43:875–8.
21. Guo GW, Sun XJ, Chen C, et al. Whole-genome and whole-exome sequencing of bladder cancer identifies frequent alterations in genes involved in sister chromatid cohesion and segregation. Nat Genet 2013;45:1459–63.
22. Cazier JB, Rao SR, McLean CM, et al. Whole-genome sequencing of bladder cancers reveals somatic CDKN1A mutations and clinicopathological associations with mutation burden. Nat Commun 2014;5:3756.
23. Kandoth C, McLellan MD, Vandin F, et al. Mutational landscape and significance across 12 major cancer types. Nature 2013;502:333–9.
24. Nik-Zainal S, Alexandrov LB, Wedge DC, et al, Breast Cancer Working Group of the International Cancer Genome Consortium. Mutational processes molding the genomes of 21 breast cancers. Cell 2012;149:979–93.
25. Roberts SA, Sterling J, Thompson C, et al. Clustered mutations in yeast and in human cancers can arise from damaged long single-strand DNA regions. Mol Cell 2012;46:424–35.
26. Hurst CD, Fiegler H, Carr P, et al. High-resolution analysis of genomic copy number alterations in bladder cancer by microarray-based comparative genomic hybridization. Oncogene 2004;23:2250–63.
27. Richter J, Beffa L, Wagner U, et al. Patterns of chromosomal imbalances in advanced urinary bladder cancer detected by comparative genomic hybridization. Am J Pathol 1998;153:1615–21.
28. Hoglund M, Sall T, Heim S, et al. Identification of cytogenetic subgroups and karyotypic pathways in transitional cell carcinoma. Cancer Res 2001;61:8241–6.

29. Sidransky D, Von Eschenbach A, Tsai YC, et al. Identification of p53 gene mutations in bladder cancers and urine samples. Science 1991;252:706–9.

30. Xu HJ, Cairns P, Hu SX, et al. Loss of RB protein expression in primary bladder cancer correlates with loss of heterozygosity at the RB locus and tumor progression. Int J Cancer 1993;53:781–4.

31. Chellappan SP, Hiebert S, Mudryj M, et al. The E2F transcription factor is a cellular target for the RB protein. Cell 1991;65:1053–61.

32. Singh D, Chan JM, Zoppoli P, et al. Transforming fusions of FGFR and TACC genes in human glioblastoma. Science 2012;337:1231–5.

33. Williams SV, Hurst CD, Knowles MA. Oncogenic FGFR3 gene fusions in bladder cancer. Hum Mol Genet 2013;22:795–803.

34. Greulich H, Kaplan B, Mertins P, et al. Functional analysis of receptor tyrosine kinase mutations in lung cancer identifies oncogenic extracellular domain mutations of ERBB2. Proc Natl Acad Sci U S A 2012;109:14476–81.

35. Jaiswal BS, Kljavin NM, Stawiski EW, et al. Oncogenic ERBB3 mutations in human cancers. Cancer Cell 2014;25:543–4.

36. Rebouissou S, Bernard-Pierrot I, de Reynies A, et al. EGFR as a potential therapeutic target for a subset of muscle-invasive bladder cancers presenting a basal-like phenotype. Sci Transl Med 2014;6:244ra91.

37. Iyer G, Hanrahan AJ, Milowsky MI, et al. Genome sequencing identifies a basis for everolimus sensitivity. Science 2012;338:221.

38. Wagle N, Grabiner BC, Van Allen EM, et al. Activating mTOR mutations in a patient with an extraordinary response on a phase I trial of everolimus and pazopanib. Cancer Discov 2014;4:546–53.

39. Shibata T, Ohta T, Tong KI, et al. Cancer related mutations in NRF2 impair its recognition by Keap1-Cul3 E3 ligase and promote malignancy. Proc Natl Acad Sci U S A 2008;105:13568.

40. Zhou JBA, Yu Q, Chng WJ. TXNIP (VDUP-1, TBP-2): a major redox regulator commonly suppressed in cancer by epigenetic mechanisms. Int J Biochem Cell Biol 2011;43:1668–73.

41. Tontonoz P, Graves RA, Budavari AI, et al. Adipocyte-specific transcription factor-ARF6 is a heterodimeric complex of 2 nuclear hormone receptors, PPAR-gamma and RXR-alpha. Nucleic Acids Res 1994;22:5628–34.

42. Taylor CF, Platt FM, Hurst CD, et al. Frequent inactivating mutations of STAG2 in bladder cancer are associated with low tumour grade and stage and inversely related to chromosomal copy number changes. Hum Mol Genet 2014;23:1964–74.

43. Balbas-Martinez C, Sagrera A, Carrillo-de-Santa-Pau E, et al. Recurrent inactivation of STAG2 in bladder cancer is not associated with aneuploidy. Nat Genet 2013;45:1464–9.

44. Solomon DA, Kim JS, Bondaruk J, et al. Frequent truncating mutations of STAG2 in bladder cancer. Nat Genet 2013;45:1428–30.

45. Lehmann AR. The xeroderma pigmentosum group D (XPD) gene: one gene, two functions, three diseases. Genes Dev 2001;15:15–23.

46. Van Allen EM, Mouw KW, Kim P, et al. Somatic ERCC2 mutations correlate with cisplatin sensitivity in muscle-invasive urothelial carcinoma. Cancer Discov 2014;4:1140–53.

47. Takata R, Katagiri T, Kanehira M, et al. Predicting response to methotrexate, vinblastine, doxorubicin, and cisplatin neoadjuvant chemotherapy for bladder cancers through genome-wide gene expression profiling. Clin Cancer Res 2005;11:2625–36.

48. Choi W, Porten S, Kim S, et al. Identification of distinct basal and luminal subtypes of muscle-invasive bladder cancer with different sensitivities to frontline chemotherapy. Cancer Cell 2014;25:152–65.
49. Damrauer JS, Hoadley KA, Chism DD, et al. Intrinsic subtypes of high-grade bladder cancer reflect the hallmarks of breast cancer biology. Proc Natl Acad Sci U S A 2014;111:3110–5.
50. Sjodahl G, Lauss M, Lovgren K, et al. A molecular taxonomy for urothelial carcinoma. Clin Cancer Res 2012;18:3377–86.
51. Sjodahl G, Lovgren K, Lauss M, et al. Toward a molecular pathologic classification of urothelial carcinoma. Am J Pathol 2013;183:681–91.

Diagnosis and Staging of Bladder Cancer

Maxine Sun, PhD[a], Quoc-Dien Trinh, MD[b],*

KEYWORDS

- Bladder cancer • Urothelial carcinoma of the bladder • Staging • Diagnosis
- Cystoscopy • Imaging • Screening • Biomarkers

KEY POINTS

- The current recommendations do not support routine bladder cancer (BCa) screening because of insufficient evidence and lack of understanding of the effects of screening in the case of overdiagnosis and overtreatment. However, the results of existing studies suggest that BCa screening may be important in high-risk populations.
- Currently, the combination of urine cytology and cystoscopy remains the gold standard for diagnosing patients with BCa. Less invasive urine biomarkers have been investigated over time, but their performance remains subpar with respect to specificity compared with cytology alone. It is unlikely that a new marker will be used to replace the conventional urine cytology and cystoscopy.
- The cornerstone of diagnosis and subsequent management of BCa is the cystoscopic examination of the lower urinary tract. Specifically, white light cystoscopy (WLC) remains the gold standard, despite its limitations. Recently, new optical diagnostic methods have been designed to improve the accuracy of WLC, such as fluorescence cystoscopy, narrow-band imaging, and optical coherence tomography; their role is currently under investigation.
- Transurethral resection of bladder tumor under regional or general anesthesia is the gold standard to excise (and potentially cure) all visible tumors and to provide specimens for staging and grading of BCa.

SCREENING, DIAGNOSIS, AND EVALUATION IN BLADDER CANCER SCREENING

Bladder cancer (BCa) is a heterogeneous disease with a variable natural history. Most patients (70%) present with superficial tumors (stages Ta, T1, or carcinoma in situ).[1]

Q.D. Trinh is supported by the Professor Walter Morris-Hale Distinguished Chair in Urologic Oncology at Brigham and Women's Hospital.
[a] Cancer Prognostics and Health Outcomes Unit, University of Montreal Health Center, Montreal, Canada; [b] Division of Urologic Surgery, Center for Surgery and Public Health, Brigham and Women's Hospital, Harvard Medical School, 45 Francis Street, ASB II-3, Boston, MA 02115, USA
* Corresponding author.
E-mail address: qtrinh@partners.org

Hematol Oncol Clin N Am 29 (2015) 205–218
http://dx.doi.org/10.1016/j.hoc.2014.10.013
0889-8588/15/$ – see front matter © 2015 Elsevier Inc. All rights reserved.

hemonc.theclinics.com

However, 3 out of 10 patients present with muscle-invasive disease (T2–4) with a high risk of death from distant metastases. Moreover, roughly between 50% and 70% of superficial tumors do recur, and approximately 10% to 20% of them progress to muscle-invasive disease.[2] However, BCa has a relatively low ratio of mortality versus incidence of new cases.[3] In consequence, there is the danger of overdiagnosis and overtreatment.

Hence, the goal and challenge of screening would be to detect the disease at an earlier stage, consequently improving morbidity and survival, but, more importantly, to be able to identify the tumors that are more likely to become muscle-invasive cancers. Such early detection of tumors could allow for earlier curative intervention and could potentially preclude the need for unnecessary surgical treatment or chemotherapy and lower the costs associated with treatment.

To date, an estimated 75,000 new cases of urinary BCa will be diagnosed in the United States (56,390 men and 18,300 women) in 2014.[4] In the same year, approximately 16,000 new deaths (11,170 men and 4410 women) are expected. BCa is the fourth most common cancer and is 3 times more common in men than in women in the United States.[5] It has also been previously reported that the age-adjusted incidence of BCa seems to be increasing over time: from 21.0 to 25.5 per 100,000 person-years between 1973 and 2009 (+0.2% per year, $P = .001$).

Two landmark studies have evaluated the effect of screening for BCa. Messing and colleagues[6] performed an important assessment based on 1575 cases ($\geq$50-year-old men screened at home using hematuria dipsticks) and 509 controls (nonscreened). Those who showed positive results underwent cystoscopy (n = 283), and 21 (7.4%) of them were diagnosed with BCa. The primary results of that study indicated that earlier detection of BCa could result in a lower proportion of invasive cancers among high-grade and/or muscle-invasive diseases in screened versus nonscreened men (10% vs 60%, $P = .002$) and a significant reduction in mortality caused by the disease (0% vs 20%, $P = .02$). Britton and colleagues[7] examined 2356 men aged 60 years and older for dipstick hematuria. The test was positive in 20% of men, and BCa was ultimately diagnosed in 17 individuals (5.3%). Of those, 9 patients had high-risk non–muscle-invasive BCa. At a 7-year follow-up, 5 out of 9 patients progressed to muscle-invasive disease and 3 out of 9 died of the disease.

Partly owning to an overall low incidence of the disease (25.5 per 100,000 person-years in 2009), screening for BCa is currently not recommended as a standard of care during routine clinical practice.[5] The challenge being that a clearly defined high-risk population needs to be identified, so as to avoid the usual harms in screening, such as unnecessary diagnostic-related treatments (ie, cystoscopy and biopsy, transurethral resection of bladder tumor [TURBT], intravesical chemotherapy), and overdiagnosis.[3,8] Wu and colleagues[9] generated a model based on large case-control data (n = 678 cases and n = 678 controls) for the prediction of BCa risk using established risk factors, such as smoking and well-known occupational exposure (eg, diesel, aromatic amines, dry cleaning fluids, radioactive materials, arsenic). At internal validation, the model demonstrated an area under the curve of 80%. However, the model is impeded by the lack of external validation.

Similarly, Vickers and colleagues[10] using data from the Prostate, Lung, Colorectal, and Ovarian Cancer Screening Trial attempted to create a risk score in order to identify those at higher risk of developing BCa. The study comprised 49,873 persons for the training set and 99,746 individuals for the external validation set. The investigators showed that the trade-off between the number of patients screened and invasive/high-grade tumors avoided was more optimal when restricting screening to a high-risk population instead of the whole population (57 vs 38 per 100,000), hence supporting the strategy to screen a high-risk population only.

Although large-scale screening programs may seem beneficial and critical, the US Preventive Services Task Force has deemed existing evidence to be insufficient in assessing the balance of benefits and harms of screening.[3] Experts have suggested that improvements have to be made with regard to the identification of what should be defined as high-risk populations before a randomized-controlled trial could be designed to validate the hypothesis of an improvement in screening.[8] It is noteworthy that in recent years, little progress in improving survival and reducing mortality for patients with muscle-invasive BCa has been seen.[11] Indeed, despite well-known risk factors (ie, smoking, occupational exposure), as well as the developments in BCa management over time, it did not lead to better cancer control outcomes. In consequence, it may be important to adequately address the challenges of screening in BCa in the near future.

FUTURE CONSIDERATIONS FOR SCREENING

Many unknowns remain before a large-scale program of BCa screening may be put forward. For one, few studies have examined the natural history of screened early stage untreated BCa. The appreciation of how such tumors behave may assist clinicians in understanding the effects of screening and overdiagnosis/overtreatment. Other randomized studies with large sample sizes that assess urine tests and the incidence of BCa, and staging, with follow-up information on clinical and cancer control outcomes are needed. A uniform definition of what constitutes a high-risk population is necessary in order to reduce the potential harms associated with overdiagnosis/overtreatment. Moreover, it may be important to invest in less invasive and costly diagnostic tools but equally sensitive and specific. For example, traditional cystoscopy may not be adequate if population-based screening is envisaged, as the procedure is invasive and not cost-efficient. In order to reduce the number cystoscopies required to diagnose one patient with BCa, the combination of dipstick testing and molecular markers have been suggested.[12] It may also be worthwhile to test the effect of less toxic treatments in patients diagnosed in the earlier stages to prevent progression versus more invasive and toxic treatments reserved for patients diagnosed in the more advanced stages. This testing may be useful in evaluating the trade-offs and costs associated with earlier treatment modalities.

PRESENTATION AND INVESTIGATION

The most common presenting symptom of BCa is gross hematuria. In patients with carcinoma in situ, additional unexplained urinary frequency, urgency, or irritative voiding symptoms may indicate the possibility of BCa. The prevalence of BCa ranges between 13% and 35% in patients presenting with gross hematuria and between 5% and 10% in patients presenting with microscopic hematuria.[13,14] The proportion of patients with asymptomatic hematuria ranges between 0.2% and 21.0%, when a direct relationship with age has been shown.[7,15]

The current practice includes urine dipstick or microscopic urinalysis for hematuria, urine cytology, and other tests for urine biomarkers, although their value has not yet been established.[1] Patients with positive results are referred for further evaluation, which generally include cystoscopy, followed by biopsy if necessary, and radiological investigation. Imaging is important in the evaluation for patients presenting with hematuria, primarily to visualize the upper urinary tract, as cystoscopy inspects the lower tracts. Options for imaging include ultrasonography, intravenous urogram (IVU), computed tomography (CT) urography, MRI, or a combination of these.

BLADDER TUMOR MARKERS

Urine cytology, a simple and noninvasive procedure, in combination with cystoscopy is superior to cystoscopy alone in identifying high-grade lesions (ie, carcinoma in situ).[16] It has a good sensitivity for detecting high-grade BCa but a poor sensitivity for detecting low-grade tumors (between 7%–17%).[16] In recent years, several novel developments of urine markers for the detection of BCa have been investigated (**Table 1**). For example, of 79 patients with BCa, the nuclear matrix protein 22 (NMP-22) assay was positive in 44 patients (sensitivity 56% and specificity 86%).[17] Similarly, fluorescence in situ hybridization (FISH, Vysis Inc., Downers Grove, IL) (ie, UroVysion assay designed to detect aneuploidy for chromosomes 3, 7, 17 and loss of the 9p21 locus via FISH) demonstrated a promising range of sensitivity (70%–86%) and specificity (66%–93%) in a pooled analysis of 4 articles as part of a meta-analysis.[18]

However, urine cytology remains superior in specificity compared with most other markers (up to 98%, see **Table 1**).[19,20] Moreover, no biomarker has demonstrated superior clinical utility over cytology and cystoscopy combined. Hence, experts agree that it is highly unlikely that a new marker could achieve the accuracy of what cytology and cystoscopy can offer. Currently, the use of urine cytology is recommended by national guidelines[5] despite the paucity of randomized trials that actually examined its use in clinical practice.[21] For patients with noninvasive disease, urine cytology also represents an important surveillance tool.

PERSPECTIVES ON SCREENING

The current recommendations do not support routine BCa screening because of insufficient evidence and lack of understanding of the effects of screening in the case of overdiagnosis and overtreatment. However, the results of existing studies suggest that BCa screening may be important in high-risk populations. The challenge remains that experts need to be able to diagnose patients at an early stage of the disease and,

Table 1
Noninvasive bladder tumor markers

	Marker	Sensitivity[a] (%)	Specificity[b] (%)
Cytology[16]	Tumor cells sloughed into urine	7–17 For low grade 53–90 For high grade	90–98
NMP-22[17,72]	Nuclear protein released during apoptosis	44–50 For non–muscle-invasive BCa 90 For muscle-invasive BCa	87
BTA Stat and BTA TRAK[73,74]	Detects urothelial basement membrane	50–80	50–75
ImmonoCyt (DiagnoCure, Inc., Québec, Canada)[75,76]	Immunofluorescence–3 monoclonal antibodies	50–74	62–73
UroVysion[18,77,78]	FISH with probes to Chr 3, 7, 17, 9p21	68–86	40–93

Abbreviation: BTA, Bladder tumor associated antigen; FISH, fluorescence in situ hybridization; NMP-22, nuclear matrix protein 22.

[a] Sensitivity: the percent of patients with the disease for whom the test is positive (true positive/total number of patients with the disease × 100).

[b] Specificity: the percent of patients without the disease in whom the test is negative (true negative/total number of individuals without the disease × 100).

at the same time, identify the tumors that are likely to progress to muscle-invasive disease. Currently, the combination of urine cytology and cystoscopy remains the gold standard for diagnosing patients with BCa. Less invasive urine biomarkers have been investigated over time, but their performance remains subpar with respect to specificity compared with cytology alone. It is unlikely that a new marker will be used to replace the conventional urine cytology and cystoscopy.

ENDOSCOPIC EXAMINATION OF THE LOWER URINARY TRACT

The cornerstone of the diagnosis and subsequent management of BCa is the cystoscopic examination of the lower urinary tract. Specifically, white light cystoscopy (WLC) remains the gold standard, despite its limitations. Recently, new optical diagnostic methods have been designed to improve the accuracy of WLC: fluorescence cystoscopy, narrow-band imaging (NBI), and optical coherence tomography (OCT).

WHITE LIGHT CYSTOSCOPY

WLC allows examination of the urethra and the bladder. It can be performed with either rigid or flexible endoscopes, depending on the clinical scenario. For screening and diagnostic office-based purposes, flexible cystoscopy is typically used. Although it is a more comfortable instrument than the rigid cystoscope, it has the disadvantages of having a small irrigation port and lacks a separate working sheath. It is also more costly and inclined to failure.

The sensitivity and specificity of WLC range from 62% to 84% and 43% to 98%, respectively.[22] Its sensitivity is lower for small papillary bladder tumors and carcinoma in situ.[22] Moreover, the accuracy of WLC has been shown to be operator dependent. Given the known drawbacks of an office-based flexible cystoscopy under local anesthesia, it is recommended to perform a thorough reassessment using the rigid cystoscope under general anesthesia when patients are brought to the operating room to resect a newly diagnosed bladder tumor.

Moreover, evidence suggests that the operator's ability to estimate the stage or grade based on the visual appearance on WLC is limited.[23] It is also difficult to differentiate inflammatory lesions because of the previous instillation therapy from carcinoma in situ (CIS), as both will present as erythema. Although WLC remains the current standard for diagnosis and follow-up, further improvements of the technique are needed.

FLUORESCENCE CYSTOSCOPY

Fluorescence cystoscopy or photodynamic diagnosis (PDD) can improve the visualization of BCa compared with conventional WLC and, consequently, reduced the rates of residual tumor at the first cystoscopy.[24–26] PPD relies on the intravesical administration of endogenous or exogenous photosensitizing agents that cause abnormal or rapidly proliferating cells to fluoresce under a specific wavelength of light. The solution containing the photosensitizing agents is instilled in the bladder thru a transurethral catheter before surgery. By illuminating the mucosa with blue-violet light, the neoplastic cells appear red or pink against a blue background. However, false or artifact fluorescence can occur with inflammation, recent TUR, or tangential illumination of the bladder mucosa.[27–30] False positives are frequent in patients who recently have had intravesical therapy, especially bacillus Calmette-Guérin.[31,32]

Multiple studies have demonstrated that PDD, in addition to WLC, improves the detection rate of BCa.[29,30,33–36] The tumor detection rate for WLC alone is 73% to 96% versus

90% to 96% for WLC plus PDD. The difference is even more striking for carcinoma in situ: 23% to 68% versus 91% to 97%, respectively. However, the false-positive detection rate of PDD is higher (9%–63% vs 7%–47%, respectively). A recent meta-analysis of 18 studies showed that the rate of residual tumor was significantly decreased after PDD (odds ratio [OR]: 0.28; 95% confidence interval [CI], 0.15–0.52; $P<.0001$), whereas the recurrence-free survival was higher at 12 and 24 months in the PDD groups relative to the WLC-only groups (log-rank = 0.00002).[37] Several researchers have also investigated the value of PDD in the evaluation of patients with positive urine cytology in the absence of disease after standard investigations. For example, Ray and colleagues[38] showed that BCa was detected by PDD in 32% of patients with confirmed positive urinary cytology and negative WLC. Finally, the same group also examined the role in the treatment of patients with multifocal tumors, who are at a 1.5-fold increased risk of recurrence.[39] They showed in a series of 18 patients that the sensitivity of PDD for the detection of tumor was 97.8% compared with 69.6% for WLC.[40]

NARROW-BAND IMAGING

For NBI, optical filters are use in the light source to narrow the bandwidth between 415 nm (blue light) and 540 nm (green light). This narrow bandwidth is strongly absorbed by hemoglobin, thus enhancing surface capillaries and blood vessels.[41] In contrast to PDD, systems integrating WLC and NBI are already available. Since its initial report in 2008,[42] several studies have examined the accuracy of NBI cystoscopy for the detection of BCa and showed improved detection for NBI over WLC. A meta-analysis including 8 studies (n = 1022) showed a sensitivity and specificity for NBI of 94.3% and 84.7%, respectively, versus 84.8% and 87.0% for WLC.[43]

OPTICAL COHERENCE TOMOGRAPHY

OCT is a noninvasive technique that provides cross-sectional imaging below the mucosal surface. OCT is analogous to ultrasound imaging, except that it is based on the depth detection of light rather than sound. For image acquisition, OCT is probe based and relies on WLC to identify suspicious areas that warrant further characterization. The sensitivity and specificity of OCT to detect BCa range from 84% to 100% and from 78% to 90%, respectively.[44–47] OCT also has demonstrated to discriminate accurately between muscle-invasive and non–muscle-invasive tumors.[45,48] Conversely, false positives may occur in the presence of scarring or inflammation of the mucosa.[44,45]

PERSPECTIVES ON ENDOSCOPIC EXAMINATION

The role of complementary approaches to endoscopic examination of the bladder remains unclear. In an era of heightened scrutiny with regard to health care costs, several investigators have hypothesized that these techniques may help in reducing the financial burden of BCa. For example, by preventing recurrences and subsequent reinterventions, PDD would potentially be cost-effective; a health technology assessment from the United Kingdom showed that management strategies involving PDD for the detection and follow-up of BCa provided some marginal financial benefits when weighing in the acquisition costs.[21]

TRANSURETHRAL RESECTION OF BLADDER TUMORS

TURBT under regional or general anesthesia is the gold standard to excise (and potentially cure) all visible tumors and to provide specimens for staging and grading of BCa.

In this section, the authors discuss the preoperative and intraoperative specifics of TURBT.

PREOPERATIVE IMAGING

Before resection, upper tract imaging is usually recommended both to identify other sources of hematuria and to assess the upper tract urothelium because of the field change nature of urothelial carcinoma that can affect such cells in all parts of the urinary tract. Such imaging studies are routinely done as part of the workup for hematuria, the most common presentation of a bladder tumor. Indeed, the American Urologic Association's best practices guidelines for asymptomatic hematuria suggest either intravenous urography or CT urography as the initial imaging test.

In the past decade, upper tract imaging is usually obtained with a CT urography, which allows the assessment of both the renal parenchyma and the upper tract urothelium. It is also able to rule out other genitourinary conditions that may cause hematuria, including urolithiasis, renal masses, urinary tract infection, and trauma. For these reasons, it is now the standard imaging modality for this indication and has completely replaced intravenous urography at Brigham and Women's Hospital since 2000. Alternatively, other diagnostic modalities of the upper tract include abdominal ultrasound, intravenous urography, magnetic resonance urography, and intraoperative retrograde pyelogram. Abdominal ultrasound is sensitive in diagnosing hydronephrosis but has a limited role to identify lesions in the ureter. Magnetic resonance provides similar information compared with CT urography, yet is less accurate for calculi,[49] takes significantly longer to perform, and costs more. However, it has the advantage of not requiring ionizing radiation. Unfortunately, there have been no direct comparisons between CT and magnetic resonance urography for the detection of urothelial carcinoma.[50] Finally, an alternative to preoperative imaging is to perform an intraoperative retrograde pyelogram. Cowan and colleagues[51] compared CT urography with retrograde pyelogram for the detection of urothelial carcinoma and found that the only false-negative CT urography was a small urothelial tumor that was not visible in a unopacified segment of the ureter.

PREOPERATIVE RISK ASSESSMENT

Basic laboratory tests should be obtained before surgery. Urine culture should be done to rule out infections, which should be treated before proceeding to this elective procedure. Complete blood count and basic metabolic profile including creatinine may provide important preoperative baseline information. A coagulation profile is often recommended and required if patients are to have the procedure under spinal anesthesia.

Preoperative risk assessment should be done meticulously, as urothelial carcinoma of the bladder is a disease of the elderly, an increasingly multi-morbid population. Patients should be assessed to ensure that they will tolerate the lithotomy position. A thorough medication history is critical. Antiplatelet agents should be discontinued 7 to 10 days before surgery when possible. In select patients, it may be necessary to continue these drugs, with an increased risk of bleeding, for medical reasons. There are data to suggest that a low dose of acetylsalicylic acid does not increase the risk of overall bleeding or reintervention.[52] Further, another study by Carmignani and colleagues[53] showed that TURBT under dual antithrombotic therapy (clopidogrel + acetylsalicylic acid) is feasible. However, there is a general consensus that warfarin should be discontinued at least 5 days prior and that the international normalized ratio should be checked the day of surgery.

SURGICAL TECHNIQUE

TURBT can be performed under local, spinal, or general anesthesia. The choice of technique will depend on several factors including the preoperative risk assessment as well as tumor characteristics (location, size, and anticipated depth of invasion). Local anesthesia TURBT should only be done to excise and fulgurate small/superficial tumors in select patients at increased risk of complications with regional/general anesthesia. Regional anesthesia in the form of spinal or epidural blockade is effective to treat tumors that are not on the lateral aspect of the bladder. This type of anesthesia provides the advantage of having a conscious patient who would present abdominal or shoulder-tip pain in the advent of an intraperitoneal perforation. Finally, general anesthesia with paralysis to prevent the obturator reflex is recommended for large, lateral bladder masses. An alternative to complete blockade is the obturator nerve block; however, this is seldom practiced. Antibiotics should be given in concordance with local and national practice guidelines.

Following anesthesia, patients are placed in a dorsal lithotomy position with padding of all pressure points. Special care should be taken to avoid foot drop because of neurapraxia of the common peroneal nerve, passing along the lateral proximal fibula.

The bladder should be inspected with a rigid cystoscope using both a 30° and a 70° lens. Cystoscopic findings should be redocumented and may differ from the office flexible cystoscopy, particularly in regard to the location of tumors. Thereafter, resection should be performed using a 30° lens placed through a resectoscope sheath. Irrigation must be used to facilitate visualization of the tumor, but efforts should be made to minimize overdistention and, consequently, the risk of bladder perforation. TURBT is usually performed in sterile water or glycine, as saline conducts electricity and scatters energy from monopolar cautery. Recently, bipolar resection has been introduced as an alternative approach using saline irrigation to minimize the risk of obturator reflex.

Tumors can be resected in a staged or en bloc fashion. Friable, low-grade tumors that are 3 cm or greater can be excised en bloc, often without electrical energy. The advantages of this approach for select tumors include decreased cautery artifact, avoidance of tumor fragmentation, and preservation of spatial orientation of the specimen. However, in most cases, the resection is performed in a staged-piecemeal fashion whereby each layer is carefully resected until the base of the tumor is reached. Staged resection minimizes the chance of bladder perforation. Moreover, using the cutting current is important to minimize cautery artifacts and, consequently, improve the pathologist's ability to assess the stage and grade. In patients with suspected involvement of the muscularis propria, following complete resection, cold cup biopsies should be obtained to determine the presence of muscle invasion of the tumor base. Failure to demonstrate invasion imposes the need for repeat resection unless the decision is made to proceed to cystectomy based on factors other than muscle invasion (such as recurrent high-grade T1).

Special attention is required in cases of tumors situated near a ureteral orifice, inside a diverticulum, or in the anterior aspect of the bladder. First, cautery should be used judiciously when resection is near the ureteral orifice. In doubt, it may be cautious to leave a ureteral stent to prevent temporary obstruction from postoperative edema. Resection of diverticular tumors presents a high risk of bladder wall perforation, and accurate staging is difficult to achieve in this circumstance because the underlying detrusor is absent. For these reasons, diverticulectomy, partial cystectomy, or radical cystectomy should be considered for large or high-grade tumors arising inside a diverticulum.

Regarding anterior tumors, minimal bladder filling combined with manual suprapubic compression to bring the tumor toward the resectoscope facilitates removal.

At the end of the procedure, bimanual examination of the bladder should be performed under anesthesia to accurately perform T staging. One hand is placed in the lower abdomen and 1 to 2 fingers of the other hand are placed in the anus (male) or vagina (female). Fixation (cT4) or persistence (cT3) of a palpable 3-dimensional mass after resection suggests locally advanced disease.

The current management guidelines from the National Comprehensive Cancer Network recommend repeat resection (within 6 weeks) in the following: (1) incomplete initial resection, (2) no muscle in original specimen for high-grade disease, (3) large or multifocal lesions, or (4) any T1 lesion. There is convincing evidence to support the use of repeat TURBT. For example, Herr[54] showed that 28 out of 96 patients with non–muscle-invasive tumors were reclassified as muscle invasive at repeat resection. A prospective trial by Divrik and colleagues[55] randomized patients with newly diagnosed T1 urothelial carcinoma of the bladder to repeat resection and adjuvant intravesical mitomycin C versus adjuvant intravesical mitomycin C without re-resection. Both the recurrence (25.7% vs 63.2%) and progression (4.1% vs 11.8%) rates were lower in patients who underwent repeat TURBT.

IMAGING

Although the gold standard of BCa diagnosis is WLC cystoscopy and subsequent TURBT, many imaging techniques have emerged to better diagnose and stage the primary lesion and regional/distant spread.

VIRTUAL CYSTOSCOPY

Virtual cystoscopy was developed in an effort to reduce discomfort and pain reported by more than one-third of patients with standard cystoscopy.[56] Two kinds of virtual cystoscopy exist: CT virtual cystoscopy and MRI virtual cystoscopy. In a meta-analysis that pooled a total of 26 studies based on 3084 patients, the pooled sensitivities of CT virtual cystoscopy and MRI virtual cystoscopy were 94% and 91%, respectively.[57] For the same groups, the pooled specificities were 98% and 95%, respectively. Although virtual cystoscopy may be less invasive compared with standard cystoscopy, the latter represents the gold standard recommended by existing guidelines.[5]

COMPUTED TOMOGRAPHY AND MRI FOR LOCALIZED BLADDER CANCER

According to the most recent version of the National Comprehensive Cancer Network's guidelines for BCa, if the cystoscopic appearance of the tumor is solid, high grade, or possibly invasive, a CT scan or MRI of the abdomen or pelvis is recommended before TURBT.[5] Previous studies have reported a sensitivity of 62% to 91% and a specificity of 63% to 95% for the detection and staging of BCa of CT scans, respectively.[58–60] Studies focusing on multidetector CT showed sensitivity ranging between 89% and 91% and specificity ranging between 92% and 95%.[59,60] Experts agree that CT cannot reliably differentiate non–muscle-invasive from muscle-invasive BCa. However, CT may be useful in detecting extravesical spread.[19]

Compared with CT, MRI seems to be superior in clinical staging of BCa.[61] On its own, staging sensitivity ranges between 68% and 80% and specificity ranges between 90% and 93%.[62,63] Compared with TURBT, MRI is unlikely to be more accurate. However, TURBT is associated with a non-negligible rate of understaging (42%),[64] whereas MRI is useful in detecting T3 to T4 disease.[19]

COMPUTED TOMOGRAPHY, MRI, AND PET FOR LYMPH NODE METASTASIS

The current conventional staging methods (ie, TUR pathology and cross-sectional imaging) may result in up to 25% of patients with lymph node metastases that are missed before surgery. In consequence, there is an obvious interest in the use of imaging tools to identify the presence of local and regional disease burden in the preoperative setting, as lymph node metastasis represents an important predictor of treatment success.

CT scans detect lymph node metastases in BCa with a sensitivity ranging between 31% and 50% and a specificity ranging between 68% and 100%.[58,65,66] What has been found in direct comparisons between CT and MRI in the detection of lymph nodes preoperatively is that MRI is in general better at finding a higher number of lymph nodes and at detecting lymph nodes that are smaller (1–5 mm).[67] Compared with CT, F-fluorodeoxyglucose PET (FDG PET) demonstrated a sensitivity of detecting metastatic disease outside of the pelvis of 54% versus 41% for CT, respectively, and comparable specificity ($\sim$97%).[68] In general, PET scan seems to be superior compared with CT or MRI in detecting lymph node metastases preoperatively.[65,68] However, the use of PET in BCa is also limited because of the urinary excretion of FDG and subsequent poor differentiation of lesions in the bladder and adjacent lymph nodes.[69]

EVALUATING CHEMOTHERAPY RESPONSE USING MRI

MRI is used after radiation for BCa to identify residual active malignancy.[70] Schrier and colleagues[71] examined 40 patients with cN1–N2 treated with chemotherapy. After patients' second and fourth chemotherapy courses, evidence of early response was assessed with dynamic-contrast-enhanced MRI. The clinical response was determined by examining the rapidity with which the tumor and lymph nodes enhanced with contrast. The results of their study suggest that if the cancerous tissue enhanced greater than 10 seconds after arterial enhancement, those individuals could be considered responders of chemotherapy. The study reported a sensitivity of 91% and a specificity of 93%.

PERSPECTIVES ON IMAGING

CT and MRI are considered options. Compared with TURBT, both CT and MRI may not be useful in staging purposes, unless it is to confirm or rule out extravesicle disease or metastatic spread. PET scan may be more accurate than CT and MRI at detecting lymph node metastases. The conjunctive use of standard CT with PET is not recommended. The use of MRI can serve as a radiographic biomarker in assessing the response to chemotherapy.

REFERENCES

1. Kaufman DS, Shipley WU, Feldman AS. Bladder cancer. Lancet 2009;374(9685): 239–49.
2. Rübben H, Lutzeyer W, Fischer N, et al. Natural history and treatment of low and high risk superficial bladder tumors. J Urol 1988;139(2):283–5.
3. Moyer VA. Screening for bladder cancer: US Preventive Services Task Force recommendation statement. Ann Intern Med 2011;155(4):246–51.
4. Siegel R, Ma J, Zou Z, et al. Cancer statistics, 2014. CA Cancer J Clin 2014;64(1): 9–29.

5. Clark PE, Agarwal N, Biagioli MC, et al. Bladder cancer. J Natl Compr Canc Netw 2013;11:446–75.
6. Messing EM, Madeb R, Young T, et al. Long-term outcome of hematuria home screening for bladder cancer in men. Cancer 2006;107(9):2173–9.
7. Britton J, Dowell A, Whelan P, et al. A community study of bladder cancer screening by the detection of occult urinary bleeding. J Urol 1992;148(3):788–90.
8. Larré S, Catto JW, Cookson MS, et al. Screening for bladder cancer: rationale, limitations, whom to target, and perspectives. Eur Urol 2013;63(6):1049–58.
9. Wu X, Lin J, Grossman HB, et al. Projecting individualized probabilities of developing bladder cancer in white individuals. J Clin Oncol 2007;25(31):4974–81.
10. Vickers AJ, Bennette C, Kibel AS, et al. Who should be included in a clinical trial of screening for bladder cancer? Cancer 2012;119(1):143–9.
11. Abdollah F, Gandaglia G, Thuret R, et al. Incidence, survival and mortality rates of stage-specific bladder cancer in United States: a trend analysis. Cancer Epidemiol 2013;37(3):219–25.
12. Lotan Y, Shariat SF, Schmitz-Dräger BJ, et al. Considerations on implementing diagnostic markers into clinical decision making in bladder cancer. Urol Oncol 2014;28(4):441–8.
13. Edwards TJ, Dickinson AJ, Gosling J, et al. Patient-specific risk of undetected malignant disease after investigation for haematuria, based on a 4-year follow-up. BJU Int 2010;107(2):247–52.
14. Mishriki SF, Nabi G, Cohen NP. Diagnosis of urologic malignancies in patients with asymptomatic dipstick hematuria: prospective study with 13 years' follow-up. Urology 2008;71(1):13–6.
15. Rodgers MA, Hempel S, Aho T, et al. Diagnostic tests used in the investigation of adult haematuria: a systematic review. BJU Int 2006;98(6):1154–60.
16. Lokeshwar VB, Soloway MS. Current bladder tumor tests: does their projected utility fulfill clinical necessity? J Urol 2001;165(4):1067–77.
17. Grossman HB, Messing E, Soloway M, et al. Detection of bladder cancer using a point-of-care proteomic assay. JAMA 2005;293(7):810–6.
18. van Rhijn BW, van der Poel HG, van der Kwast TH. Urine markers for bladder cancer surveillance: a systematic review. Eur Urol 2005;47(6):736–48.
19. Kamat AM, Hegarty PK, Gee JR, et al. ICUD-EAU International Consultation on Bladder Cancer 2012: screening, diagnosis, and molecular markers. Eur Urol 2013;63(1):4–15.
20. Tilki D, Burger M, Dalbagni G, et al. Urine markers for detection and surveillance of non muscle invasive bladder cancer. Eur Urol 2011;60(3):484–92.
21. Mowatt G, Zhu S, Kilonzo M, et al. Systematic review of the clinical effectiveness and cost-effectiveness of photodynamic diagnosis and urine biomarkers (FISH, ImmunoCyt, NMP22) and cytology for the detection and follow-up of bladder cancer. Health Technol Assess 2010;14(4):1–331, iii–iv.
22. Jocham D, Stepp H, Waidelich R. Photodynamic diagnosis in urology: state-of-the-art. Eur Urol 2008;53(6):1138–48.
23. Cina SJ, Epstein JI, Endrizzi JM, et al. Correlation of cystoscopic impression with histologic diagnosis of biopsy specimens of the bladder. Hum Pathol 2001;32(6):630–7.
24. Riedl CR, Daniltchenko D, Koenig F, et al. Fluorescence endoscopy with 5-aminolevulinic acid reduces early recurrence rate in superficial bladder cancer. J Urol 2001;165(4):1121–3.
25. Kriegmair M, Zaak D, Rothenberger KH, et al. Transurethral resection for bladder cancer using 5-aminolevulinic acid induced fluorescence endoscopy versus white light endoscopy. J Urol 2002;168(2):475–8.

26. Filbeck T, Pichlmeier U, Knuechel R, et al. Clinically relevant improvement of recurrence-free survival with 5-aminolevulinic acid induced fluorescence diagnosis in patients with superficial bladder tumors. J Urol 2002;168(1):67–71.

27. Hungerhuber E, Stepp H, Kriegmair M, et al. Seven years' experience with 5-aminolevulinic acid in detection of transitional cell carcinoma of the bladder. Urology 2007;69(2):260–4.

28. Zaak D, Kriegmair M, Stepp H, et al. Endoscopic detection of transitional cell carcinoma with 5-aminolevulinic acid: results of 1012 fluorescence endoscopies. Urology 2001;57(4):690–4.

29. Fradet Y, Grossman HB, Gomella L, et al. A comparison of hexaminolevulinate fluorescence cystoscopy and white light cystoscopy for the detection of carcinoma in situ in patients with bladder cancer: a phase III, multicenter study. J Urol 2007;178(1):68–73 [discussion: 73].

30. Grossman HB, Gomella L, Fradet Y, et al. A phase III, multicenter comparison of hexaminolevulinate fluorescence cystoscopy and white light cystoscopy for the detection of superficial papillary lesions in patients with bladder cancer. J Urol 2007;178(1):62–7.

31. Draga RO, Grimbergen MC, Kok ET, et al. Photodynamic diagnosis (5-aminolevulinic acid) of transitional cell carcinoma after bacillus Calmette-Guerin immunotherapy and mitomycin C intravesical therapy. Eur Urol 2010;57(4):655–60.

32. Grimbergen MC, van Swol CF, Jonges TG, et al. Reduced specificity of 5-ALA induced fluorescence in photodynamic diagnosis of transitional cell carcinoma after previous intravesical therapy. Eur Urol 2003;44(1):51–6.

33. Schmidbauer J, Witjes F, Schmeller N, et al. Improved detection of urothelial carcinoma in situ with hexaminolevulinate fluorescence cystoscopy. J Urol 2004; 171(1):135–8.

34. Jichlinski P, Guillou L, Karlsen SJ, et al. Hexyl aminolevulinate fluorescence cystoscopy: new diagnostic tool for photodiagnosis of superficial bladder cancer–a multicenter study. J Urol 2003;170(1):226–9.

35. Jocham D, Witjes F, Wagner S, et al. Improved detection and treatment of bladder cancer using hexaminolevulinate imaging: a prospective, phase III multicenter study. J Urol 2005;174(3):862–6 [discussion: 866].

36. Denzinger S, Burger M, Walter B, et al. Clinically relevant reduction in risk of recurrence of superficial bladder cancer using 5-aminolevulinic acid-induced fluorescence diagnosis: 8-year results of prospective randomized study. Urology 2007;69(4):675–9.

37. Kausch I, Sommerauer M, Montorsi F, et al. Photodynamic diagnosis in non-muscle-invasive bladder cancer: a systematic review and cumulative analysis of prospective studies. Eur Urol 2010;57(4):595–606.

38. Ray ER, Chatterton K, Khan MS, et al. Hexylaminolaevulinate 'blue light' fluorescence cystoscopy in the investigation of clinically unconfirmed positive urine cytology. BJU Int 2009;103(10):1363–7.

39. Sylvester RJ, van der Meijden AP, Oosterlinck W, et al. Predicting recurrence and progression in individual patients with stage Ta T1 bladder cancer using EORTC risk tables: a combined analysis of 2596 patients from seven EORTC trials. Eur Urol 2006;49(3):466–77.

40. Ray ER, Chatterton K, Thomas K, et al. Hexylaminolevulinate photodynamic diagnosis for multifocal recurrent nonmuscle invasive bladder cancer. J Endourol 2009;23(6):983–8.

41. Kuznetsov K, Lambert R, Rey JF. Narrow-band imaging: potential and limitations. Endoscopy 2006;38(1):76–81.

42. Bryan RT, Billingham LJ, Wallace DM. Narrow-band imaging flexible cystoscopy in the detection of recurrent urothelial cancer of the bladder. BJU Int 2008;101(6): 702–5 [discussion: 705–6].

43. Zheng C, Lv Y, Zhong Q, et al. Narrow band imaging diagnosis of bladder cancer: systematic review and meta-analysis. BJU Int 2012;110(11 Pt B):E680–7.

44. Ren H, Waltzer WC, Bhalla R, et al. Diagnosis of bladder cancer with microelectromechanical systems-based cystoscopic optical coherence tomography. Urology 2009;74(6):1351–7.

45. Goh AC, Tresser NJ, Shen SS, et al. Optical coherence tomography as an adjunct to white light cystoscopy for intravesical real-time imaging and staging of bladder cancer. Urology 2008;72(1):133–7.

46. Hermes B, Spoler F, Naami A, et al. Visualization of the basement membrane zone of the bladder by optical coherence tomography: feasibility of noninvasive evaluation of tumor invasion. Urology 2008;72(3):677–81.

47. Manyak MJ, Gladkova ND, Makari JH, et al. Evaluation of superficial bladder transitional-cell carcinoma by optical coherence tomography. J Endourol 2005; 19(5):570–4.

48. Zagaynova EV, Streltsova OS, Gladkova ND, et al. In vivo optical coherence tomography feasibility for bladder disease. J Urol 2002;167(3):1492–6.

49. Regan F, Kuszyk B, Bohlman ME, et al. Acute ureteric calculus obstruction: unenhanced spiral CT versus HASTE MR urography and abdominal radiograph. Br J Radiol 2005;78(930):506–11.

50. Silverman SG, Leyendecker JR, Amis ES Jr. What is the current role of CT urography and MR urography in the evaluation of the urinary tract? Radiology 2009; 250(2):309–23.

51. Cowan NC, Turney BW, Taylor NJ, et al. Multidetector computed tomography urography for diagnosing upper urinary tract urothelial tumour. BJU Int 2007;99(6): 1363–70.

52. Picozzi S, Marenghi C, Ricci C, et al. Risks and complications of transurethral resection of bladder tumor among patients taking antiplatelet agents for cardiovascular disease. Surg Endosc 2014;28(1):116–21.

53. Carmignani L, Picozzi S, Stubinski R, et al. Endoscopic resection of bladder cancer in patients receiving double platelet antiaggregant therapy. Surg Endosc 2011;25(7):2281–7.

54. Herr HW. The value of a second transurethral resection in evaluating patients with bladder tumors. J Urol 1999;162(1):74–6.

55. Divrik RT, Yildirim U, Zorlu F, et al. The effect of repeat transurethral resection on recurrence and progression rates in patients with T1 tumors of the bladder who received intravesical mitomycin: a prospective, randomized clinical trial. J Urol 2006 May;175(5):1641–4.

56. van der Aa M, Steyerberg E, Sen E, et al. Patients' perceived burden of cystoscopic and urinary surveillance of bladder cancer: a randomized comparison. BJU Int 2008;101(9):1106–10.

57. Qu X, Huang X, Wu L, et al. Comparison of virtual cystoscopy and ultrasonography for bladder cancer detection: a meta-analysis. Eur J Radiol 2011;80(2):188–97.

58. Baltaci S, Resorlu B, Yagci C, et al. Computerized tomography for detecting perivesical infiltration and lymph node metastasis in invasive bladder carcinoma. Urol Int 2008;81(4):399–402.

59. Kim J, Park S, Ahn H, et al. Bladder cancer: analysis of multi-detector row helical CT enhancement pattern and accuracy in tumor detection and perivesical staging. Radiology 2004;231(3):725–31.

60. Koplay M, Kantarci M, Güven F, et al. Diagnostic efficiency of multidetector computed tomography with multiplanar reformatted imaging and virtual cystoscopy in the assessment of bladder tumors after transurethral resection. J Comput Assist Tomogr 2010;34(1):121–6.
61. Fernandez Mena F, Moreno-Torres Y. Bladder cancer. Arch Esp Urol 2001;54(6): 493–510.
62. Tillou X, Gardel E, Fourmarier M, et al. Can MRI be used to distinguish between superficial and invasive transitional cell bladder cancer? Prog Urol 2008;18(7):440–4.
63. Watanabe H, Kanematsu M, Kondo H, et al. Preoperative T staging of urinary bladder cancer: does diffusion-weighted MRI have supplementary value? AJR Am J Roentgenol 2009;192(5):1361–6.
64. Shariat SF, Palapattu GS, Karakiewicz PI, et al. Discrepancy between clinical and pathologic stage: impact on prognosis after radical cystectomy. Eur Urol 2007; 51(1):137–49 [discussion: 149–51].
65. Lodde M, Lacombe L, Friede J, et al. Evaluation of fluorodeoxyglucose positron-emission tomography with computed tomography for staging of urothelial carcinoma. BJU Int 2010;106(5):658–63.
66. Picchio M, Treiber U, Beer AJ, et al. Value of 11C-choline PET and contrast-enhanced CT for staging of bladder cancer: correlation with histopathologic findings. J Nucl Med 2006;47(6):938–44.
67. Saokar A, Islam T, Jantsch M, et al. Detection of lymph nodes in pelvic malignancies with computed tomography and magnetic resonance imaging. Clin Imaging 2010;34(5):361–6.
68. Goodfellow H, Viney Z, Hughes P, et al. Role of fluorodeoxyglucose positron emission tomography (FDG PET)-computed tomography (CT) in the staging of bladder cancer. BJU Int 2014;114:389–95.
69. Shvarts O, Han KR, Seltzer M, et al. Positron emission tomography in urologic oncology. Cancer Control 2002;9(4):335–42.
70. Donaldson S, Bonington S, Kershaw L, et al. Dynamic contrast-enhanced MRI in patients with muscle-invasive transitional cell carcinoma of the bladder can distinguish between residual tumour and post-chemotherapy effect. Eur J Radiol 2013;82:2161–8.
71. Schrier BP, Peters M, Barentsz JO, et al. Evaluation of chemotherapy with magnetic resonance imaging in patients with regionally metastatic or unresectable bladder cancer. Eur Urol 2006;49(4):698–703.
72. Grossman HB, Soloway M, Messing E, et al. Surveillance for recurrent bladder cancer using a point-of-care proteomic assay. JAMA 2006;295(3):299–305.
73. Irani J, Desgrandchamps F, Millet C, et al. BTA stat and BTA TRAK: a comparative evaluation of urine testing for the diagnosis of transitional cell carcinoma of the bladder. Eur Urol 1999;35(2):89–92.
74. Glas AS, Roos D, Deutekom M, et al. Tumor markers in the diagnosis of primary bladder cancer. A systematic review. J Urol 2003;169(6):1975–82.
75. Vriesema J, Atsma F, Kiemeney L, et al. Diagnostic efficacy of the ImmunoCyt test to detect superficial bladder cancer recurrence. Urology 2001;58(3):367–71.
76. Têtu B, Tiguest R, Harel F, et al. ImmunoCyt/uCyt+ improves the sensitivity of urine cytology in patients followed for urothelial carcinoma. Mod Pathol 2005;18(1):83–9.
77. Hajdinjak T. UroVysion FISH test for detecting urothelial cancers: meta-analysis of diagnostic accuracy and comparison with urinary cytology testing. Urol Oncol 2008;26(6):646–51.
78. Ferra S, Denley R, Herr HW, et al. Reflex UroVysion testing in suspicious urine cytology cases. Cancer 2009;117(1):7–14.

Management of Low-risk and Intermediate-risk Non–Muscle-invasive Bladder Carcinoma

Yme Weijers, MD, Harm C. Arentsen, MD, PhD,
Tom J.H. Arends, MD, J. Alfred Witjes, MD, PhD*

KEYWORDS

- Non–muscle-invasive bladder cancer • Risk groups • Intermediate risk • Low risk
- Treatment

KEY POINTS

- Bladder cancer is a frequent and expensive malignancy with high rates of recurrence.
- Good initial transurethral resection of the bladder tumor is crucial for adequate staging and prognosis.
- In low-risk and intermediate-risk non–muscle-invasive bladder cancer, 1 immediate instillation of chemotherapy is recommended.
- Adherence to international guidelines remains insufficient, resulting in high recurrence rates. New safe and effective therapies are needed.

INTRODUCTION

Bladder cancer (BC) is a frequent and costly disease: it is reported to be the most expensive cancer per patient, and it is the 11th most commonly diagnosed cancer and the 14th leading cause of cancer deaths worldwide.[1,2] In the United States in 2012, there were an estimated 73,510 cases of BC, with 55,600 and 17,910 cases in men and women, respectively.[3] Risk factors for BC include tobacco use (50%), exposure to aromatic amines and polycyclic aromatic hydrocarbons other than in tobacco (10%), and genetic predisposition and aging.[1,4,5] The most common histologic subtype of BC is urothelial carcinoma, accounting for more than 90% of all bladder tumors.[6] Approximately 75% of patients with BC present with non–muscle-invasive BC (NMIBC), ie, Ta (70%), T1 (20%), and carcinoma in situ (CIS; 10%). The

Disclosures: J.A. Witjes is an advisor for Photocure and Ipsen.
Department of Urology, RadboudUMC, PO Box 9101, Nijmegen 6500 HB, The Netherlands
* Corresponding author.
E-mail address: fred.witjes@radboudumc.nl

Hematol Oncol Clin N Am 29 (2015) 219–225
http://dx.doi.org/10.1016/j.hoc.2014.11.001
0889-8588/15/$ – see front matter © 2015 Elsevier Inc. All rights reserved.

remainder of patients present with tumors invading the detrusor muscle (stage T2), the perivesical tissue (T3), the organs surrounding the bladder (T4), or metastatic disease.[5,7]

NON–MUSCLE-INVASIVE BLADDER CANCER

Stage Ta tumors have a papillary configuration, are confined to the urothelium, and do not penetrate into the lamina propria or detrusor muscle. Stage T1 tumors originate from the urothelium but penetrate the basement membrane separating the urothelium from the deeper layers. They invade into the lamina propria, but do not reach the detrusor muscle.

At present, 2 classifications are used for grading of papillary NMIBC (World Health Organization [WHO] 1973 and 2004; **Box 1**).[8] 1973 WHO grade 1 carcinomas have been reassigned to papillary urothelial neoplasms of low malignant potential and low-grade carcinomas in the 2004 WHO classification. It is a subject of controversy that grade 2 carcinomas have been eliminated in the 2004 WHO classification and reassigned to either low-grade or high-grade carcinomas. The 2004 WHO classification contains a detailed histologic description of the various grades in order to minimize diagnostic variability among pathologists. However, so far, published comparisons do not clearly confirm better reproducibility for the WHO 2004 classification compared with the 1973 WHO classification.[9,10]

Several studies have compared the two classifications concerning prognostic implications with conflicting results.[10–14] Until the prognostic role of this classification has been validated by more prospective trials with sufficient follow-up, both classifications should be used, because it is indicated by the 2014 European Association of Urology (EAU) guideline on NMIBC as a grade A recommendation.[15] Moreover, most clinical trials published so far have been performed using the 1973 WHO classification, meaning that recommendations from current guidelines are still based on this version.

CIS is a high-grade carcinoma confined to the urothelium, but with a flat nonpapillary configuration. Unlike a papillary tumor, CIS appears as reddened and velvety mucosa and is slightly elevated, although sometimes it is not visible. The diagnosis of CIS is based on the histology of biopsies from the bladder wall.

Box1
WHO grading 1973 and 2004

1973 WHO grading

Urothelial papilloma

Grade 1: well differentiated

Grade 2: moderately differentiated

Grade 3: poorly differentiated

2004 WHO grading

Urothelial papilloma

Papillary urothelial neoplasm of low malignant potential

Low-grade papillary urothelial carcinoma

High-grade papillary urothelial carcinoma

From Babjuk M, Burger M, Zigeuner R, et al. EAU guidelines on non-muscle-invasive urothelial carcinoma of the bladder: update 2013. Eur Urol 2013; 64:639–53; with permission.

The standard initial therapy for Ta and T1 papillary bladder tumors is a visually complete transurethral resection (TURBT) including a part of the underlying muscle.[16,17] This resection allows for the initial staging that is critical for further management decisions, and the TURBT is a first and important step in the treatment of the disease. A reresection is advised if there is any doubt about the completeness of the initial TURBT, or if there was no muscle in the specimen (with the exception of Ta grade 1 tumors and primary CIS). A restaging second TURBT within 2 to 6 weeks after the initial TURBT is necessary in all T1 and/or grade 3 tumors, except for tumors in patients with CIS alone.[18]

Another means to improve the completeness of the initial TURBT is the use of fluorescence techniques (photodynamic diagnosis [PDD]) or narrow band imaging. Of these two techniques PDD is the best studied. The most recent review by Burger and colleagues[19] clearly confirmed that PDD-guided cystoscopy significantly improves the detection of bladder tumors, leading to a significant and clinically meaningful reduction of recurrence at 9 to 12 months, but it has no impact on progression. The benefit is independent of the patient's risk category, and is evident in patients with Ta, T1, CIS, primary, and recurrent cancer.

Because there is considerable risk for recurrence and/or progression of tumors after TURBT, perioperative and/or adjuvant intravesical instillation therapy is recommended. Risk stratification depends on clinical (number of tumors, tumor size, prior recurrence rate), and pathologic (T category, CIS, grade) factors. The European Organization for Research and Treatment of Cancer Genitourinary group has developed a scoring system and risk tables that predict separately the risks of recurrence and progression in individual patients at different intervals after TURBT.[20] This scoring system and the corresponding risk tables have been used for several years to categorize patients and were the basis for risk-adapted treatment recommendations. However, in 2013 this scoring system was left and the risk group classification was simplified. The current EAU guideline recommends stratification of patients into 3 risk groups and provides practical treatment recommendations (**Table 1**). The stratification is based on an overview of the International Bladder Cancer Group, which reviewed several international guidelines to give best practice recommendations for the management of patients with NMIBC.[21] This recommendation resulted in a

Table 1
Treatment recommendations in NMIBC according to risk group stratification

Risk Category	Definition	Treatment Recommendation
Low	Primary, solitary, Ta, G1 (low grade), <3 cm, no CIS	One immediate instillation of chemotherapy
Intermediate	All cases not defined in the 2 adjacent categories	One immediate instillation of chemotherapy followed by further instillations, either chemotherapy for a maximum of 1 y or 1 y full-dose BCG
High	Any of the following: • T1 • G3 (high grade) • CIS • Multiple and recurrent and large (>3 cm) TaG1–2 tumors (all conditions must be presented)	Full-dose BCG instillations for 1–3 y or cystectomy (in highest risk tumors)

Abbreviations: BCG, bacillus Calmette-Guérin; TaG, tumor stage "a" grade.

more uniform work-up to NMIBC management, and the EAU risk group classification is now similar to the American Urological Association (AUA) risk group stratification.[22]

Patients at low risk for both recurrence and progression, with a primary, solitary, small (<3 cm), low-grade Ta tumor without CIS, should receive immediate single post-TURBT intravesical instillation (SPI) with a chemotherapeutic agent (ie, mitomycin C, epirubicin).[22] Further treatment is not recommended until recurrence. In daily practice a SPI is not always done. Burks and colleagues[23] recently reported the use of a SPI in the United States. The study period was between June 2011 and January 2012. They defined ideal candidates for an SPI from their total cohort (n = 1931) as those patients with 1 to 2 completely resected papillary tumors (n = 718). Between 27% and 50% of these ideal patients had an SPI, compared with 9% to 24% of nonideal patients. There were several reasons for not giving an SPI in ideal patients, such as logistic factors in 24%, doubt about the benefit of a SPI in 20%, resection aspects (not complete or fear for a perforation) in 17%, and patient factors (malignancy uncertain, other therapy planned) in 54%. In an more recent study, Barocas and colleagues[24] also studied SPI in clinical US practice. They reported on 2794 cases treated between September 2010 and July 2012. An SPI was given to ideal candidates in 35% to 38%, and in nonideal candidates in 12% to 15%. However, in most instances, nonuse represented appropriate clinical judgment, and overall judicious use of chemotherapy ranged from 83% to 85.7%. In all, although an SPI is the standard recommendation in low-risk patients after the initial TURBT, it seems to be done in a minority of patients, but usually with understandable arguments.

The EAU guideline recommends the use of 1 immediate postoperative instillation in patients with intermediate-risk tumors (ie, all cases between categories of low and high risk). However, the SPI should be followed by additional instillations, and this recommendation is not supported by consistent evidence.[25] Adjuvant intravesical therapy is necessary but consensus regarding the optimal drug and the most appropriate scheme is lacking. Intravesical immunotherapy with 1 year of bacillus Calmette-Guérin (BCG) maintenance therapy shows a better reduction of the recurrence rate, but the impact on tumor progression is uncertain.[26–30] Moreover, BCG-related side effects are more severe and occur more often than with chemotherapy.[31,32] In case adjuvant intravesical chemotherapy is administered, different schedules are possible, but duration of treatment should not exceed 1 year.[33]

However, a substantial percentage of treated patients still experience tumor recurrences or even progression to muscle-invasive BC (MIBC). This suboptimal treatment outcome can partly be attributed to inadequate adherence of BC guidelines. For example, Witjes and colleagues[34] found a marked underuse of guideline-recommended adjuvant intravesical therapy in patients with intermediate-risk and high-risk NMIBC in a retrospective chart review study. In intermediate-risk patients, only 47% received adjuvant intravesical therapy as recommended in AUA or EAU guidelines. Twenty-four percent of intermediate-risk patients and 9% of high-risk patients received TURBT only, with no further intravesical therapy. These findings are consistent with other studies that have found poor adherence to BC guidelines and underuse of BCG.[35–39]

Gemcitabine, taxanes, interferon alfa in addition to BCG, and chemohyperthermia are new intravesical treatment options in NMIBC. These therapies are not elucidated in this article, because most are only applied in high-risk patients with recurrence or relapse after BCG.

In conclusion, initial therapy for NMIBC is a good and radical transurethral resection, followed by intravesical chemotherapeutic or immunotherapeutic therapy. Drugs and treatment schedules are risk group adapted and described in guidelines. However, because of a limited guideline adherence, even with the use of adjuvant intravesical instillations, a substantial percentage of treated patients still experience tumor recurrences or even progression to MIBC. In patients failing on intravesical BCG there is no accepted standard alternative conservative approach. Moreover, current intravesical therapy can be accompanied by serious local and systemic adverse effects. Therefore, current intravesical treatment strategies against NMIBC are suboptimal and, in order to reduce toxicity and to enhance efficacy, improved new intravesical treatment modalities are urgently needed.

REFERENCES

1. Sievert K, Amend B, Nagele U, et al. Economic aspects of bladder cancer: what are the benefits and costs? World J Urol 2009;27:295–300.
2. Botteman MF, Pashos CL, Redaelli A, et al. The health economics of bladder cancer. A comprehensive review of the published literature. Pharmacoeconomics 2003;21:1315–30.
3. Siegel R, Naishadham D, Jemal A. Cancer statistics, 2012. CA Cancer J Clin 2012;62:10–29.
4. Rafnar T, Vermeulen SH, Sulem P, et al. European genome-wide association study identifies SLC14A1 as a new urinary bladder cancer susceptibility gene. Hum Mol Genet 2011;20(21):4268–81.
5. Burger M, Catto JW, Dalbagni G, et al. Epidemiology and risk factors of urothelial bladder cancer. Eur Urol 2013;63(2):234–41.
6. Ploeg M, Aben KK, Hulsbergen-Van de Kaa CA, et al. The clinical epidemiology of non-urothelial bladder cancer. J Urol 2010;183:915–20.
7. Sobin LH, Gospodarowicz MK, Wittekind C. TNM classification of malignant tumors (UICC International Union Against Cancer). 7th edition. New York: Wiley-Blackwell; 2009. p. 262–5.
8. Epstein JI, Amin MB, Reuter VR, et al. The World Health Organization International Society of Urological Pathology consensus classification of urothelial (transitional cell) neoplasms of the urinary bladder. Am J Surg Pathol 1998;22: 1435–48.
9. Van Rhijn BW, van Leenders GJ, Ooms BC, et al. The pathologist's mean grade is constant and individualizes the prognostic value of bladder cancer grading. Eur Urol 2010;57:1052–7.
10. May M, Brookman-Amissah S, Roigas J, et al. Prognostic accuracy of individual uropathologists in noninvasive urinary bladder carcinoma: a multicentre study comparing the 1973 and 2004 World Health Organisation classifications. Eur Urol 2010;57:850–8.
11. Cao D, Vollmer RT, Luly J, et al. Comparison of 2004 and 1973 World Health Organization grading systems and their relationship to pathologic staging for predicting long-term prognosis in patients with urothelial carcinoma. Urology 2010; 76:593–9.
12. Pellucchi F, Freschi M, Ibrahim B, et al. Clinical reliability of the 2004 WHO histological classification system compared with the 1973 WHO system for Ta primary bladder tumors. J Urol 2011;186:2194–9.
13. Otto W, Denzinger S, Fritsche HM, et al. The WHO classification of 1973 is more suitable than the WHO classification of 2004 for predicting survival in pT1 urothelial bladder cancer. BJU Int 2010;107:404–8.
14. Chen Z, Ding W, Xu K, et al. The 1973 WHO classification is more suitable than the 2004 WHO classification for predicting prognosis in non-muscle-invasive

bladder cancer. PLoS One 2012;7:e47199. http://dx.doi.org/10.1371/journal. pone.0047199.

15. Babjuk M, Bohle A, Burger M, et al. EAU guidelines on non-muscle invasive bladder cancer (Ta, T1 and CIS)-limited text update April 2014. Available at: http://www. uroweb.org/guidelines/online-guidelines/.

16. Brausi M, Collette L, Kurth K, et al, EORTC Genito-Urinary Tract Cancer Collaborative Group. Variability in the recurrence rate at first follow-up cystoscopy after TUR in stage Ta T1 transitional cell carcinoma of the bladder: a combined analysis of seven EORTC studies. Eur Urol 2002;41:523–31.

17. Mariappan P, Zachou A, Grigor KM. Detrusor muscle in the first, apparently complete transurethral resection of bladder tumour specimen is a surrogate marker of resection quality, predicts risk of early recurrence, and is dependent on operator experience. Eur Urol 2010;57:843–9.

18. Divrik RT, Şahin AF, Yildirim Ü, et al. Impact of routine second transurethral resection on the long-term outcome of patients with newly diagnosed pT1 urothelial carcinoma with respect to recurrence, progression rate, and disease-specific survival: a prospective randomised clinical trial. Eur Urol 2010;58:185–90.

19. Burger M, Grossman HB, Droller M, et al. Photodynamic diagnosis of non-muscle-invasive bladder cancer with hexaminolevulinate cystoscopy: a meta-analysis of detection and recurrence based on raw data. Eur Urol 2013;64(5): 846–54.

20. Sylvester RJ, van der Meijden AP, Oosterlinck W, et al. Predicting recurrence and progression in individual patients with stage TaT1 bladder cancer using EORTC risk tables: a combined analysis of 2596 patients from seven EORTC trials. Eur Urol 2006;49:466–77.

21. Brausi M, Witjes JA, Lamm D, et al. A review of current guidelines and best practice recommendations for the management of nonmuscle invasive bladder cancer by the International Bladder Cancer Group. J Urol 2011;186:2158–67.

22. Hall MC, Chang SS, Dalbagni G, et al. Guideline for the management of non-muscle invasive bladder cancer (stages Ta, T1, and Tis): 2007 update. J Urol 2007;178:2314–30.

23. Burks FN, Liu AB, Suh RS, et al. Understanding the use of immediate intravesical chemotherapy for patients with bladder cancer. J Urol 2012;188(6):2108–13.

24. Barocas DA, Liu A, Burks FN, et al. Practice based collaboration to improve the use of immediate intravesical therapy after resection of nonmuscle invasive bladder cancer. J Urol 2013;190(6):2011–6.

25. Gudjonsson S, Adell L, Merdasa F, et al. Should all patients with non-muscle-invasive bladder cancer receive early intravesical chemotherapy after transurethral resection? The results of a prospective randomized multicentre study. Eur Urol 2009;55:773–80.

26. Sylvester RJ, Oosterlinck W, van der Meijden AP. A single immediate postoperative instillation of chemotherapy decreases the risk of recurrence in patients with stage Ta T1 bladder cancer: a meta-analysis of published results of randomized clinical trials. J Urol 2004;171:2186–90.

27. Sylvester RJ, van der Meijden AP, Lamm DL. Intravesical bacillus Calmette-Guérin reduces the risk of progression in patients with superficial bladder cancer: a meta-analysis of the published results of randomized clinical trials. J Urol 2002; 168:1964–70.

28. Böhle A, Bock PR. Intravesical bacille Calmette-Guérin versus mitomycin C in superficial bladder cancer: formal meta-analysis of comparative studies on tumor progression. Urology 2004;63:682–7.

29. Malmström PU, Sylvester RJ, Crawford DE, et al. An individual patient data meta-analysis of the long-term outcome of randomised studies comparing intravesical mitomycin C versus bacillus Calmette-Guérin for non-muscle-invasive bladder cancer. Eur Urol 2009;56:247–56.

30. Sylvester RJ, Brausi MA, Kirkels WJ, et al. Long-term efficacy results of EORTC Genito-Urinary Group randomized phase 3 study 30911 comparing intravesical instillations of epirubicin, bacillus Calmette-Guérin, and bacillus Calmette-Guérin plus isoniazid in patients with intermediate- and high-risk stage Ta T1 urothelial carcinoma of the bladder. Eur Urol 2010;57:766–73.

31. Böhle A, Jocham D, Bock PR. Intravesical bacillus Calmette-Guérin versus mitomycin C for superficial bladder cancer: a formal meta-analysis of comparative studies on recurrence and toxicity. J Urol 2003;169:90–5.

32. Van der Meijden AP, Sylvester RJ, Oosterlinck W, et al. Maintenance bacillus Calmette-Guerin for TaT1 bladder tumors is not associated with increased toxicity: results from a European Organisation for Research and Treatment of Cancer Genito-Urinary Group phase III trial. Eur Urol 2003;44:429–34.

33. Sylvester RJ, Oosterlinck W, Witjes JA. The schedule and duration of intravesical chemotherapy in patients with non-muscle-invasive bladder cancer: a systematic review of the published results of randomized clinical trials. Eur Urol 2008;53:709–19.

34. Witjes JA, Palou J, Soloway M, et al. Current clinical practice gaps in the treatment of intermediate- and high-risk non-muscleinvasive bladder cancer (NMIBC) with emphasis on the use of bacillus Calmette-Guérin (BCG): results of an international individual patient data survey (IPDS). BJU Int 2013. http://dx.doi.org/10.1111/bju.12012.

35. Chamie K, Saigal CS, Lai J, et al, The Urologic Diseases in America Project. Compliance with guidelines for patients with bladder cancer: variation in the delivery of care. Cancer 2011;117:5392–401.

36. Gontero P, Oderda M, Altieri V, et al. Are referral centers for non-muscle-invasive bladder cancer compliant to EAU guidelines? A report from the Vesical Antiblastic Therapy Italian Study. Urol Int 2011;86:19–24.

37. Adiyat KT, Katkoori D, Soloway CT, et al. Complete transurethral resection of bladder tumor: are the guidelines being followed? Urology 2010;75:365–9.

38. Skolarus TA, Ye Z, Montgomery JS, et al. Use of restaging bladder tumor resection for bladder cancer among Medicare beneficiaries. Urology 2011;78:1345–50.

39. Madeb R, Golijanin D, Noyes K, et al. Treatment of nonmuscle invading bladder cancer: do physicians in the United States practice evidence based medicine? Cancer 2009;115:2660–70.

High-Risk Nonmuscle Invasive Bladder Cancer

 CrossMark

Anna Orsola, MD, PhD[a],*, Joan Palou, MD, PhD[b], Eduardo Solsona, MD, PhD[c]

KEYWORDS

- Nonmuscle invasive bladder cancer • High-risk bladder cancer • High-grade T1
- HGT1 • Carcinoma in situ • CIS • TUR • reTUR

KEY POINTS

- Advanced age ($\geq$70 years), female sex, larger tumor size, and multiple tumors are associated with increased progression and, for some of these factors, also decreased cancer-specific survival. Bacillus Calmette-Guérin has also been shown to impact progression and also recently on cancer-specific survival.
- Updated information on large series and a meta-analysis has helped set the risk of progression in 20% of high-grade T1 cases.
- Deep lamina propria invasion combined with age, tumor size, associated carcinoma in situ and other risk factors described should be used for patient stratification in future clinical trials. Future research should attempt to combine these prognostic factors into a risk-prediction nomogram in which validation in a prospective cohort would also be of value.
- Identifying that 20% of patients with risk of progression would allow to indicate selectively both repeat transurethral resection and early cystectomy, preserving bladders in less-risk cases.

INTRODUCTION

Approximately 75% of the 386,000 new cases of bladder cancer diagnosed worldwide annually are nonmuscle invasive bladder cancer (NMIBC). In the United States, there are currently 500,000 survivors of bladder cancer, mainly of this NMIBC subtype.[1] It is still unclear what clicks the progression and makes 20% of high-risk NMIBC[2] progress to an invasive and extremely aggressive tumor. Expert recommendations on the optimal treatment strategy for patients within this category range from conservative therapy to early radical cystectomy.[3,4] There is a strong claim to reexamine the

The authors have nothing to disclose.
[a] Bladder Cancer Center, Dana Farber Cancer Institute, Harvard Medical School, 450 Brookline Avenue, Boston, MA 02115, USA; [b] Urology Department, Fundacio Puigvert, Cartagena 340-350, Barcelona 08025, Spain; [c] Urology Department, Instituto Valenciano de Oncologia, Calle del Profesor Beltrán Bàguena, 8, València 46009, Spain
* Corresponding author.
E-mail address: annaorsola@gmail.com

treatment algorithm for these patients, to improve risk stratification, and to find the tools to identify this 20% with the potential of invasiveness.

The first issue to overcome when addressing high-risk bladder cancer is the mere definition of this category. There is no consensus among guidelines as to the risk-level definitions. As a consequence, an international committee of experts on bladder cancer management, the International Bladder Cancer Group (IBCG), reviewed all of these guidelines and published in 2008[5] and updated in 2011[6] their take on these variations. Their recommendation was to include as high-risk NMIBC any T1, G3, and/or carcinoma in situ (CIS). Originally, the European Association of Urology's (EAU) guidelines (2001) included as high-risk NMIBC all T1, G3 (multifocal or highly recurrent), and CIS.[7] With the introduction of the European Organization for Research and Treatment of Cancer's (EORTC) risk tables, an attempt was made in the 2011 version of the guidelines to use the risk calculator.[8] Currently, the definition of high-risk NMIBC for this association has, in part, gone back to the original definition and considers any of the following to be a high-risk NMIBC: T1 tumor or G3 (high grade) tumor or CIS, together with any multiple, recurrent, and large (>3 cm) Ta G1G2 tumors, if all conditions are present. This definition is quite similar (though not exact) to the definition recommended by the IBCG and, as in that case, involves using the old World Health Organization's (WHO) grading system (G1, G2, G3) instead of the updated high and low grade.

Throughout the past 2 decades, the variability in the definition of risk levels, together with the changes in the WHO's grading system and the staging system, has introduced elements of bias. Besides, there are variations in definitions of outcomes or prognostic factors, which might also lead to heterogeneity.[9] Finally, there is a lack in the literature of randomized data and large studies for HGT1 bladder cancer since the advent of bacillus Calmette-Guérin (BCG) in the early 1990s. Most of these studies are retrospective observational studies, which, compared with randomized controlled trials, are subject to various selection biases, carrying a higher risk of uncontrolled confounding factors, with potential preferential reporting of positive findings.

Regardless of the definition used, the clinical care of high-risk NMIBC is directed at preventing progression to muscle invasion because this event marks a dramatic increase in the risk of metastasis and disease-specific mortality. This is as opposed to low- and intermediate-risk NMIBC, for which the focus is on cost and quality-of-life issues. In this update, to keep a focus on progression, prognostic factors, and treatment strategies, the authors use the more restricted definition of high-risk NMIBC contemplating only HG cases, mainly HGT1 and CIS, as well as the more rare case of HGTa.

PROGNOSTIC FACTORS

Classically, around 30% of these tumors have been considered to progress,[10] with this being part of the currently outdated rule of thirds for HGT1. A new lower cutoff of 21% has been established in a meta-analysis based on more than 12,000 HGT1 cases,[11] consistent with a previous review of high-risk NMIBC based on 3088 patients from 19 trials[2] and a recent multicenter study of 2451 HGT1 cases.[12] Compared with other HGT1 reports with higher progression estimates of up to 40%,[3,13,14] this lower rate may represent true improvements in HGT1 prognosis over time[11] and, in part, may also reflect a shift in the definition mentioned in the earlier section. Along the same line, the rates of mortality for this group of bladder cancer were reported to reach 34%[3]; but these recent reports show a 9% to 14% mortality,[2,11,12] with 79% of patients retaining their bladders.[12]

These favorable outcomes confirm that most HGT1 tumors can be safely managed conservatively with standard treatment with first-line BCG.[15,16] Prognostic factors that might aid in the identification of 20% of HGT1 tumors at higher risk of progression and hence those would benefit most from a repeat transurethral resection (reTUR) and/or an early radical cystectomy are desperately needed. Unfortunately for high-risk NMIBC, the predictive value of the EORTC and club urológico español de tratamiento oncológico (CUETO) scoring systems[10,17] has been shown to be limited with poor discriminating ability, limited predictive value, and a tendency to overestimate progression.[18,19]

Pathologic Prognostic Factors

The depth/extent of invasion is the basis of all TNM classification; the importance of *substaging* results to prognosis in HGT1 disease is a risk factor proposed almost 20 years ago,[20–22] with more than 2500 published cases substaged according to invasion of the muscularis mucosae.[23] Martin-Doyle and colleagues'[11] meta-analysis identified deep lamina propria invasion as having the largest negative impact in both progression and cancer specific survival (CSS) in HGT1. Because this evaluation is subject to interobserver and intraobserver variability, it has faced this criticism for the last 2 decades; but there is growing evidence on its reproducibility.[23,24] Additional work is needed to identify the optimal method to quantify the depth of invasion because other methods for substaging HGT1 that is not yet externally validated have been described.[25–28]

CIS is also a strong and independent prognostic factor, showing a hazard ratio of 1.24 (confidence interval 1.09–1.4)[12] to a 2-fold increase[11] in the risk of progression. This prognostic factor is limited by the fact that CIS is a microscopic lesion with an incidence in large series around 24%.[12] Its diagnosis can be optimized by additional random bladder biopsies,[29] increasing the incidence to up to 65%.[30,31]

The *involvement of the prostatic urethra and ducts by CIS* in male patients with NMIBC has been reported; the risk is higher if the tumor is located on the trigone or bladder neck, in the presence of bladder CIS, and in multiple tumors.[8,30] In these cases and when cytology is positive with no evidence of tumor in the bladder or when abnormalities of prostatic urethra are visible, loop biopsies of the prostatic urethra are recommended.

The presence of *lymphovascular invasion* also significantly predicts outcomes (ref WMD[11]), but the incidence is relatively low (under 15%); further work has to be done to strengthen the evidence. Finally, when *micropapillary histology* has evaluated specifically within HGT1,[11] it has not been found to carry a significant effect on either recurrence or progression. But this was based on only 2 identified studies meeting the criteria of at least 75 cases of HGT1 and at least 75% of HGT1.[32,33] Given the conflicting findings on the impact of micropapillary histology,[34–37] the association of this factor with the prognosis deserves further evaluation, specifically in the HGT1 population.

Clinical Prognostic Factors

The recent report by Gontero and colleagues[12] proposes the combination of age of 70 years and older, size of 3 cm or greater, and the presence of CIS as the highest risk of progression, reaching 52% within this group compared with 17% in the group without any of the 3 risk factors. *Advanced age* (≥70 years) has been associated with a higher bladder cancer–related mortality[11,12,17] and suggests that BCG may be less effective in elderly patients. However, other reports point to advancing age (>70 years) as being associated with a statistically significant lower hazard of progression in HGT1.[14]

Female sex was found to increase the risk of progression but not recurrence or cancer-specific survival by Martin-Doyle and colleagues[11] and Gontero and colleagues,[12] but additional data may be required to confirm this finding. The underlying factors driving this sex disparity are poorly understood and have been hypothesized to include hormonal, anatomic, and societal factors, including sex differences in the immunologic response to BCG.[17,30,38]

Both larger *tumor size* and *multiple tumors* are associated with an increased recurrence and progression and decreased cancer-specific survival,[11,12] which is consistent with these factors' relevance in the broader NMIBC population.[10]

In the broader bladder cancer population, *recurrent tumors* have also been found to impact negatively when compared with the initial tumor[10,17]; but this finding has yet to be confirmed in the restricted group of HGT1.[11,12]

BCG has a known impact on progression and also recently on cancer-specific survival in HGT1 disease.[11,12] *Maintenance BCG* also seems to have a significant positive impact on all outcome measures,[12] strengthening the evidence base for existing recommendations to use BCG in high-risk NMIBC.[39,40] *Besides, the response to BCG has been known for a long time to predict progression.*[41]

Chromosomal Alterations and Molecular Markers

Because clinical and pathologic variables alone are inadequate to predict progression in HGT1 bladder cancer, the search for tissue-based biomarkers is an ongoing area of effort even though no marker has been validated thus far. Recent evidence suggests that histopathologic classification into pTa, pT1a, and pT1b can be translated into a molecular signature, reflecting progressive deregulation to more invasive stages.[42]

Altered protein expression of p53, p21, pRb, and p27 has been shown to correlate negatively with outcomes.[43,44] The value of p53 expression as a prognostic factor in T1G3 disease, however, is controversial.[45,46] There has also been several articles reporting the ability of microRNAs to help evaluate patients with NMIBC, even though future work is needed to validate the potential clinical utility.[47] Also, the epidermal growth factor receptor[48] as well as the cell cycle regulators, including cyclin D1, cyclin D3, and p53, may have therapeutic importance in T1G3 disease.[49]

Another interesting approach is the search for markers of the BCG response, such as ezrin[50] or cathepsin E, maspin, Plk1, and survivin.[51] All of these markers have been shown to predict progression in a wider population of NMIBC and are in the process of being externally validated in the near future.

TREATMENT OPTIONS

Standard initial treatment is based on endoscopic TUR and intravesical immunotherapy with BCG. A good quality TUR as described in detail in the updated version of the EAU's guidelines is critical.[39] It includes a thorough evaluation of the bladder, a staged TUR with separate inclusion of the underlying bladder wall and tumor edges, and cold cup biopsies if indicated. Because this is subject to interpretation, an alternative approach is to proceed with these biopsies either in a standardized manner at the initial TUR or at the time of reTUR,[29–31,52] even though its usefulness in the broad population of NMIBC is controversial.[53]

BCG instillations are classically given according to the empirical 6-weekly induction schedule. There is currently no agreement on the optimal BCG maintenance schedule; the Southwest Oncology Group recommends a regimen of 3 weekly instillations at 3 and 6 months after induction and every 6 months thereafter for up to 3 years, and the EAU's guidelines recommend at least 1 year of BCG maintenance therapy. Recent evidence contributes to decision making when dosing BCG.[54]

Residual tumor has been a point of wide debate in NMIBC because of the variability among different surgeons and the severe impact on outcomes.[55] Because of the risk of residual tumor and of understaging, guidelines recommend a second TUR should be performed when a high-grade non–muscle-invasive tumor or a T1 tumor is detected at the initial TUR.[39,40] However, for an array of reasons, reTUR remains underutilized, with no higher than 7.7% of patients with HGT1 disease reportedly undergoing this second procedure.[56] ReTUR may improve outcomes[57] but adds morbidity and is probably unnecessary in more than 60% of cases.[58,59]

Because both substaging and associated CIS are such strong prognostic factors, one alternative approach is to proceed with a reTUR in deeply invasive cases (T1b) and search for CIS actively by taking multiple bladder biopsies at the time of reTUR. Positive findings could then direct patients toward an early curative radical cystectomy. Conversely, less invasive cases (T1a) could be safely managed conservatively with BCG and reTUR could be spared, particularly in the case of single tumors less than 3 cm in size. This approach has been the basis of a prospective study initiated in 2005 that shows consistently that T1b cases have a much deleterious prognosis even though they undergo a more aggressive treatment.[29,33,60]

Prolongation of conservative treatment and deferring radical cystectomy may allow progression and decrease cancer-specific survival.[59,61] The decision to proceed with immediate radical cystectomy is undertaken under various criteria and is one of the most difficult clinical decisions in urology and an ongoing area of controversy.[62–64] This major surgical procedure requires urinary diversion, is associated with substantial morbidity (50%–67% complication rate) and up to 9% mortality,[65] and may represent overtreatment.[16] However, in patients at the highest risk of tumor progression and those that have failed BCG, immediate radical cystectomy should be considered, as recommended by guidelines.

FUTURE IMPLICATIONS/DIRECTIONS

As opposed to other cancers, progress has been extremely slow in the search of tissue-based biomarkers and novel therapies for high-risk NMIBC. Among them, targeted therapy that improves the efficacy and decreases the side effects of antineoplastic agents might be implemented in NMIBC. Nanoparticles improving the delivery of these agents to tumor cells and gene therapy might be another strategy to induce an antitumor response. Another novel approach encompasses the engineering of the BCG vaccine to minimize side effects.[66]

However, updated information on large series and a meta-analysis has helped set the risk of progression in 20% of HGT1 cases. Deep lamina propria invasion combined with age, tumor size, associated CIS, and the other risk factors described should be used for patient stratification in future clinical trials. Future research should attempt to combine these prognostic factors into a risk-prediction nomogram in which validation in a prospective cohort would also be of value. These results could individualize decision making, identifying those cases of HGT1 suitable for organ preservation and differentiating them from those that will benefit most from an early cystectomy.

Finally, some of the issues that need to be addressed in this area include

- Improve quality and standardization of TUR
- Unify definitions of risk groups and the definition of progression
- Improve public awareness and interest on NMIBC and bladder cancer in general
- Increase funding for clinical and basic research

REFERENCES

1. Ploeg M, Aben KK, Kiemeney LA. The present and future burden of urinary bladder cancer in the world. World J Urol 2009;27(3):289–93. http://dx.doi.org/10.1007/s00345-009-0383-3 Epub 2009/02/17.
2. van den Bosch S, Alfred Witjes J. Long-term cancer-specific survival in patients with high-risk, non-muscle-invasive bladder cancer and tumour progression: a systematic review. Eur Urol 2011;60(3):493–500. http://dx.doi.org/10.1016/j.eururo.2011.05.045 Epub 2011/06/15.
3. Kulkarni GS, Hakenberg OW, Gschwend JE, et al. An updated critical analysis of the treatment strategy for newly diagnosed high-grade T1 (previously T1G3) bladder cancer. Eur Urol 2010;57(1):60–70. http://dx.doi.org/10.1016/j.eururo.2009.08.024 Epub 2009/09/11.
4. Daneshmand S. Determining the role of cystectomy for high-grade T1 urothelial carcinoma. Urol Clin North Am 2013;40(2):233–47. http://dx.doi.org/10.1016/j.ucl.2013.01.003 Epub 2013/04/02.
5. Lamm D, Colombel M, Persad R, et al. Clinical practice recommendations for the management of non-muscle invasive bladder cancer. Eur Urol Suppl 2008; 7:651.
6. Brausi M, Witjes JA, Lamm D, et al. A review of current guidelines and best practice recommendations for the management of nonmuscle invasive bladder cancer by the International Bladder Cancer Group. J Urol 2011;186(6): 2158–67. http://dx.doi.org/10.1016/j.juro.2011.07.076.
7. Oosterlinck W, Lobel B, Jakse G, et al. Guidelines on bladder cancer. Eur Urol 2002;41(2):105–12.
8. Babjuk M, Oosterlinck W, Sylvester R, et al. EAU guidelines on non-muscle-invasive urothelial carcinoma of the bladder, the 2011 update. Actas Urol Esp 2012;36(7):389–402. http://dx.doi.org/10.1016/j.acuro.2011.12.001 [in Spanish].
9. Lamm D, Persad R, Brausi M, et al. Defining progression in nonmuscle invasive bladder cancer: it is time for a new, standard definition. J Urol 2014;191(1):20–7. http://dx.doi.org/10.1016/j.juro.2013.07.102.
10. Sylvester RJ, van der Meijden AP, Oosterlinck W, et al. Predicting recurrence and progression in individual patients with stage Ta T1 bladder cancer using EORTC risk tables: a combined analysis of 2596 patients from seven EORTC trials. Eur Urol 2006;49(3):466–75. http://dx.doi.org/10.1016/j.eururo.2005.12.031 [discussion: 475–7].
11. Improving selection criteria for early cystectomy in high-grade T1 bladder cancer: A meta-analysis of 15,215 patients. William Martin-Doyle, Jeffrey J. Leow, Anna Orsola, Steven L. Chang, Joaquim Bellmunt. JCO accepted, in press.
12. Gontero P, Sylvester R, Pisano F, et al. Prognostic factors and risk groups in T1G3 non-muscle-invasive bladder cancer patients initially treated with bacillus Calmette-Guérin: results of a retrospective multicenter study of 2451 patients. Eur Urol 2014. http://dx.doi.org/10.1016/j.eururo.2014.06.040.
13. van Rhijn BW, Burger M, Lotan Y, et al. Recurrence and progression of disease in non-muscle-invasive bladder cancer: from epidemiology to treatment strategy. Eur Urol 2009;56(3):430–42. http://dx.doi.org/10.1016/j.eururo.2009.06.028 Epub 2009/07/07.
14. Chamie K, Litwin MS, Bassett JC, et al. Recurrence of high-risk bladder cancer: a population-based analysis. Cancer 2013;119(17):3219–27. http://dx.doi.org/10.1002/cncr.28147.

15. Jakse G, Algaba F, Malmström P, et al. A second-look TUR in T1 transitional cell carcinoma: why? Eur Urol 2004;45(5):539–46. http://dx.doi.org/10.1016/j.eururo. 2003.12.016 [discussion: 546]. pii:S0302283804000053.

16. Pansadoro V, Emiliozzi P, de Paula F, et al. Long-term follow-up of G3T1 transitional cell carcinoma of the bladder treated with intravesical bacille Calmette-Guérin: 18-year experience. Urology 2002;59(2):227–31.

17. Fernandez-Gomez J, Solsona E, Unda M, et al. Prognostic factors in patients with non-muscle-invasive bladder cancer treated with bacillus Calmette-Guerin: multivariate analysis of data from four randomized CUETO trials. Eur Urol 2008;53(5): 992–1001. http://dx.doi.org/10.1016/j.eururo.2007.10.006 Epub 2007/10/24.

18. Xylinas E, Kent M, Kluth L, et al. Accuracy of the EORTC risk tables and of the CUETO scoring model to predict outcomes in non-muscle-invasive urothelial carcinoma of the bladder. Br J Cancer 2013;109(6):1460–6. http://dx.doi.org/10. 1038/bjc.2013.372 Epub 2013/08/29.

19. van Rhijn BW, Liu L, Vis AN, et al. Prognostic value of molecular markers, substage and European Organisation for the Research and Treatment of Cancer risk scores in primary T1 bladder cancer. BJU Int 2012;110(8):1169–76. http:// dx.doi.org/10.1111/j.1464-410X.2012.10996.x Epub 2012/03/28.

20. Holmang S, Hedelin H, Anderstrom C, et al. The importance of the depth of invasion in stage T1 bladder carcinoma: a prospective cohort study. J Urol 1997;157(3):800–3 [discussion: 804]. Epub 1997/03/01.

21. Smits G, Schaafsma E, Kiemeney L, et al. Microstaging of pT1 transitional cell carcinoma of the bladder: identification of subgroups with distinct risks of progression. Urology 1998;52(6):1009–13 [discussion: 1013–4]. Epub 1998/12/04.

22. Cheng L, Weaver AL, Neumann RM, et al. Substaging of T1 bladder carcinoma based on the depth of invasion as measured by micrometer: a new proposal. Cancer 1999;86(6):1035–43 Epub 1999/09/24.

23. Rouprêt M, Seisen T, Compérat E, et al. Prognostic interest in discriminating muscularis mucosa invasion (T1a vs T1b) in nonmuscle invasive bladder carcinoma: French national multicenter study with central pathology review. J Urol 2013;189(6):2069–76. http://dx.doi.org/10.1016/j.juro.2012.11.120.

24. Cottrell L, Nairn ER, Hair M. Consistency of microstaging pT1 bladder transitional cell carcinoma. J Clin Pathol 2007;60(6):735–6.

25. Bertz S, Denzinger S, Otto W, et al. Substaging by estimating the size of invasive tumour can improve risk stratification in pT1 urothelial bladder cancer-evaluation of a large hospital-based single-centre series. Histopathology 2011;59(4): 722–32. http://dx.doi.org/10.1111/j.1365-2559.2011.03989.x.

26. Cheng L, Neumann RM, Weaver AL, et al. Predicting cancer progression in patients with stage T1 bladder carcinoma. J Clin Oncol 1999;17(10):3182–7.

27. van der Aa MN, van Leenders GJ, Steyerberg EW, et al. A new system for substaging pT1 papillary bladder cancer: a prognostic evaluation. Hum Pathol 2005;36(9):981–6. http://dx.doi.org/10.1016/j.humpath.2005.06.017.

28. van Rhijn BW, van der Kwast TH, Alkhateeb SS, et al. A new and highly prognostic system to discern T1 bladder cancer substage. Eur Urol 2012;61(2): 378–84. http://dx.doi.org/10.1016/j.eururo.2011.10.026.

29. Orsola A, Cecchini L, Raventos CX, et al. Risk factors for positive findings in patients with high-grade T1 bladder cancer treated with transurethral resection of bladder tumour (TUR) and bacille Calmette-Guerin therapy and the decision for a repeat TUR. BJU Int 2010;105(2):202–7. http://dx.doi.org/10.1111/j.1464-410X.2009.08694.x Epub 2009/06/30.

30. Palou J, Sylvester RJ, Faba OR, et al. Female gender and carcinoma in situ in the prostatic urethra are prognostic factors for recurrence, progression, and disease-specific mortality in T1G3 bladder cancer patients treated with bacillus Calmette-Guerin. Eur Urol 2012;62(1):118–25. http://dx.doi.org/10.1016/j.eururo.2011.10.029 Epub 2011/11/22.

31. Millan-Rodriguez F, Chechile-Toniolo G, Salvador-Bayarri J, et al. Multivariate analysis of the prognostic factors of primary superficial bladder cancer. J Urol 2000;163(1):73–8 Epub 1999/12/22.

32. Brimo F, Wu C, Zeizafoun N, et al. Prognostic factors in T1 bladder urothelial carcinoma: the value of recording millimetric depth of invasion, diameter of invasive carcinoma, and muscularis mucosa invasion. Hum Pathol 2013;44(1): 95–102. http://dx.doi.org/10.1016/j.humpath.2012.04.020 Epub 2012/09/04.

33. Orsola A, Raventos C, Allue M, et al. Optimizing therapeutic strategies in initial high grade T1 bladder cancer: post-BCG second TUR according to lamina propria invasion microstaging (T1 A/B). J Urol 2011;185(4):e703.

34. Kamat AM, Gee JR, Dinney CP, et al. The case for early cystectomy in the treatment of nonmuscle invasive micropapillary bladder carcinoma. J Urol 2006;175(3 Pt 1):881–5. http://dx.doi.org/10.1016/s0022-5347(05)00423-4 Epub 2006/02/14.

35. Kamat AM, Dinney CP, Gee JR, et al. Micropapillary bladder cancer: a review of the University of Texas M. D. Anderson Cancer Center experience with 100 consecutive patients. Cancer 2007;110(1):62–7. http://dx.doi.org/10.1002/cncr.22756 Epub 2007/06/02.

36. Comperat E, Roupret M, Yaxley J, et al. Micropapillary urothelial carcinoma of the urinary bladder: a clinicopathological analysis of 72 cases. Pathology 2010;42(7): 650–4. http://dx.doi.org/10.3109/00313025.2010.522173 Epub 2010/11/18.

37. Spaliviero M, Dalbagni G, Bochner BH, et al. Clinical outcome of patients with T1 micropapillary urothelial carcinoma of the bladder. J Urol 2014. http://dx.doi.org/10.1016/j.juro.2014.02.2565. Epub 2014/03/08.

38. Rodriguez Faba O, Palou J. Predictive factors for recurrence progression and cancer specific survival in high-risk bladder cancer. Curr Opin Urol 2012;22(5): 415–20. http://dx.doi.org/10.1097/MOU.0b013e328356ac20 Epub 2012/07/25.

39. Babjuk M, Burger M, Zigeuner R, et al. EAU guidelines on non-muscle-invasive urothelial carcinoma of the bladder: update 2013. Eur Urol 2013;64(4):639–53. http://dx.doi.org/10.1016/j.eururo.2013.06.003 Epub 2013/07/06.

40. American Urological Association. Guidelines for the management of non-muscle invasive bladder cancer (stages Ta, T1, and TIS): 2007 update Linthicum, MD2007 [12 January 2014]. Available at: http://www.auanet.org/common/pdf/education/clinical-guidance/Bladder-Cancer.pdf. Accessed January 12, 2014.

41. Ojea A, Nogueira JL, Solsona E, et al. A multicentre, randomised prospective trial comparing three intravesical adjuvant therapies for intermediate-risk superficial bladder cancer: low-dose bacillus Calmette-Guerin (27 mg) versus very low-dose bacillus Calmette-Guerin (13.5 mg) versus mitomycin C. Eur Urol 2007; 52(5):1398–406. http://dx.doi.org/10.1016/j.eururo.2007.04.062.

42. Descotes F, Dessen P, Bringuier PP, et al. Microarray gene expression profiling and analysis of bladder cancer supports the sub classification of the T1 tumours in T1a and T1b stages. BJU Int 2013. http://dx.doi.org/10.1111/bju.12364.

43. Chatterjee SJ, Datar R, Youssefzadeh D, et al. Combined effects of p53, p21, and pRb expression in the progression of bladder transitional cell carcinoma. J Clin Oncol 2004;22(6):1007–13. http://dx.doi.org/10.1200/JCO.2004.05.174.

44. Shariat SF, Ashfaq R, Sagalowsky AI, et al. Predictive value of cell cycle bio-markers in nonmuscle invasive bladder transitional cell carcinoma. J Urol 2007; 177(2):481–7. http://dx.doi.org/10.1016/j.juro.2006.09.038 [discussion: 487].
45. Lebret T, Becette V, Barbagelatta M, et al. Correlation between p53 over expression and response to bacillus Calmette-Guerin therapy in a high risk select population of patients with T1G3 bladder cancer. J Urol 1998;159(3):788–91.
46. Peyromaure M, Weibing S, Sebe P, et al. Prognostic value of p53 overexpression in T1G3 bladder tumors treated with bacillus Calmette-Guérin therapy. Urology 2002;59(3):409–13.
47. Noon AP, Catto JW. Noncoding RNA in bladder cancer: a specific focus upon high-risk nonmuscle invasive disease. Curr Opin Urol 2014. http://dx.doi.org/10.1097/MOU.0000000000000090.
48. Mellon K, Wright C, Kelly P, et al. Long-term outcome related to epidermal growth factor receptor status in bladder cancer. J Urol 1995;153(3 Pt 2):919–25.
49. Lopez-Beltran A, Luque RJ, Alvarez-Kindelan J, et al. Prognostic factors in stage T1 grade 3 bladder cancer survival: the role of G1-S modulators (p53, p21Waf1, p27kip1, Cyclin D1, and Cyclin D3) and proliferation index (ki67-MIB1). Eur Urol 2004;45(5):606–12. http://dx.doi.org/10.1016/j.eururo.2003.11.011.
50. Palou J, Algaba F, Vera I, et al. Protein expression patterns of ezrin are predictors of progression in T1G3 bladder tumours treated with nonmaintenance bacillus Calmette-Guérin. Eur Urol 2009;56(5):829–36. http://dx.doi.org/10.1016/j.eururo.2008.09.062.
51. Fristrup N, Ulhøi BP, Birkenkamp-Demtröder K, et al. Cathepsin E, maspin, Plk1, and survivin are promising prognostic protein markers for progression in nonmuscle invasive bladder cancer. Am J Pathol 2012;180(5):1824–34. http://dx.doi.org/10.1016/j.ajpath.2012.01.023.
52. Orsola A, Trias I, Raventos CX, et al. Initial high-grade T1 urothelial cell carcinoma: feasibility and prognostic significance of lamina propria invasion microstaging (T1a/b/c) in BCG-treated and BCG-non-treated patients. Eur Urol 2005; 48(2):231–8. http://dx.doi.org/10.1016/j.eururo.2005.04.013 [discussion: 238]. Epub 2005/06/21.
53. Kiemeney LA, Witjes JA, Heijbroek RP, et al. Should random urothelial biopsies be taken from patients with primary superficial bladder cancer? A decision analysis. Br J Urol 1994;73(2):164–71.
54. Solsona E. Words of wisdom. Re: Final results of an EORTC-GU cancers group randomized study of maintenance bacillus Calmette-Guérin in intermediate- and high-risk Ta, T1 papillary carcinoma of the urinary bladder: one-third dose versus full dose and 1 year versus 3 years of maintenance. Eur Urol 2014; 65(4):847–8. http://dx.doi.org/10.1016/j.eururo.2013.12.034.
55. Brausi M, Collette L, Kurth K, et al. Variability in the recurrence rate at first follow-up cystoscopy after TUR in stage Ta T1 transitional cell carcinoma of the bladder: a combined analysis of seven EORTC studies. Eur Urol 2002;41(5):523–31.
56. Skolarus TA, Ye Z, Montgomery JS, et al. Use of restaging bladder tumor resection for bladder cancer among Medicare beneficiaries. Urology 2011;78(6): 1345–9. http://dx.doi.org/10.1016/j.urology.2011.05.071.
57. Herr HW, Donat SM, Dalbagni G. Can restaging transurethral resection of T1 bladder cancer select patients for immediate cystectomy? J Urol 2007;177(1): 75–9. http://dx.doi.org/10.1016/j.juro.2006.08.070 [discussion: 79].
58. Sfakianos JP, Kim PH, Hakimi AA, et al. The effect of restaging transurethral resection on recurrence and progression rates in patients with nonmuscle

invasive bladder cancer treated with intravesical bacillus Calmette-Guérin. J Urol 2014;191(2):341–5. http://dx.doi.org/10.1016/j.juro.2013.08.022.

59. Divrik RT, Sahin AF, Yildirim U, et al. Impact of routine second transurethral resection on the long-term outcome of patients with newly diagnosed pT1 urothelial carcinoma with respect to recurrence, progression rate, and disease-specific survival: a prospective randomised clinical trial. Eur Urol 2010;58(2):185–90. http://dx.doi.org/10.1016/j.eururo.2010.03.007.

60. Orsola A, Werner L, Torres ID, et al, editors. An optimized treatment strategy for HGT1 bladder cancer based on microstaging: results at 6 years follow-up in 200 patients. AUA Annual Meeting, abstract book. Orlando, May 16-21, 2014.

61. Raj GV, Herr H, Serio AM, et al. Treatment paradigm shift may improve survival of patients with high risk superficial bladder cancer. J Urol 2007;177(4):1283–6. http://dx.doi.org/10.1016/j.juro.2006.11.090 [discussion: 1286].

62. Thalmann GN, Markwalder R, Shahin O, et al. Primary T1G3 bladder cancer: organ preserving approach or immediate cystectomy? J Urol 2004;172(1):70–5. http://dx.doi.org/10.1097/01.ju.0000132129.87598.3b Epub 2004/06/18.

63. Denzinger S, Fritsche HM, Otto W, et al. Early versus deferred cystectomy for initial high-risk pT1G3 urothelial carcinoma of the bladder: do risk factors define feasibility of bladder-sparing approach? Eur Urol 2008;53(1):146–52. http://dx.doi.org/10.1016/j.eururo.2007.06.030 Epub 2007/07/13.

64. Badalato GM, Gaya JM, Hruby G, et al. Immediate radical cystectomy vs conservative management for high grade cT1 bladder cancer: is there a survival difference? BJU Int 2012;110(10):1471–7. http://dx.doi.org/10.1111/j.1464-410X.2012.11116.x Epub 2012/04/11.

65. Aziz A, May M, Burger M, et al. Prediction of 90-day mortality after radical cystectomy for bladder cancer in a prospective European multicenter cohort. Eur Urol 2013. http://dx.doi.org/10.1016/j.eururo.2013.12.018.

66. Weintraub MD, Li QQ, Agarwal PK. Advances in intravesical therapy for the treatment of non-muscle invasive bladder cancer (review). Mol Clin Oncol 2014;2(5):656–60. http://dx.doi.org/10.3892/mco.2014.314.

Nonurothelial Bladder Cancer and Rare Variant Histologies

Daniel Willis, MD, FACS, Ashish M. Kamat, MD, MBBS*

KEYWORDS

- Urothelial carcinoma • Variant histology • Micropapillary bladder cancer
- Radical cystectomy • Chemotherapy • Treatment guidelines

KEY POINTS

- At present, radical cystectomy is a mainstay in the management of all bladder cancers, whether of conventional urothelial histology or variant.
- In some variants, it is clearly not enough and multimodal therapy is imperative; in other cases, systemic therapy might be ineffective or even detrimental if it leads to delay in surgery.
- Identification of variant histology is a critical part of bladder cancer staging because such histology may require appropriately tailored therapy.

INTRODUCTION

Although approximately 80% of bladder cancer is caused by "conventional" urothelial carcinoma (UC), the remaining 10% to 25% is the result of nonurothelial and "variants" of UC.[1,2] Although the term "variant histology" can sometimes be used in a variety of different capacities, for the current discussion variant histology refers to any bladder malignancy other than pure UC. This simplification includes UC with aberrant differentiation in which the tumor arises from a common urothelial stem cell as well as "nonurothelial" carcinoma, which is the result of metaplasia. In reality, these histologic descriptions are based on morphologic features from hematoxylin and eosin–stained pathologic sections with little insight into their biologic derivative. Furthermore, mixed histologies are often present (including so-called urothelial and nonurothelial carcinomas), for which the term variant histology is generally used. **Box 1** describes the

Disclosure: Dr Kamat: FKD Industries Research Funding, Photocure Advisory Board, Bioniche Consultant, Sanofi Advisory Board, Merck Advisory Board, Abbott Molecular Consultant, Theralese Consultant, Heat Biologics Research Funding.
The University of Texas MD Anderson Cancer Center, 1515 Holcombe Boulevard, Unit 1373 Houston, TX 77030, USA
* Corresponding author. The University of Texas MD Anderson Cancer Center, 1515 Holcombe Boulevard, Unit 1373, Houston, TX 77030, USA.
E-mail address: akamat@mdanderson.org

Hematol Oncol Clin N Am 29 (2015) 237–252
http://dx.doi.org/10.1016/j.hoc.2014.10.011
0889-8588/15/$ – see front matter © 2015 Elsevier Inc. All rights reserved.

hemonc.theclinics.com

Box 1
Histologic classification of tumors of the urinary tract

Infiltrating Urothelial Tumors	Squamous Neoplasms	Melanocytic Tumors
With squamous differentiation	Squamous cell carcinoma	Malignant melanoma
With glandular differentiation	Verrucous carcinoma	Nevus
With trophoblastic differentiation	Squamous cell papilloma	**Mesenchymal Tumors**
Nested	**Glandular Neoplasms**	Rhabdomyosarcoma
Microcystic	Adenocarcinoma	Leiomyosarcoma
Micropapillary	Enteric	Angiosarcoma
Lymphoepithelioma-like	Mucinous	Osteosarcoma
Lymphoma-like	Signet-ring cell	Malignant fibrous histiocytoma
Plasmacytoid	Clear cell	Leiomyoma
Sarcomatoid	Villous adenoma	Hemangioma
Giant Cell	**Neuroendocrine Tumors**	**Hematopoietic and Lymphoid Tumors**
Undifferentiated	Small cell carcinoma	Lymphoma
	Carcinoid	Plasmacytoma
	Paraganglioma	

Adapted from Eble JN, Sauter G, Epstein JI, et al. World Health Organization Classification of Tumours. Pathology and Genetics of Tumours of the Urinary System and Male Genital Organs. Lyon: IARC Press; 2004. p.90; with permission.

---

histologic classification of tumors arising from the urinary tract and was adapted from the 2004 World Health Organization Classification of Tumors.[3]

CHALLENGES IN THE STUDY OF VARIANT HISTOLOGY

Studying the clinical significance of variant histology can be difficult as a result of subjectivity and challenges with diagnosis and cell type identification. As a result of sampling error and tumor heterogeneity, transurethral resection (TUR) has been reported to detect only 39% of variant cancers that present within the bladder.[4,5] Adding to the inherent difficulty with detection, it has been estimated that up to 44% of cases of histologic variants are not recognized or documented by community pathologists, which further leads to underreporting and the potential for mismanagement of patients. Initial reports also suggested that variant tumors were uniformly present at a high stage with invasion into muscularis propria.[1] However, since that time, multiple studies have been published showing variant histology present within non–muscle-invasive (NMI) tumors.[6–12] This is likely a reflection of increased awareness and recognition within the scientific community. In fact, in a large registry with more than 28,000 bladder cancer patients from The Netherlands, 23% of all variant tumors identified within the registry presented with NMI disease.[13]

Another issue complicating the study of variant histology is whether the extent of variant histology (ie, focal vs extensive) effects patient outcomes. Most studies do not control for this fact in their design. Some have explored relevant cutoffs, as was the case of 1 early study proposing that 20% variant histology was associated with worse survival outcomes.[14] However, no consistency has been shown among subsequent studies and it has become apparent that each bladder cancer variant behaves differently and needs to be addressed individually to assess its impact on the overall biology of the disease. The significance of the extent of each specific variant remains an area under investigation and study.

These diagnostic challenges underscore the difficulty in studying variant histology. Without consistent and reliable diagnosis, it will be difficult to reliably determine the biologic origins of variant bladder tumors, or how they might respond to therapy compared with conventional UC. In an effort to combat these challenges, many groups are attempting to outline standards and guidelines formally to aid in the identification and reporting of variant histology.[5] With the incorporation of collaborative efforts and centralized pathologic review, it is hoped that a better understanding of variant bladder cancer will result.

SIGNIFICANCE OF VARIANT HISTOLOGY

Several retrospective studies have suggested that variant histology portends worse clinical outcomes. Collectively, this is thought to be the result of a higher propensity of locally aggressive disease, higher rates of distant metastasis, and a different response to chemotherapy or radiotherapy compared with conventional UC. In a study of 448 consecutive TUR bladder tumor cases with 295 subsequent cystectomies, mixed histology was present in 25%, and the presence of variant architecture almost uniformly predicted the presence of locally advanced disease at cystectomy.[1] A separate group observed that, among 600 cystectomy patients, variant histology (defined as squamous, glandular, or other) predicted upstaging at the time of cystectomy with an odds ratio of 2.77.[15] The presence of variant histology has also been found to be associated with increased rates of pathologic lymph node metastasis in several multivariate analyses leading to worse survival outcomes.[16,17] Finally, a multi-institutional study with approximately 1000 patients found that patients with adenocarcinoma, small cell carcinoma, or other histologic subtypes had worse disease specific survival compared with conventional UC, even after accounting for stage, adjunct treatment, and lymphovascular invasion on multivariate analyses.[18]

However, other studies have presented conflicting evidence that these trends may not be true for all variants types of bladder cancer. A secondary analysis of the Southwest Oncology Group randomized trial S8710 was performed after the original study that showed increased survival for neoadjuvant methotrexate, vincristine, adriamycin, and cisplatin (MVAC) plus cystectomy over cystectomy alone in patients with locally advanced (cT2–T4a) bladder cancer.[19] This secondary analysis showed that patients with mixed histology (squamous and glandular differentiation) had improved survival rates after neoadjuvant MVAC chemotherapy as well as a higher rate of pT0 downstaging (34%) versus cystectomy alone (4%). This correlated with improved survival rates for patients with mixed histology after neoadjuvant chemotherapy, although statistical significance was not attained. This secondary analysis that was based on high-quality clinical trial data opposes the idea that all variant histology leads to a worse overall prognosis and outcome.

NON–MUSCLE-INVASIVE VARIANT BLADDER CANCER

There is some controversy regarding NMI bladder cancer with variant histology, both in terms of diagnosis and the role of intravesical therapy. A critical issue in considering therapy for NMI variant bladder cancer is that of correct staging. Although this is the case for conventional UC as well, some argue that because variant tumors notoriously are associated with advanced disease, there may be a potentially greater risk of understaging variant tumors. In such situations, intravesical therapy would be less effective. Retrospective studies looking at cT1 NMI variant bladder cancer have reported local understaging rates of 27% to

57%.[1,5,20] Rates of occult metastatic disease have also been reported as high as 27% to 44% among NMI variant tumors,[6] and in several multivariate analyses, divergent histology has been associated with the presence of lymph node metastasis and decreased survival.[21,22] This evidence of relatively high rates of understaged, locally advanced disease or occult metastatic disease raises the concern that even in the setting of NMI disease, a more aggressive treatment strategy is warranted. However, others have reported progression rates of approximately 40% (similar to conventional UC with high-risk features) and similar survival and response rates with induction and maintenance Bacillus Calmette-Guerin (BCG) treatment compared with control groups of conventional UC tumors.[6,12,13,23] These studies included tumors with squamous or glandular differentiation, nested variant (NV), and micropapillary disease. Thus, a thoughtful approach to management of NMI variant bladder cancer should be employed because of the morbidity associated with radical cystectomy. In general, the role of intravesical treatment for variant NMIBC should be considered based on the unique subtype and should be weighed against the risk of understaging.

MANAGEMENT OF VARIANT BLADDER CANCER

Based on existing studies, variant histology has been proposed as a clinical feature that identifies "high-risk" bladder cancer, and subsequent treatment algorithms have been presented.[13] Conceptually, if variant histology signals high risk for advanced bladder cancer, one could argue that the mere presence of variant architecture justifies an aggressive treatment algorithm that might depart from the standard treatment for conventional UC and warrant a multimodality approach to treatment.[24] However, if variant architecture confers resistance to chemotherapy or radiation therapy, then delaying surgery for ineffective neoadjuvant therapy may also lead to adverse events.

The reality for variant bladder cancer is that each histologic subtype (see **Box 1**) should be addressed individually because each may differ in their predisposition for metastasis and sensitivity to systemic treatment. For that reason, the common variant subtypes are addressed individually as they appear in **Box 1** with an emphasis on both muscle-invasive disease and NMI disease. Treatment algorithms are summarized in **Figs. 1** and **2**.

SQUAMOUS/GLANDULAR DIFFERENTIATION

Because the biologic origins of variant tumors are still in question, squamous and glandular differentiation have been included in the present discussion of variant histology. Each is typically present in the background of conventional UC in varying degrees. Squamous and glandular differentiation are discussed together here because many studies have commonly grouped them as "mixed" histology in the current literature. In reality, squamous differentiation is more prevalent and dominates studies with "mixed" histology. In fact, squamous differentiation has been reported to be present in as many as 60% of urothelial tumors specimens,[25,26] although it is less likely to be reported unless the architecture predominates the specimen as low proportions of squamous differentiation have not been shown to be clinically relevant. Glandular differentiation has not been adequately studied independently to allow any conclusions. Interestingly, in many postcystectomy bladder cancer series, squamous differentiation correlates with advanced stage and poor prognosis in multivariate models, suggesting it is a clinically relevant entity.[27,28] However, most studies are retrospective in nature and many other conflicting reports exist.

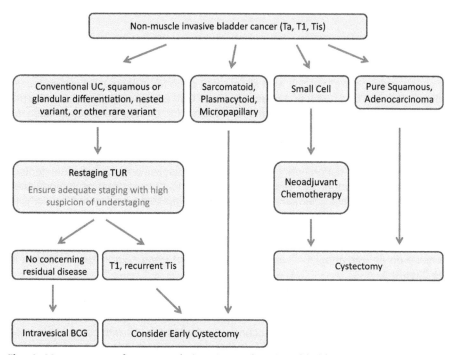

Fig. 1. Management of non–muscle-invasive and variant bladder cancer. BCG, Bacillus Calmette-Guerin; TUR, transurethral resection; UC, urothelial carcinoma.

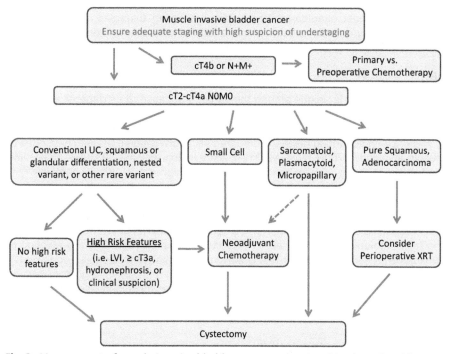

Fig. 2. Management of muscle-invasive bladder cancer and variant histology. Consider neoadjuvant chemotherapy for select patients. LVI, lymphatic invasion; UC, urothelial carcinoma; XRT, x-ray therapy.

As mentioned, secondary analysis of the Southwest Oncology Group neoadjuvant MVAC trial shows relatively high rates of response to neoadjuvant chemotherapy among tumors with squamous/glandular differentiation.[19] Separate, large, retrospective, case control studies also shown that despite an increased rate of locally advance tumors and nodal metastasis, patients with squamous/glandular differentiation had similar survival rates after controlling for clinical parameters such as T stage.[29,30] One study even stratified by the extent of differentiation and found no survival difference between tumors with less than 30% versus 30% or greater squamous differentiation.[29] In general, based on the current evidence, squamous or glandular differentiation may indicate advanced disease or a risk for understaging. However, these tumors are thought to respond to current treatment modalities, including neoadjuvant chemotherapy, and so they should be treated similarly to stage matched conventional UC. It has been suggested that extensive squamous differentiation may clinically resemble pure squamous cell carcinoma (SCC) with a predisposition for local recurrence, for which other treatment algorithms could be considered (ie, radiation),[27,31] although this has not been reliably demonstrated in the literature.

Although the majority of tumors with squamous and glandular differentiation present with muscle-invasive disease (70%),[27,28] there is no evidence to suggest that NMI tumors with squamous or glandular differentiation do not respond to intravesical treatments. Most studies have shown outcomes similar to pure UC with comparable rates of recurrence and progression.[13,32] It is therefore acceptable to pursue intravesical therapy for NMI tumors with "mixed histology" with the caveat that close surveillance and a high suspicion for understaging be maintained. Patients with low-volume, completely resected tumors with a small focus of squamous or glandular elements would be the best candidates for bladder preserving therapies. One should be cautious to delay definitive treatment in the form of radical cystectomy for those patients not responding to intravesical treatments.

NESTED VARIANT

NV bladder cancer is unique among the variants because of its deceptively benign appearance, which can easily be confused with von Brunn nests.[5] As has been consistent with other variants of bladder cancer, most studies show a predisposition to present with advanced disease compared with conventional UC with high rates of muscle invasion at TUR (70% vs 31%), extravesical disease (83% vs 33%), and metastasis (67% vs 19%) when compared with high-grade UC, respectively.[33,34] Nevertheless, stage for stage, NV does not seem to be any more aggressive than conventional UC with matched cohort analyses (n = 52) showing that, despite high rates of locally advanced (69%) and node-positive (19%) disease (10-year cancer-specific survival of 41%), NV has equivalent survival outcomes after controlling for pathologic stage.[32] There is very little published regarding the efficacy of neoadjuvant chemotherapy for NV. Unfortunately, little work has been done on NV bladder cancer and there is little evidence to support a treatment algorithm outside that employed for high-risk conventional UC for either muscle invasive or NMI NV. However, the high rates of extravesical and metastatic disease suggest a need for multimodal therapy.

MICROPAPILLARY BLADDER CANCER

Micropapillary bladder cancer (MPBC) has been a recent interest of many groups and a host of studies have been published. Uniquely, the micropapillary morphology has been identified in tumors from other organ sites, such as breast and ovarian cancer, with aggressive behavior in other tissue sites. Although MPBC is typically found in the background of conventional UC, it can also be associated with SCC of the bladder,[35] adenocarcinoma,[36] small cell carcinoma,[37] and sarcomatoid carcinoma.[38] The attention that MPBC has garnered has helped to bring to light many of the challenges associated with the study of variant histology. For example, published literature has shown that MPBC has a relatively poor recognition in community practices. Furthermore, in a study designed around expert genitourinary trained pathologist, a great deal of variability existed regarding the histologic diagnosis of micropapillary architecture with only classical cases of MPBC among showing consensus. The interobserver agreement among this group was modest at best with a kappa of 0.54.[39]

The majority of studies consistently show that muscle-invasive MPBC is associated with high rates of locally advanced and distant disease and is associated with poor overall survival.[7,9,36–38,40] Early studies even showed that small amounts of micropapillary component within the tumor was clinically significant with greater than 10% MPBC being associated with worse clinical outcomes.[26,40] The largest single institution series to date from MD Anderson Cancer Center (n = 100) demonstrated that the overall prognosis of MPBC was poor in this cohort with 5- and 10-year overall survival rates of 54% and 27%, respectively,[23] despite a relatively high proportion of NMI MPBC disease at presentation (44%). In this series, there were high rates of upstaging at the time of radical cystectomy (52.7%) and occult lymph node metastases were found in 27.3% of patients. Others have reported rates of occult metastatic disease as high as 35%[8] and 86%.[7] In the MD Anderson cohort, lymph node metastases were often reported to contain micropapillary features, even if it only represented a small fraction of the primary tumor, suggesting a propensity of MPBC to spread by lymphatic invasion. As has been the case with other variant tumors, case-matched studies with conventional UC that control for pathologic parameters show that stage for stage, there is no survival difference in MPBC and conventional UC.[41,42]

A recent study published a survey on MPBC given to the Society of Urologic Oncology. Among the "experts" in the field of urologic oncology, there was surprisingly very little consensus regarding the clinical management of MPBC.[43] For example, approximately one half of the surveyed physicians felt that muscle-invasive MPBC responded to chemotherapy and utilized it in their treatment algorithms, whereas the other half considered it to be a chemoresistant variant and did not utilize systemic treatment routinely. The MD Anderson cohort first suggested that MPBC might not respond to chemotherapy with worse survival identified among those receiving neoadjuvant chemotherapy after controlling for stage.[23] However, others have argued that, based on the high rates of upstaging at surgery and high rates of lymph node metastasis, systemic chemotherapy should be incorporated, especially because many of the lymph node metastases occur outside of accepted lymphadenectomy templates.[7] A recent retrospective cohort (n = 40) reported a 45% pathologic pT0 downstaging rate among MPBC patients after neoadjuvant chemotherapy compared with a 13% downstaging rate in the upfront cystectomy cohort. A corresponding survival advantage with neoadjuvant chemotherapy was also reported for patients who were downstaged.[44] Although there are limitations to all of these studies, including small sample size, relatively short follow-up, and few quality controls for the chemotherapy regimens, the role of neoadjuvant chemotherapy for organ-confined MPBC remains controversial.

The initial MD Anderson study was one of the first to help develop an awareness of variant histology among NMI tumors. From the same institution, a 44-patient study with NMI MPBC compared patients treated with intravesical BCG versus upfront radical cystectomy.[6] Sixty-seven percent showed cancer progression in the BCG group, including 22% who developed metastasis. Patients that underwent delayed cystectomy after BCG failure were found to have worse disease specific survival rates compared with upfront radical cystectomy. In a 72-patient follow-up study with an emphasis on cT1 MPBC comparing primary cystectomy with intravesical BCG, 35% of the BCG cohort developed lymph node metastasis, whereas 20% of the upfront cystectomy cohort still showed occult metastatic disease. In these studies, the authors concluded that because of the high rates of occult metastatic disease and the poor prognosis associated with BCG failure, that upfront radical cystectomy was the treatment of choice for cT1 MPBC. These findings coincide with a recent Surveillance, Epidemiology and End Results 17–based study that identified 120 patients with MPBC. After controlling for TNM staging, no difference in survival between MPBC and conventional UC was identified except among patients with NMI micropapillary disease, where worse survival outcomes were reported.[9]

Other authors have presented conflicting views on NMI MPBC, suggesting that intravesical BCG might be an appropriate therapy. In a recent publication from Memorial Sloan Kettering, equivalent survival outcomes between intravesical BCG and upfront radical cystectomy were reported in a 36 patient cohort with 3 years of follow-up. Although no survival difference was reported, a 21% incidence of metastasis was described in the BCG cohort with a 27% rate of occult metastatic disease in the upfront cystectomy cohort.[45] Other smaller reports made similar conclusions regarding intravesical BCG, including one that suggested that BCG might be appropriate in patients with a small percentage of micropapillary component in the tumor.[10,11]

Although no universal guidelines exist for the management of micropapillary bladder cancer, because of the predisposition for metastasis, expedient cystectomy is encouraged for invasive disease, leaving physicians to their own judgment over how to incorporate chemotherapy. Although conflicting evidence exists regarding NMI MPBC, many experts still favor upfront radical cystectomy over BCG because of the high rates of distant metastasis and poor survival after BCG failure.[46] This recommendation is supported by the survey to the Society of Urologic Oncology, which reported that 80.5% of its members would recommend upfront cystectomy for cT1 MPBC.[43]

LYMPHOEPITHELIOMA-LIKE CARCINOMA OF THE BLADDER

Lymphoepithelioma-like carcinoma of the bladder is a rare, undifferentiated carcinoma and is pure in approximately one half of all cases. One of the largest reported series (30 patients) suggests that patients with this variant have outcomes similar to conventional UC after radical cystectomy.[47] In tumors with pure or predominant lymphoepithelioma-like histology (lacking a significant conventional UC component), case series have suggested that these tumors are quite chemosensitive. However, without studies with larger sample sizes, no other treatment paradigms have been proven and so patients with this histologic subtype should be treated based on standard treatment algorithms.

PLASMACYTOID UROTHELIAL CARCINOMA

Although plasmacytoid UC (PUC) is uncommon, it exhibits a unique clinical behavior. As is the case with the prior variants, PUC is associated with advanced local and distant disease at presentation. Interestingly, however, even in the setting of negative surgical margins, the peritoneum remains a site of major recurrence. Because of this predisposition for peritoneal metastasis, carcinoembryonic antigen, cancer antigen (CA) 125, and CA19-9 have been incorporated as tumor markers for the disease.[48,49] Although few studies on PUC exist, a 31-patient case series has been published in patients with greater than 50% PUC at the time of TUR to determine the utility of neoadjuvant chemotherapy.[49] In that study, no survival difference was noted between those receiving neoadjuvant chemotherapy and those proceeding to upfront cystectomy, although some chemotherapeutic responses were observed. Because of the aggressive nature of PUC and the high rates of peritoneal metastasis, aggressive therapy incorporating radical cystectomy is likely required for both invasive and NMI forms of PUC.

SARCOMATOID CARCINOMA OF THE BLADDER

The 2004 World Health Organization definition of sarcomatoid carcinoma of the bladder now includes what used to be called carcinosarcoma as well as sarcomatoid carcinoma in prior versions of the World Health Organization nomenclature. Sarcomatoid bladder cancer now refers to any tumor possessing mesenchymal-like spindle cells or sarcomatous elements with or without (previously referred to as carcinosarcoma) epithelial markers. When discussing sarcomatoid carcinoma, studies using both terms are included. Similar to other variants, sarcomatoid carcinoma also tends to present with advanced stage, distant metastasis, and local progression.[12,50] However, even in these studies, after controlling for stage, patients with sarcomatoid disease had a worse survival and higher disease-specific mortality (almost 2-fold greater) than those with conventional UC. This difference was most pronounced at earlier stages. Response to chemotherapy and radiation remains controversial because no large series are available for review, but the aggressive nature of the disease favors a multimodal approach.[31,51,52] As a result, no formal treatment recommendations can be made, except that based on the aggressive nature of the disease, early radical cystectomy should be incorporated for all stages. The 1 patient with sarcomatoid disease who received intravesical BCG reported in the literature progressed on therapy after 1 year and unfortunately died from metastasis at 3 years.[13]

PURE SQUAMOUS CELL CARCINOMA

Pure SCC of the bladder is classically categorized into bilharzial and nonbilharzial forms. In the United States, nonbilharzial SCC (NBSCC) predominates and typically presents as muscle-invasive disease. A large, population-based study with more than 12,000 patients found, that after comparing 614 cases with NBSCC of the bladder with the remaining conventional UC controls, NBCSS presented more often with locally advanced disease (72% vs 52%).[22] Furthermore, despite negative surgical margins, SCC has shown a tendency for local recurrence, which can occur in as many as 75% of patients. However, after controlling for stage and other-cause mortality, a competing risks analysis showed no cancer-specific survival differences between NBSCC and conventional UC in a multivariate competing risks analysis.[22] Despite a similar survival after controlling for stage, the important difference between conventional UC and NBSCC is the tendency for local recurrence, which occurs more often in NBSCC than UC. In fact, 1 study reported a median survival of 9 months after pelvic recurrence after radical cystectomy versus 86.7 months without. This underscores the need to address the high rates of local recurrence into treatment algorithms for pure SCC of the bladder.[53]

Extrapolating from SCC of other organ sites, the role of radiation therapy has been studied for both bilharzial SCC and NBSCC. One retrospective study (n = 25) showed increased rates of downstaging (40%) and no rates of recurrence with 50 Gy of neoadjuvant radiation therapy before cystectomy after limited follow-up.[53] Adjuvant radiation therapy has also been studied for pure SCC of the bladder, albeit in the bilharzial setting. Many of the bilharzial studies have been extrapolated to NBSCC for the sake of this discussion. A prospective trial with 236 patients with pT2b–4a cancer showed that postoperative radiotherapy improved 5-year disease-free survival rates by 44% to 49% versus 25% after cystectomy alone. This was likely the result of improved rates of local control/recurrence with adjuvant radiation leading to local control rates of 87% to 93% versus 50% alone in the cystectomy only group.[54] A recent Egyptian, prospective, randomized trial has further compared preoperative and postoperative radiation with cystectomy (46% with SCC) and showed comparable rates of locoregional control (89% vs 81%) and disease-free survival (47% vs 34%) at 3 years.[55] Despite relatively good data on the effect of radiation treatment on local control for SCC of the bladder, radiation therapy has been avoided in the United States owing to a paucity of SCC cases and concerns for small bowel complications in the postoperative setting. Despite these treatment trends, most studies suggest that providers should strongly consider the role of perioperative radiation therapy for patients with pure SCC of the bladder.

SCC of the bladder also seems to differ from conventional UC in its response to systemic chemotherapy. Unfortunately, most traditional chemotherapeutic and experimental agents have mostly been ineffective in improving survival and local recurrence rates for BSCC in various Egyptian trials.[56] There is some evidence that gemcitabine–cisplatin may lead to improved rates of downstaging; however, no significant differences in survival have been reported.[56]

In the United States, NMI SCC of the bladder represents only about 2.6% of reported cases.[21] In a Surveillance, Epidemiology and End Results analysis looking at trends among patients with T1 disease, pure SCC remained an independent predictor of mortality with patients with T1 NMI bladder cancer who did not undergo upfront radical cystectomy as part of their initial treatment. Based on the rarity of pure SCC, the importance of local control, and the high rates of locally advanced disease, we recommend early cystectomy for patients presenting with NMI SCC of the bladder.

ADENOCARCINOMA

Nonurachal adenocarcinoma (primary bladder adenocarcinoma) also tends to be high grade and to present at an advanced stage at presentation.[57] Adenocarcinoma of the bladder (AC) is characterized by relatively high rates of local recurrence (30%) and metastasis. Based on these facts, retrospective case series have reported improved rates of local control (96% vs 53%) and improved 5-year disease-specific survival (61% vs 37%) with the use of adjuvant radiation therapy compared with cystectomy alone.[58] However, no other controlled trials exist to date and there is currently no evidence of effective chemotherapy that improves outcome for primary bladder adenocarcinoma. For nonurachal AC, it has been shown that patients treated with cystectomy have better survival than those treated with TUR alone,[59] and among 7 documented patients treated with radical cystectomy for T1 NMI AC, all benefitted with a 100% 5-year disease-free survival. Based on limited current evidence, definitive surgery with radical cystectomy for patients with resectable disease is advocated followed by consideration of adjuvant radiation therapy for improved local control.[24,53]

Urachal adenocarcinoma is defined by its location at the dome of the bladder and accounts for approximately 10% of bladder adenocarcinoma cases.[59] It seems to behave differently than its nonurachal counterpart and primarily affects younger women and African Americans. Approximately two thirds are low grade. Owing to its lower malignant potential (15% rate of metastasis), favorable location, and lack of field defect, urachal adenocarcinoma can be successfully managed with partial cystectomy. For urachal AC, negative surgical margins and adequate local control are essential; salvage surgery has poor outcomes.[58,60] Thus, attention to surgical technique is critical and should include removal of the umbilical stalk, closed surgical technique, and attention to surgical margins to provide oncologic efficacy. In the setting of metastatic disease, a clinical trial does exist on this variant that demonstrated the utility of a chemotherapy regimen composed of gemcitabine, 5-flurouracil, leucovorin, and cisplatin. This chemotherapy regimen showed a 30% to 40% objective response rate and an increase of median survival to 24 months (compared with 12 months).[60] Based on these results, one could hypothesize that neoadjuvant chemotherapy could benefit patients with clinically advanced disease, and adjuvant therapy might benefit those with a high likelihood of relapse (positive margins, lymph node/peritoneal involvement, no resection of umbilicus). Thus, based on the biology of this disease, even for presumed NMI forms of urachal AC, the gold standard treatment involves partial cystectomy with en bloc resection of the urachal ligament and umbilicus with pelvic lymph node dissection with the intent of cure. No standards exist to indicate when to incorporate chemotherapy, but patients are likely to benefit from systemic treatment when applied to cases of advanced disease.

SMALL CELL CARCINOMA

Small cell carcinoma of the bladder is a variant that seems to differ biologically from conventional UC. It is characterized by early metastasis, unique metastatic sites (brain and bone), and rapid progression. In fact, among patients with organ-confined small cell carcinoma, approximately 50% of patients were found to have occult metastasis after radical cystectomy.[61] Because of the high rates of metastatic disease and the unique sites, neurologic imaging and bone imaging should be incorporated into small cell staging protocols as appropriate. Furthermore, any degree of small cell component seems to confer aggressive biology. Because of this predisposition for metastatic spread, small cell carcinoma can almost be approached as a systemic disease; metastasis may be presumed. For that reason, chemotherapy plays an essential role in treatment. A recent clinical trial with a neuroendocrine chemotherapy regimen with ifosfomide, doxorubicin, etoposide, and cisplatin compared upfront cystectomy with cystectomy plus neoadjuvant chemotherapy. The neoadjuvant cohort demonstrated a dramatically improved overall survival (median 159.5 vs 18.3 months; $P<.001$) and disease-specific survival (5-year 79% vs 20%; $P<.001$), as well as improved downstaging rates (62% vs 9%).[62] Neuroendocrine chemotherapy regimens have elsewhere been confirmed to have superior pT0 rates compared with conventional urothelial regimens with small cell carcinoma of the bladder. In contrast, in studies where initial surgery was followed by adjuvant chemotherapy for patients with small cell components, survival was dismal, with rates as low as 10% at 5 years.[63] For patients unable to undergo cystectomy, combined chemoradiotherapy has been proposed as an alternative with fairly equivalent outcomes based on small retrospective cohorts with short follow-up.[64,65]

Because of the need for systemic treatment for small cell carcinoma of the bladder, intravesical therapy for NMI small disease conceptually is inappropriate. Although this has never been officially reported, we advocate primary chemotherapy with a small cell–specific regimen (ie, cisplatin with etoposide) followed by surgical extirpation as the mainstay of treatment for any degree of small cell carcinoma at any stage. Others have even proposed prophylactic radiation to the brain as a result of the propensity of the tumor to recur intracranially, even when pT0 after surgery. However, these results are not yet published and this practice remains investigational at this time.

FUTURE THERAPY

Appropriate management of variant bladder cancer depends on precise diagnosis, accurate staging, and a pretherapy prediction of sensitivity to nonoperative therapy (ie, chemotherapy, BCG, radiation therapy). However, insight is lacking in all of these areas, because limitations with each makes the diagnosis and management of variant bladder cancer challenging. It is hoped that, through future research, improved diagnostics will result from a development of reproducible pathologic criteria as well as molecular diagnostics in conjunction with improved tissue sampling techniques. To adequately characterize the role of medical therapy for variant tumors, studies must be appropriately powered to control for stage, differences in treatment, and other confounders so prevalent among current studies. Small, confounded studies only lead to confusion and collaborative and multi-institutional efforts will likely be necessary to move the field forward.

SUMMARY

At present, radical cystectomy is a mainstay in the management of all bladder cancers, whether of conventional urothelial histology or variant. However, in the case of some variants, it is clearly not enough and multimodal therapy is an imperative. In other cases, systemic therapy might be ineffective or even detrimental if it leads to delay in surgery (ie, SCC). Thus, identification of variant histology is a critical part of bladder cancer staging as such histology may require appropriately tailored therapy.

REFERENCES

1. Wasco MJ, Daignault S, Zhang Y, et al. Urothelial carcinoma with divergent histologic differentiation (mixed histologic features) predicts the presence of locally advanced bladder cancer when detected at transurethral resection. Urology 2007;70(1):69–74.
2. Kantor AF, Hartge P, Hoover RN, et al. Epidemiological characteristics of squamous cell carcinoma and adenocarcinoma of the bladder. Cancer Res 1988; 48(13):3853–5.
3. Eble JN, Sauter G, Epstein JI, et al. World Health Organization Classification of Tumours. Pathology and Genetics of Tumours of the Urinary System and Male Genital Organs. Lyon, France: IARC Press; 2004. p. 1–354.
4. Abd El-Latif A, Watts KE, Elson P, et al. The sensitivity of initial transurethral resection or biopsy of bladder tumor(s) for detecting bladder cancer variants on radical cystectomy. J Urol 2012;189(4):1263–7.
5. Hansel DE, Amin MB, Comperat E, et al. A contemporary update on pathology standards for bladder cancer: transurethral resection and radical cystectomy specimens. Eur Urol 2013;63(2):321–32.
6. Kamat AM, Gee JR, Dinney CP, et al. The case for early cystectomy in the treatment of nonmuscle invasive micropapillary bladder carcinoma. J Urol 2006;175: 881–5.

7. Ghoneim IA, Miocinovic R, Stephenson AJ, et al. Neoadjuvant systemic therapy or early cystectomy? Single-center analysis of outcomes after therapy for patients with clinically localized micropapillary urothelial carcinoma of the bladder. Urology 2011;77:867–70.

8. Comperat E, Roupret M, Yaxley J, et al. Micropapillary urothelial carcinoma of the urinary bladder: a clinicopathological analysis of 72 cases. Pathology 2010;42: 650–4.

9. Vourganti S, Harbin A, Singer EA, et al. Low grade micropapillary urothelial carcinoma, does it exist? - analysis of management and outcomes from the surveillance, epidemiology and end results (SEER) database. J Cancer 2013;4:336–42.

10. Amin A, Epstein JI. Noninvasive micropapillary urothelial carcinoma: a clinicopathologic study of 18 cases. Hum Pathol 2012;43:2124–8.

11. Gaya JM, Palou J, Algaba F, et al. The case for conservative management in the treatment of patients with non-muscle-invasive micropapillary bladder carcinoma without carcinoma in situ. Can J Urol 2010;17:5370–6.

12. Wright JL, Black PC, Brown GA, et al. Differences in survival among patients with sarcomatoid carcinoma, carcinosarcoma and urothelial carcinoma of the bladder. J Urol 2007;178:2302–6.

13. Shapur NK, Katz R, Pode D, et al. Is radical cystectomy mandatory in every patient with variant histology of bladder cancer. Rare Tumors 2011;3:e22.

14. Jozwicki W, Domaniewski J, Skok Z, et al. Usefulness of histologic homogeneity estimation of muscle-invasive urinary bladder cancer in an individual prognosis: a mapping study. Urology 2005;66(5):1122–6.

15. Turker P, Bostrom PJ, Wroclawski ML, et al. Upstaging of urothelial cancer at the time of radical cystectomy: factors associated with upstaging and its effect on outcome. BJU Int 2012;110(6):804–11.

16. Kassouf W, Agarwal PK, Grossman HB, et al. Outcome of patients with bladder cancer with pN+ disease after preoperative chemotherapy and radical cystectomy. Urology 2009;73(1):147–52.

17. Domanowska E, Jozwicki W, Domaniewski J, et al. Muscle-invasive urothelial cell carcinoma of the human bladder: multidirectional differentiation and ability to metastasize. Hum Pathol 2007;38(5):741–6.

18. Rogers CG, Palapattu GS, Shariat SF, et al. Clinical outcomes following radical cystectomy for primary nontransitional cell carcinoma of the bladder compared to transitional cell carcinoma of the bladder. J Urol 2006;175(6):2048–53.

19. Scosyrev E, Ely BW, Messing EM, et al. Do mixed histological features affect survival benefit from neoadjuvant platinum-based combination chemotherapy in patients with locally advanced bladder cancer? A secondary analysis of Southwest Oncology Group-Directed Intergroup Study (S8710). BJU Int 2011;108(5): 693–9.

20. Weizer AZ, Wasco MJ, Wang R, et al. Multiple adverse histological features increase the odds of under staging T1 bladder cancer. J Urol 2009;182:59–65.

21. El-Sebaie M, Zaghloul MS, Howard G, et al. Squamous cell carcinoma of the bilharzial and non-bilharzial urinary bladder: a review of etiological features, natural history, and management. Int J Clin Oncol 2005;10(1):20–5.

22. Abdollah F, Sun M, Jeldres C, et al. Survival after radical cystectomy of non-bilharzial squamous cell carcinoma vs urothelial carcinoma: a competing-risks analysis. BJU Int 2012;109(4):564–9.

23. Kamat AM, Dinney CP, Gee JR, et al. Micropapillary bladder cancer: a review of the University of Texas M. D. Anderson Cancer Center experience with 100 consecutive patients. Cancer 2007;110(1):62–7.

24. Willis DL, Porten SP, Kamat AM. Should histologic variants alter definitive treatment of bladder cancer? Curr Opin Urol 2013;23:435–43.
25. Martin JE, Jenkins BJ, Zuk RJ, et al. Clinical importance of squamous metaplasia in invasive transitional cell carcinoma of the bladder. J Clin Pathol 1989;42(3):250–3.
26. Lopez-Beltran A, Cheng L. Histologic variants of urothelial carcinoma: differential diagnosis and clinical implications. Hum Pathol 2006;37(11):1371–88.
27. Ehdaie B, Maschino A, Shariat SF, et al. Comparative outcomes of pure squamous cell carcinoma and urothelial carcinoma with squamous differentiation in patients treated with radical cystectomy. J Urol 2012;187(1):74–9.
28. Antunes AA, Nesrallah LJ, Dall'Oglio MF, et al. The role of squamous differentiation in patients with transitional cell carcinoma of the bladder treated with radical cystectomy. Int Braz J Urol 2007;33(3):339–45.
29. Kim SP, Frank I, Cheville JC, et al. The impact of squamous and glandular differentiation on survival after radical cystectomy for urothelial carcinoma. J Urol 2012;188(2):405–9.
30. Mitra AP, Bartsch CC, Bartsch G Jr, et al. Does presence of squamous and glandular differentiation in urothelial carcinoma of the bladder at cystectomy portend poor prognosis? An intensive case-control analysis. Urol Oncol 2014;32(2):117–27.
31. Black PC, Brown GA, Dinney CP. The impact of variant histology on the outcome of bladder cancer treated with curative intent. Urol Oncol 2009;27(1):3–7.
32. Miller JS, Epstein JI. Noninvasive urothelial carcinoma of the bladder with glandular differentiation: report of 24 cases. Am J Surg Pathol 2009;33:1241–8.
33. Linder BJ, Frank I, Cheville JC, et al. Outcomes following radical cystectomy for nested variant of urothelial carcinoma: a matched cohort analysis. J Urol 2013; 189:1670–5.
34. Wasco MJ, Daignault S, Bradley D, et al. Nested variant of urothelial carcinoma: a clinicopathologic and immunohistochemical study of 30 pure and mixed cases. Hum Pathol 2010;41(2):163–71.
35. Holmang S, Thomsen J, Johansson SL. Micropapillary carcinoma of the renal pelvis and ureter. J Urol 2006;175(2):463–6.
36. Johansson SL, Borghede G, Holmang S. Micropapillary bladder carcinoma: a clinicopathological study of 20 cases. J Urol 1999;161(6):1798–802.
37. Alvarado-Cabrero I, Sierra-Santiesteban FI, Mantilla-Morales A, et al. Micropapillary carcinoma of the urothelial tract. A clinicopathologic study of 38 cases. Ann Diagn Pathol 2005;9(1):1–5.
38. Baschinsky DY, Chen JH, Vadmal MS, et al. Carcinosarcoma of the urinary bladder–an aggressive tumor with diverse histogenesis. A clinicopathologic study of 4 cases and review of the literature. Arch Pathol Lab Med 2000; 124(8):1172–8.
39. Sangoi AR, Beck AH, Amin MB, et al. Interobserver reproducibility in the diagnosis of invasive micropapillary carcinoma of the urinary tract among urologic pathologists. Am J Surg Pathol 2010;34(9):1367–76.
40. Samaratunga H, Khoo K. Micropapillary variant of urothelial carcinoma of the urinary bladder; a clinicopathological and immunohistochemical study. Histopathology 2004;45(1):55–64.
41. Wang JK, Boorjian SA, Cheville JC, et al. Outcomes following radical cystectomy for micropapillary bladder cancer versus pure urothelial carcinoma: a matched cohort analysis. World J Urol 2012;30(6):801–6.
42. Fairey AS, Daneshmand S, Wang L, et al. Impact of micropapillary urothelial carcinoma variant histology on survival after radical cystectomy. Urol Oncol 2013; 32(3):110–6.

43. Willis DL, Flaig TW, Hansel DE, et al. Micropapillary bladder cancer: current treatment patters and review of the literature. Urol Oncol 2014;32(6):826–32.
44. Meeks JJ, Taylor JM, Matsushita K, et al. Pathological response to neoadjuvant chemotherapy for muscle-invasive micropapillary bladder cancer. BJU Int 2013;111(8):E325–30.
45. Spaliviero M, Dalbagni G, Bochner BH, et al. Clinical outcome of patients with T1 micropapillary urothelial carcinoma of the bladder. J Urol 2014;192(3):702–7.
46. Porten SP, Willis D, Kamat AM. Variant histology: role in management and prognosis of nonuscle invasive bladder cancer. Curr Opin Urol 2014;24(5):517–23.
47. Tamas EF, Nielsen ME, Schoenberg MP, et al. Lymphoepithelioma-like carcinoma of the urinary tract: a clinicopathological study of 30 pure and mixed cases. Mod Pathol 2007;20(8):828–34.
48. Topalak O, Saygili U, Soyturk M, et al. Serum, pleural effusion, and ascites CA-125 levels in ovarian cancer and nonovarian benign and malignant diseases: a comparative study. Gynecol Oncol 2002;85(1):108–13.
49. Dayyani F, Czerniak BA, Sircar K, et al. Plasmacytoid urothelial carcinoma, a chemosensitive cancer with poor prognosis, and peritoneal carcinomatosis. J Urol 2013;189(5):1656–61.
50. Wang J, Wang FW, Lagrange CA, et al. Clinical features of sarcomatoid carcinoma (carcinosarcoma) of the urinary bladder: analysis of 221 cases. Sarcoma 2010. Epub 2010 Jul 18.
51. Ikegami H, Iwasaki H, Ohjimi Y, et al. Sarcomatoid carcinoma of the urinary bladder: a clinicopathologic and immunohistochemical analysis of 14 patients. Hum Pathol 2000;31(3):332–40.
52. Lopez-Beltran A, Pacelli A, Rothenberg HJ, et al. Carcinosarcoma and sarcomatoid carcinoma of the bladder: clinicopathological study of 41 cases. J Urol 1998;159(5):1497–503.
53. Swanson DA, Liles A, Zagars GK. Preoperative irradiation and radical cystectomy for stages T2 and T3 squamous cell carcinoma of the bladder. J Urol 1990;143(1):37–40.
54. Zaghloul MS, Awwad HK, Akoush HH, et al. Postoperative radiotherapy of carcinoma in bilharzial bladder: improved disease free survival through improving local control. Int J Radiat Oncol Biol Phys 1992;23(3):511–7.
55. El-Monim HA, El-Baradie MM, Younis A, et al. A prospective randomized trial for postoperative vs. preoperative adjuvant radiotherapy for muscle-invasive bladder cancer. Urol Oncol 2013;31(3):359–65.
56. Khaled HM. Systemic management of bladder cancer in Egypt: revisited. J Egypt Natl Canc Inst 2005;17(3):127–31.
57. Lughezzani G, Sun M, Jeldres C, et al. Adenocarcinoma versus urothelial carcinoma of the urinary bladder: comparison between pathologic stage at radical cystectomy and cancer-specific mortality. Urology 2010;75(2):376–81.
58. Zaghloul MS, Nouh A, Nazmy M, et al. Long-term results of primary adenocarcinoma of the urinary bladder: a report on 192 patients. Urol Oncol 2006;24(1):13–20.
59. Wright JL, Porter MP, Li CI, et al. Differences in survival among patients with urachal and nonurachal adenocarcinomas of the bladder. Cancer 2006;107(4):721–8.
60. Siefker-Radtke AO, Gee J, Shen Y, et al. Multimodality management of urachal carcinoma: the M. D. Anderson Cancer Center experience. J Urol 2003;169(4):1295–8.
61. Cheng L, Pan CX, Yang XJ, et al. Small cell carcinoma of the urinary bladder: a clinicopathologic analysis of 64 patients. Cancer 2004;101(5):957–62.

62. Lynch SP, Shen Y, Kamat A, et al. Neoadjuvant chemotherapy in small cell urothelial cancer improves pathologic downstaging and long-term outcomes: results from a Retrospective Study at the MD Anderson Cancer Center. Eur Urol 2013; 64(2):307–13.

63. Quek ML, Nichols PW, Yamzon J, et al. Radical cystectomy for primary neuroendocrine tumors of the bladder: the University of Southern California experience. J Urol 2005;174(1):93–6.

64. Bex A, de Vries R, Pos F, et al. Long-term survival after sequential chemoradiation for limited disease small cell carcinoma of the bladder. World J Urol 2009;27(1): 101–6.

65. Schreiber D, Rineer J, Weiss J, et al. Characterization and outcomes of small cell carcinoma of the bladder using the surveillance, epidemiology, and end results database. Am J Clin Oncol 2013;36(2):126–31.

New Trends in the Surgical Management of Invasive Bladder Cancer

Mark A. Preston, MD, MPH[a],*, Seth P. Lerner, MD[b],
Adam S. Kibel, MD[c]

KEYWORDS

- Robotic-assisted radical cystectomy • Lymph node dissection • Surgical trends
- Centralization • ERAS

KEY POINTS

- Use of robotic-assisted radical cystectomy has increased steadily during past decade, with comparable short-term surgical quality metrics and functional and complication outcomes compared with open radical cystectomy. Ongoing randomized trials are needed to demonstrate durable oncologic efficacy and equivalence to open surgery.
- Bilateral dissection of the primary pelvic lymph node drainage system is a critical part of the surgical approach; however, the proximal extent of the dissection is currently being evaluated in phase III trials.
- Enhanced recovery after surgery protocols show tremendous potential in the perioperative management of patients undergoing radical cystectomy, reducing complications and length of hospital stay through targeted interventions aimed at ensuring that patients' medical status is optimized before surgery and that they return to baseline function as soon as possible postoperatively.
- Alvimopan has been shown in randomized controlled trials to provide quicker return of gastrointestinal function.
- Improved perioperative morbidity and mortality are seen with centralization of radical cystectomy in high-volume centers and with high-volume surgeons.

Disclosure: Board member—BCAN; Consultant—BioCancell and Vaxxion; Expert Advisor—Genentech, Merck, Sitka, Neuclexx; Grants/Research—ENDO, FKD grant NCT01687244 (S.P. Lerner).
[a] Harvard Medical School; Division of Urology, Brigham and Women's Hospital, Boston, MA 02115, USA; [b] Beth and Dave Swalm Chair in Urologic Oncology, Scott Department of Urology; Director of Urologic Oncology; Director of the Multidisciplinary Bladder Cancer Program; Faculty Group Practice Medical Director, Baylor College of Medicine Medical Center, Houston, TX 77030, USA; [c] Harvard Medical School; Division of Urology, Brigham and Women's Hospital, Boston, MA 02115, USA
* Corresponding author.
E-mail address: MPRESTON1@PARTNERS.ORG

Hematol Oncol Clin N Am 29 (2015) 253–269
http://dx.doi.org/10.1016/j.hoc.2014.10.010
0889-8588/15/$ – see front matter © 2015 Elsevier Inc. All rights reserved.

hemonc.theclinics.com

INTRODUCTION

Radical cystectomy with bilateral pelvic lymph node dissection (PLND) and urinary diversion is the gold standard for management of clinical stage T2 through 4a bladder cancer that is not metastatic and for non–muscle-invasive high-grade urothelial carcinoma that is refractory to intravesical therapy, and for palliation in patients with severe local symptoms.[1–4] Open radical cystectomy (ORC) has been the mainstay of curative treatment for decades, with modifications including nerve-sparing continent urinary diversion and proximal extent of PLND. During the preceding 30 years, 5-year trends in relative survival of bladder cancer have only improved marginally, from 72% in 1975 through 1977 to 80% in 2003 through 2009.[5] Although survival rates have not shifted dramatically, complication rates have improved but remain high, with rates up to 60% and prolonged hospital stays still common.[4,5] Thus, novel technology, techniques, and management strategies have continually been sought to improve surgical outcomes after radical cystectomy.

This article discusses several modifications in surgical care. First, traditional ORC is performed via an open, infraumbilical midline incision. Surgeons continue to innovate and lengths of stay have steadily decreased. However, the introduction of robotic-assisted radical cystectomy (RARC) offers the hope of a less morbid surgical approach.[6–8] Although uptake has not been as rapid as robotic-assisted laparoscopic prostatectomy (RALP), it is increasingly being used.[7] Second, extended PLND was introduced. Although strong evidence exists for the benefit of bilateral PLND, the relative extent of lymphadenectomy, standard versus extended, is currently under investigation. Third, enhanced recovery after surgery (ERAS) protocols have emerged, with initial evidence from colorectal surgery showing tremendous potential in the perioperative management of patients undergoing radical cystectomy. Studies suggest that these protocols have reduced complications and length of hospital stay through targeted interventions aimed at ensuring that patients' medical status is optimized before surgery and that they return to baseline function as soon as possible postoperatively. Fourth, level I evidence supports the use of alvimopan for earlier return of bowel function, and this agent is commonly incorporated within an ERAS protocol. Finally, the benefits of radical cystectomy centralization in high-volume surgical centers are reviewed.

ROBOTIC-ASSISTED LAPAROSCOPIC CYSTECTOMY

Although laparoscopic cystectomy was first reported in the literature in the early 90s, it was not widely embraced because of the high technical skill required.[9] The robotic platform, however, provides the benefits of a magnified 3-dimensional image; the ability to use an EndoWrist, which allows superior motion over laparoscopic instruments; and a more ergonomic position that effectively makes minimally invasive radical cystectomy a viable alternative for surgeons with advanced laparoscopic and robotic experience. Potential benefits include reduced blood loss, fewer transfusions, lower narcotic requirements, quicker return of bowel function, shortened length of stay and improved cosmesis.[8,10–12] These perceived advantages are offset by longer operative times and a lack of tactile feedback, which is typically a mainstay of ORC in determining resectability and the presence of extravesical disease.[13] Furthermore, in a value-based purchasing environment, cost must be accounted for in the evaluation of the relative advantages and disadvantages associated with these 2 approaches. In addition, RARC may be limited in patients with multiple prior abdominal surgeries or in those who cannot tolerate the pneumoperitoneum or steep Trendelenburg position required because of body habitus or comorbidities.

The technique for RARC initially developed through replicating the steps and principles of the open procedure. In addition, the preexisting and widespread uptake of RALP certainly aided in the advancement and modification of RARC, specifically shortening operative times, reducing blood loss, and improving lymph node yield.[14]

Complications

Radical cystectomy with PLND is a morbid operation, with complication rates up to 60% and mortality rates of 1% to 7%.[3,4,15,16] A driving force behind adoption of RARC was the belief that the minimally invasive approach would lessen the burden of these complications through reduced blood loss, decreased need for transfusion, and absence of a large, midline incision. A small pilot randomized controlled trial (n = 40) found that the RARC group (400 mL; interquartile range [IQR], 300.0–762.5) had a decreased estimated blood loss compared with the ORC group (800 mL; IQR, 400–1100) but similar blood transfusion rates and no significant reduction in "excessive length of stay" (>5 days; 65% vs 90%; P = .11) compared with the ORC group.[17] Blood transfusion rates in radical cystectomy series range from 42% to 60% because of intraoperative blood loss and preoperative anemia secondary to deconditioning, hematuria, and use of neoadjuvant chemotherapy.[18] Retrospective studies also suggest that transfusions are associated with worse outcomes in patients with bladder cancer who are undergoing radical cystectomy.[18,19]

It is important to note when comparing RARC with ORC that most studies are retrospective or prospective in nature and randomized trials are limited. Memorial Sloan Kettering Cancer Center (MSKCC) recently published results of a randomized trial of 118 patients assessing whether RARC would be associated with a lower rate of perioperative complications than open surgery, with extracorporeal urinary diversion (ECUD) being used in both arms.[12] In the intention-to-treat analysis, the investigators reported that 37 patients (62%) who underwent RARC and 38 (66%) who underwent open surgery had a grade 2 to 5 complication (P = .66), and that rates of high-grade complications were also similar (P = .90).[12] Intraoperative blood loss was less in the RARC group (mean difference, 159 cm^3), but length of surgery was significantly shorter in the open-surgery group (mean difference, 127 minutes; P<.001). The mean length of hospital stay was similar in the RARC and ORC arms (8 days; P = .53). This trial was stopped early because interim analysis showed that outcomes had met predefined criteria for futility in showing a difference in complications between ORC and RARC. Unfortunately, details on types and severity of complications were limited. Randomized data are still not available for investigating oncologic and pain control outcomes and whether intracorporeal urinary diversion (ICUD) affects any of the perioperative morbidity or functional outcomes.

A recent meta-analysis[10,13] showed that patients undergoing RARC experienced fewer overall perioperative complications (P = .04), had less estimated blood loss (P<.001), required fewer perioperative transfusions (P<.001), and had a shorter length of hospital stay (P<.001). These findings provide at best level III evidence, which is not sufficient to support meaningful comparisons, as evidenced by the data from the randomized trials reported earlier. Long-term studies are needed to determine complication rates beyond the perioperative period, including complications associated with urinary diversion that may take months or years to present.

Oncologic Outcomes

Margin status at radical cystectomy is a short-term oncologic marker known to affect cancer-specific survival. Studies seem to show equivalent rates of positive surgical margins between ORC and RARC, ranging from 0% to 9% (**Table 1**).[8,10,12,17,20–26]

Table 1
Summary of published studies on robotic-assisted radical cystectomy

Author	Institution	Level of Evidence	Number of Patients	Lymph Node Yield	Positive Surgical Margins	Median Estimated Blood Loss (mL)	Median Operative Time (min)	Length of Stay (d)	Overall Complications	Ileal Conduit	CSS (2-y)	OS (2-y)
Parekh et al,[17] 2013	University of Texas Southwestern	2	20	11 (median)	5%	400	300	6.0	25% (>grade 2)	N/A	N/A	N/A
Nix et al,[10] 2010	University of North Carolina	2	21	19 (mean)	0%	200	252	4.0	33%	50%	N/A	N/A
Kader et al,[20] 2013	Wake Forest	3	100	18 (mean)	11%	423 (mean)	451 (mean)	6.0	35% (90 d)	97%	N/A	N/A
Knox et al,[21] 2013	University of Alabama	3	58	21 (mean)	7%	276 (mean)	468 (mean)	6.3 (mean)	43% (30 d)	91%	N/A	N/A
Nepple et al,[22] 2013	Washington University	3	36	17 (median)	14%	675 (mean)	410 (mean)	7.9 (mean)		81%	73%	68%
Ng et al,[23] 2010	Weill Cornell	3	83	16 (median)	7%	460 (mean)	365 (mean)	5.5	48% (90 d)	56%	N/A	N/A
Kauffman et al,[24] 2011	Weill Cornell	4	85	17 (median)	6%	400	360	N/A		71%	85%	79%
Pruthi et al,[25] 2010	University of North Carolina	4	100	19 (mean)	0%	250	258	4.9 (mean)	8% (>grade 3)	61%	94% (18 mo)	91% (18 mo)
Guru et al,[26] 2009	Roswell Park	4	100	17–26 (mean)	3%	598 (mean)	343 (mean)	N/A	38%	93%	N/A	N/A
Bochner et al,[12] 2014	Memorial Sloan Kettering	2	60	N/A	N/A	N/A	456 (mean)	8 (mean)	62% (≥grade 2)	N/A	N/A	N/A

Abbreviations: CSS, cancer-specific survival; N/A, not applicable; OS, overall survival; RARC, robotic-assisted radical cystectomy.

Adapted from Liss MA, Kader AK. Robotic-assisted laparoscopic radical cystectomy: history, techniques and outcomes. World J Urol 2013;31:489–97; with permission.

One of the few randomized trials comparing ORC and RARC observed no significant differences between oncologic outcomes of positive margins (5% each; $P = .50$) or number of lymph nodes removed (n = 23 vs 11, respectively; IQR, 15.00–28.00 vs 8.75–21.50, respectively; $P = .135$).[17] However, only 40 patients were randomized, thus limiting definitive conclusions. A second small randomized controlled trial (n = 41) found similar median nodal yields between ORC and RARC (18 ORC vs 18 RARC; $P = .515$).[10] Oncology outcomes from the MSKCC randomized trial have not yet been published.[12] Although most of the technical hurdles have been overcome for RARC with respect to many quality metrics by advanced laparoscopic/robotic surgeons, no level I evidence yet supports a claim that RARC is better than, worst than, equivalent to, or noninferior to ORC with respect to probability of progression, cancer-specific survival, or overall survival.

One retrospective series reported on long-term oncologic outcomes in 121 patients who underwent RARC, with a median follow-up of 5.5 years.[11] They found that 24 patients (20.0%) had node-positive disease and 8 patients (6.6%) had positive soft tissue margins. The 5-year actuarial overall, cancer-specific, and recurrence-free survival rates were 48%, 71%, and 65%, respectively.[11] However, 56% of patients in this cohort had pT2 through pT4 cancers, indicating that almost 50% had low-volume disease.

The challenge of accurately assessing the oncologic outcome of RARC in the absence of large well-designed randomized controlled trials is largely caused by selection bias present in nonrandomized studies. Although more of a factor in earlier series, older, more complex patients with higher-stage disease are still more likely to undergo open than robotic surgery. Statistical analysis can only partially compensate for this.

Although short-term outcomes and pathologic findings between ORC and RARC may be comparable, long-term outcomes and results of ongoing larger randomized controlled trials are required before equivalence can be properly assessed.[12] Oncologic principles remain true regardless of surgical modality, and radical cystectomy with bilateral PLND, including external and internal iliac and obturator nodes, should be performed in a timely fashion in all patients with muscle-invasive bladder cancer, and radical cystectomy should be considered for primary therapy in higher-risk patients with pT1G3 bladder cancer.[2,27]

Extracorporeal Versus Intracorporeal Urinary Diversion

On completion of the bladder removal and lymph node dissection, incontinent cutaneous (ileal conduit), continent cutaneous diversion, or orthotopic urinary diversion can be conducted either extracorporeally or intracorporeally. In early experience, ECUD was more commonly used because of the increased complexity and prolonged operative times of ICUD. However, intracorporeal diversion is gaining popularity because of increasing experience and potential benefits, including decreased bowel exposure and handling, reduced risk of fluid imbalance, reduced pain, and smaller incision.[28,29] Novel devices, such as the robotic vessel-sealing instruments and staplers, have potential to improve operative times and ease of procedure but at a substantial additional expense.

A recent study from the International Robotic Cystectomy Consortium reported on 768 patients who had ECUD (570 conduits, 198 neobladders) and 167 who had ICUD (106 conduits, 61 neobladders).[28] The investigators reported that operative time was similar (414 minutes; $P > .05$) and that patients receiving ICUD were less likely to experience a 90-day postoperative complication compared with those undergoing ECUD (41% vs 49%; $P = .05$).[28] Limitations of this retrospective study include only reporting 90-day outcomes and that ICUD were more likely to be performed on healthier patients and by more experienced practitioners. Gore and colleagues[30] previously reported in 2010 that perioperative complications were similar between patients receiving either an ileal conduit or a continent diversion, but did not comment on whether open or robotic surgery was used.

Ongoing randomized trials will help determine whether robotic approaches can improve oncologic and functional outcomes. The largest trial currently underway is randomized open versus robotic cystectomy (RAZOR) (ClinicalTrials.gov identifier: NCT01157676)[31]; this is a multi-institutional noninferior phase III trial that will randomize patients with T1–T4, N0–1, M0 bladder cancer to undergo either open or robotic surgery, with approximately 160 patients in each arm. The purpose of this trial is to compare open versus RARC, PLND, and urinary diversion in terms of oncologic outcomes, complications, and quality-of-life measures, with a primary end point of 2-year progression-free survival. Full data from the RAZOR trial are not expected until 2016 to 2017.

EXTENDED LYMPH NODE DISSECTION

A bilateral PLND is an important component of a radical cystectomy, because the lymph nodes may be the only site of metastases. Thus, pelvic lymphadenectomy can be both prognostic and therapeutic.[32,33] Studies show that positive pelvic lymph nodes are found in 21% to 35% of patients.[11,34,35] Stein and colleagues[1] reported on 246 patients who had positive lymph nodes at the time of radical cystectomy and PLND, noting 5- and 10-year recurrence-free survival rates of 35% and 34%, respectively.

The minimum requirement for bilateral (standard) lymphadenectomy includes all lymphatic tissue distal to the common iliac bifurcation, and includes the external iliac, internal iliac, and obturator fossa extending to the Cooper ligament distally, the pelvis sidewall laterally, and the bladder medially. An extended pelvic lymphadenectomy includes the lymph nodes at least up to the aortic bifurcation, and includes the bilateral common iliac, presacral, and presciatic (or fossa of Marseilles) nodes and the nodal regions of standard dissection. Some surgeons extend the dissection above the aortic bifurcation up to the origin of the inferior mesenteric artery. Retrospective data suggest that the proximal extent of node dissection and individual surgeon's experience may have a beneficial impact on the therapeutic outcome and overall survival.[36] The limits of node dissection do not differ between open and RARC. Repeat studies have shown that RARC lymph node yields can equal those of ORC with adequate surgeon effort and case volume.[10,37,38]

Studies of efficacy of extended lymph node dissection are complicated by the fact that lymph node yield depends on node viability, method of submission (en bloc or separate), and processing technique.[39,40] Furthermore, in routine clinical practice, lymphadenectomy is less commonly performed and lymph node yields have been lower than those reported in published studies.[41,42] Although thorough, extended node dissection adds time to an already lengthy procedure; however, current evidence supports a survival benefit, and therefore it should be performed when possible.[43]

Most studies are retrospective or provide insufficient quality of evidence to make definitive conclusions regarding extent of node dissection. The Southwest Oncology Group has initiated a randomized trial to compare disease-free survival of patients with muscle-invasive urothelial carcinoma of the bladder undergoing radical cystectomy with extended PLND versus standard pelvic lymphadenectomy (ClinicalTrials.gov identifier: NCT01224665). The estimated enrollment is 620 patients; accrual began in 2011, with estimated completion in 2022.

ENHANCED RECOVERY AFTER SURGERY PROTOCOLS

The ERAS protocol is a multimodal perioperative care pathway designed to attenuate a patient's stress response during a surgical procedure (**Fig. 1**) through facilitating the maintenance of preoperative bodily compositions and organ function, and thereby achieving early recovery.[44–46] Evidence for ERAS in the urologic literature remains limited, but the data published, and those extrapolated from colorectal studies, are very promising.[44] Given the well-established morbidity of radical cystectomy and complex perioperative care, this procedure is perfectly suited for evidence-based patient care, with the most potential for benefit. ERAS protocols, by design, necessitate a multidisciplinary approach, with surgeons, anesthesia, nursing, nutrition, and other support services collaborating closely in patient care.

Behaviors and patient care interventions are targeted in the preoperative, intraoperative, and postoperative setting (see **Fig. 1**). Key interventions in the preoperative period are different from traditional management and include no prolonged fasting, high-concentration carbohydrate loading, and no bowel preparation, because level I evidence suggests that bowel preparations do not improve operative outcomes.[47–51] Intraoperative interventions are characterized by short-acting epidural agents, avoidance of salt and water overload, normothermia, and use of an epidural.[52] ERAS is based on randomized data and meta-analyses that perioperative care improves with appropriate management. For instance, a Cochrane meta-analysis investigating early nasogastric tube removal in patients undergoing abdominal procedures included 33 randomized controlled trials and showed more postoperative complications and no

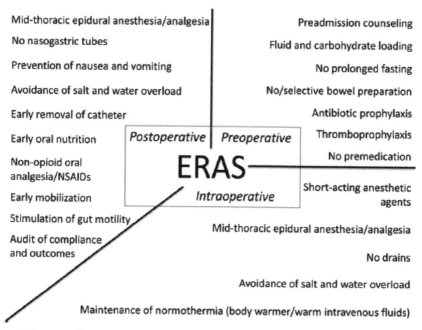

Fig. 1. Preoperative, intraoperative, and postoperative components of enhanced recovery after surgery (ERAS) protocols. NSAID, nonsteroidal anti-inflammatory drug. (*From* Varadhan KK, Lobo DN, Ljungqvist O. Enhanced recovery after surgery: the future of improving surgical care. Crit Care Clin 2010;26:527–47, with permission.)

advantage to maintaining prophylactic nasogastric tube after surgery.[53] Early naso-gastric tube removal (defined typically as removal immediately postoperatively or within 12 hours vs removal at first flatus) reduced morbidity, bowel recovery time, and length of hospital stay.[54,55] Postoperative interventions include early postopera-tive feeding, early mobilization, and gum chewing to promote a quicker return of bowel function, and prevention of nausea and vomiting.[49,50,54,56,57] These evidence-based steps have been included in ERAS protocols to improve patient care, and early results showed marked benefit.

Daneshmand and colleagues[49] reported on the use of an ERAS protocol among a prospective group of 110 patients who underwent ORC and urinary diversion (68% continent diversion). A bowel movement occurred in 82% of patients by postoperative day 2. Median length of stay was 4 days, with a 30-day readmission rate of 21% (n = 23). The most common reasons for readmission were urinary tract infection and dehydration.

Although much evidence for ERAS protocols can be extrapolated from the wealth of evidence in the colorectal literature, important differences should be noted, including the presence of small bowel anastomoses, urine within the peritoneal cavity, both extraper-itoneal and intraperitoneal access, longer operative times, and increased risk of blood loss and transfusion.[54] It is certainly plausible that ERAS protocols may have a greater impact on length of stay and complications than surgical modality alone (**Table 2**).[50]

ALVIMOPAN, μ-OPIOID RECEPTOR ANTAGONIST

Radical cystectomy with urinary diversion is a prolonged procedure, with complica-tions and increased length of stay commonly caused by delayed return of gastrointes-tinal function. Improving speed of gastrointestinal recovery is thus the focus of intervention after radical cystectomy, whether this occurs through ERAS protocols or other strategies. One new medication with much potential is alvimopan. Alvimopan is a peripheral μ-opioid receptor antagonist that has been shown in multiple random-ized trials to accelerate gastrointestinal activity after bowel resection.[58,59]

A multicenter, randomized, placebo-controlled phase IV trial studied the efficacy of alvimopan in accelerating gastrointestinal recovery after radical cystectomy.[59] They found that the alvimopan cohort experienced quicker gastrointestinal recovery (5.5 vs 6.8 days; hazard ratio, 1.8; $P<.0001$), shorter mean length of stay (7.4 vs 10.1 days; $P = .0051$), and fewer episodes of postoperative ileus-related morbidity (8.4% vs 29.1%; $P<.001$). The study was conducted in mostly high-volume centers using open cystectomy without the use of epidurals, and safety was found to be com-parable with that of placebo.[59] A modified ERAS protocol including the use of alvimo-pan and no epidural is used at the University of Southern California, with a reported 4-day median length of stay.[50]

RADICAL CYSTECTOMY VOLUME AND CENTRALIZATION IN CENTERS OF EXCELLENCE

It has been previously established that hospitals and surgeons with higher surgical volumes typically have better outcomes than those with lower volumes.[60,61] This cor-relation is especially pertinent in more complex operations. Radical cystectomy is one of the most complex urologic procedures, whether performed open or robotically. The learning curve is steep, perioperative care and management of complications is critical, and experience matters. Studies have shown that most cystectomies are conducted by urologists who perform very few procedures each year. Konety and colleagues,[62] using the Nationwide Inpatient Sample, identified 13,964 patients under-going radical cystectomy between 1988 and 1999, and ranked hospitals into tertiles

Table 2
Enhanced recovery after surgery (ERAS) elements applied to radical cystectomy

ERAS Item	Summary	Specifics for Patients Undergoing Radical Cystectomy	Evidence for Cystectomy/Rectal Surgery	Recommendation Grade
1. Preoperative counseling and education	Patients should receive dedicated preoperative counseling and education	Provide surgical details, hospital stay, and discharge criteria in oral and written form Stoma education Address patient expectations	NA/low	Strong
2. Preoperative medical optimization	Preoperative optimization of medical conditions should be recommended Preoperative nutritional support should be considered, especially for malnourished patients	Correction of anemia and comorbidities Nutritional support Smoking cessation and alcohol reduction 4 wk before surgery Encourage physical exercise	NA/moderate NA/high NA/moderate NA/very low	Strong Strong Strong Strong
3. Oral mechanical bowel preparation	Preoperative bowel preparation can be safely omitted		Moderate/high	Strong
4. Preoperative carbohydrate loading	Preoperative oral carbohydrate loading should be administered to all patients without diabetes		NA/low	Strong
5. Preoperative fasting	Clear fluid intake until 2 h and solid food until 6 h before general anesthesia		NA/moderate	Strong
6. Preanesthesia medication	Long-acting sedatives should be avoided		NA/moderate	Strong

(continued on next page)

Table 2
(continued)

ERAS Item	Summary	Specifics for Patients Undergoing Radical Cystectomy	Evidence for Cystectomy/Rectal Surgery	Recommendation Grade
7. Thrombosis prophylaxis	Patients should wear well-fitting compression stockings and receive pharmacologic prophylaxis with LMWH Leave 12-h interval between injections and epidural manipulation	Patients are considered at high risk	NA/high	Strong
	LMWH extended prophylaxis should be given for 4 wk in patients at risk	Prolonged prophylaxis should be administered	NA/high	Strong
8. Epidural analgesia	Thoracic epidural analgesia is superior to systemic opioids in relieving pain and should be continued for 72 h		NA/high	Strong
9. Minimally invasive approach	Should be attempted in a trial setting Long-term oncologic results are awaited	Laparoscopic/robotic cystectomy is recommended inside a trial setting until long-term results are available	Low/moderate	Strong
10. Resection site drainage	Perianastomotic and/or pelvic drain can be safely omitted	Because of urine leak, drainage might be required	NA/low	Weak
11. Antimicrobial prophylaxis and skin preparation	Patient should receive a single dose of antimicrobial prophylaxis 1 h before skin incision Skin preparation with chlorhexidine-alcohol prevents/decreases surgical site infection		NA/high NA/moderate	Strong Strong
12. Standard anesthetic protocol	To attenuate the surgical stress response, intraoperative maintenance of adequate hemodynamic control, central and peripheral oxygenation, muscle relaxation, depth of anesthesia, and appropriate analgesia are recommended		NA/moderate	Strong

Item	Recommendation	Evidence level/Recommendation grade	
13. Perioperative fluid management	Fluid balance should be optimized by targeting cardiac output using the esophageal Doppler system; avoid overhydration / Judicious use of vasopressors is recommended with arterial hypotension	Low/moderate	Strong
14. Preventing intraoperative hypothermia	Normal body temperature should be maintained perioperatively and postoperatively	NA/high	Strong
15. Nasogastric intubation	Postoperative nasogastric intubation should not be used routinely	Low/high	Strong
16. Urinary drainage	Transurethral catheter is removed as early as possible after pelvic surgery in patients with a low risk of urinary retention	Very low/low	Weak
	Ureteral stents and transurethral neobladder catheter should be used / The optimal duration of ureteral stenting (at least until POD 5) and transurethral catheterization is unknown		
	No transurethral catheter if ileal conduit	Very low/low	Strong
17. Prevention of postoperative ileus	Multimodal approach to optimize gut function / Gum chewing and oral magnesium required	Moderate/moderate	Strong
18. Prevention of PONV	Multimodal PONV prophylaxis in all patients with ≥2 risk factors	Very low/low (high in high-risk patients)	Strong
19. Postoperative analgesia	Multimodal postoperative analgesia, include thoracic epidural analgesia	NA/high	Strong
20. Early mobilization	Early mobilization should be encouraged / 2 h out of bed same day of surgery (POD 0) / 6 h out of bed POD 1	NA/low	Strong
21. Early oral diet	Oral nutrition started 4 h after surgery	NA/moderate	Strong
22. Audit	All patients should be audited for compliance and outcomes / Audit outcomes, cost-effectiveness, compliance, and protocol changes	NA/low	Strong

Abbreviations: LMWH, low-molecular-weight heparin; NA, not applicable (missing); NGT, nasogastric tube; POD, postoperative day; PONV, postoperative nausea and vomiting.

From Cerantola Y, Valerio M, Persson B, et al. Guidelines for perioperative care after radical cystectomy for bladder cancer: Enhanced Recovery After Surgery (ERAS(®)) society recommendations. Clin Nutr 2013;32:879–87; with permission.

according to average number of postcystectomy discharges reported per year. Low-volume centers performed fewer than 1.5 cystectomies per year and high-volume centers performed 2.75 cystectomies or greater per year.[62]

Additional studies support the conclusion that perioperative morbidity and mortality are improved with centralization of radical cystectomy in high-volume centers and with high-volume surgeons.[62–66] Kulkarni and colleagues[66] studied the impact of surgeon volume on long-term mortality rates independent of short-term postoperative mortality. From 1992 to 2004, radical cystectomy was performed by 199 surgeons in 90 hospitals across Ontario, Canada. The average annual surgeon volumes per quartile were 0.96 (range, 0.77–1.54), 2.05 (range, 1.67–2.54), 4.44 (range, 2.63–8.08), and 11.56 (range, 8.11–16.71) cases per year for quartiles 1, 2, 3, and 4, respectively.[66] They found that high-volume providers were associated with improved long-term mortality rates compared with low-volume providers. Patients treated by high-volume providers were also more likely to receive adjuvant chemotherapy. This finding suggests that the beneficial effects of higher volume may extend beyond just improved surgical technique with experience. The additional benefit may be from more use of neoadjuvant and adjuvant chemotherapy, involvement of medical oncology, postoperative surveillance for recurrence, and screening for complications of urinary diversion.

The increased use of robotics is also contributing to the centralization of radical cystectomy care. Monn and colleagues[7] found that, compared with patients undergoing ORC, those undergoing RARC were more likely to have a higher median income and be managed at a teaching hospital. Although RALP experienced a rapid uptake in nonacademic centers, the increased complexity of RARC together with increased awareness of the costs and challenges of robotic surgery, along with availability of surgical trainees to assist in care, has likely led to more cystectomies being conducted in academic centers.

Maintaining an appropriate level of expertise among the whole care team requires a certain number of cases. However, case volume is not the only factor. Past results and access to available support services (eg, intensive care unit, medical consultants, interventional radiology) must also be considered. Although perioperative mortality may be explained by several factors, including patient and disease characteristics and surgical technique, the quality of postoperative care is equally important. Trinh and colleagues[67] outline the importance of rapid recognition of adverse events and their appropriate management in minimizing the consequences of postoperative complications.

SUMMARY

The surgical management of invasive bladder cancer continues to evolve. Ongoing randomized trials will help determine whether extended lymph node dissection and robotic approaches truly improve oncologic and functional outcomes. Improvements in perioperative care and referrals to high-volume centers may be as responsible for better outcomes as intraoperative technical advances.

REFERENCES

1. Stein JP, Lieskovsky G, Cote R, et al. Radical cystectomy in the treatment of invasive bladder cancer: long-term results in 1,054 patients. J Clin Oncol 2001; 19:666–75.
2. Herr HW, Sogani PC. Does early cystectomy improve the survival of patients with high risk superficial bladder tumors? J Urol 2001;166:1296–9.

3. Novotny V, Hakenberg OW, Wiessner D, et al. Perioperative complications of radical cystectomy in a contemporary series. Eur Urol 2007;51:397–401. http://dx.doi.org/10.1016/j.eururo.2006.06.014 [discussion: 401–2].

4. Shabsigh A, Korets R, Vora KC, et al. Defining early morbidity of radical cystectomy for patients with bladder cancer using a standardized reporting methodology. Eur Urol 2009;55:164–74. http://dx.doi.org/10.1016/j.eururo.2008.07.031.

5. Siegel R, Ma J, Zou Z, et al. Cancer statistics, 2014. CA Cancer J Clin 2014;64: 9–29. http://dx.doi.org/10.3322/caac.21208.

6. Menon M, Hemal AK, Tewari A, et al. Nerve-sparing robot-assisted radical cystoprostatectomy and urinary diversion. BJU Int 2003;92:232–6.

7. Monn MF, Cary KC, Kaimakliotis HZ, et al. National trends in the utilization of robotic-assisted radical cystectomy: an analysis using the nationwide inpatient sample. Urol Oncol 2014. http://dx.doi.org/10.1016/j.urolonc.2014.04.007.

8. Liss MA, Kader AK. Robotic-assisted laparoscopic radical cystectomy: history, techniques and outcomes. World J Urol 2013;31:489–97. http://dx.doi.org/10.1007/s00345-013-1053-z.

9. Parra RO, Andrus CH, Jones JP, et al. Laparoscopic cystectomy: initial report on a new treatment for the retained bladder. J Urol 1992;148:1140–4.

10. Nix J, Smith A, Kurpad R, et al. Prospective randomized controlled trial of robotic versus open radical cystectomy for bladder cancer: perioperative and pathologic results. Eur Urol 2010;57:196–201. http://dx.doi.org/10.1016/j.eururo.2009.10.024.

11. Snow-Lisy DC, Campbell SC, Gill IS, et al. Robotic and laparoscopic radical cystectomy for bladder cancer: long-term oncologic outcomes. Eur Urol 2014;65: 193–200. http://dx.doi.org/10.1016/j.eururo.2013.08.021.

12. Bochner BH, Sjoberg DD, Laudone VP, Memorial Sloan Kettering Cancer Center Bladder Cancer Surgical Trials Group. A randomized trial of robot-assisted laparoscopic radical cystectomy. N Engl J Med 2014;371:389–90. http://dx.doi.org/10.1056/NEJMc1405213.

13. Li K, Lin T, Fan X, et al. Systematic review and meta-analysis of comparative studies reporting early outcomes after robot-assisted radical cystectomy versus open radical cystectomy. Cancer Treat Rev 2013;39:551–60. http://dx.doi.org/10.1016/j.ctrv.2012.11.007.

14. Hayn MH, Hellenthal NJ, Hussain A, et al. Does previous robot-assisted radical prostatectomy experience affect outcomes at robot-assisted radical cystectomy? Results from the International Robotic Cystectomy Consortium. Urology 2010;76: 1111–6. http://dx.doi.org/10.1016/j.urology.2010.05.010.

15. Novara G, De Marco V, Aragona M, et al. Complications and mortality after radical cystectomy for bladder transitional cell cancer. J Urol 2009;182:914–21. http://dx.doi.org/10.1016/j.juro.2009.05.032.

16. Tang K, Xia D, Li H, et al. Robotic vs. open radical cystectomy in bladder cancer: a systematic review and meta-analysis. Eur J Surg Oncol 2014. http://dx.doi.org/10.1016/j.ejso.2014.03.008.

17. Parekh DJ, Messer J, Fitzgerald J, et al. Perioperative outcomes and oncologic efficacy from a pilot prospective randomized clinical trial of open versus robotic assisted radical cystectomy. J Urol 2013;189:474–9. http://dx.doi.org/10.1016/j.juro.2012.09.077.

18. Linder BJ, Frank I, Cheville JC, et al. The impact of perioperative blood transfusion on cancer recurrence and survival following radical cystectomy. Eur Urol 2013;63:839–45. http://dx.doi.org/10.1016/j.eururo.2013.01.004.

19. Morgan TM, Barocas DA, Chang SS, et al. The relationship between perioperative blood transfusion and overall mortality in patients undergoing radical

cystectomy for bladder cancer. Urol Oncol 2013;31:871–7. http://dx.doi.org/10. 1016/j.urolonc.2011.07.012.

20. Kader AK, Richards KA, Krane LS, et al. Robot-assisted laparoscopic vs open radical cystectomy: comparison of complications and perioperative oncological outcomes in 200 patients. BJU Int 2013;112:E290–4. http://dx.doi.org/10.1111/ bju.12167.

21. Knox ML, El-Galley R, Busby JE. Robotic versus open radical cystectomy: identification of patients who benefit from the robotic approach. J Endourol 2013;27: 40–4. http://dx.doi.org/10.1089/end.2012.0168.

22. Nepple KG, Strope SA, Grubb RL 3rd, et al. Early oncologic outcomes of robotic vs. open radical cystectomy for urothelial cancer. Urol Oncol 2013;31:894–8. http://dx.doi.org/10.1016/j.urolonc.2011.06.009.

23. Ng CK, Kauffman EC, Lee MM, et al. A comparison of postoperative complications in open versus robotic cystectomy. Eur Urol 2010;57:274–81. http://dx.doi. org/10.1016/j.eururo.2009.06.001.

24. Kauffman EC, Ng CK, Lee MM, et al. Early oncological outcomes for bladder urothelial carcinoma patients treated with robotic-assisted radical cystectomy. BJU Int 2011;107:628–35. http://dx.doi.org/10.1111/j.1464-410X.2010.09577.x.

25. Pruthi RS, Nielsen ME, Nix J, et al. Robotic radical cystectomy for bladder cancer: surgical and pathological outcomes in 100 consecutive cases. J Urol 2010;183:510–4. http://dx.doi.org/10.1016/j.juro.2009.10.027.

26. Guru KA, Perlmutter AE, Butt ZM, et al. The learning curve for robot-assisted radical cystectomy. JSLS 2009;13:509–14. http://dx.doi.org/10.4293/108680809X 12589998404128.

27. Gore JL, Lai J, Setodji CM, et al, Urologic Diseases in America Project. Mortality increases when radical cystectomy is delayed more than 12 weeks: results from a surveillance, epidemiology, and end results-medicare analysis. Cancer 2009; 115:988–96. http://dx.doi.org/10.1002/cncr.24052.

28. Ahmed K, Khan SA, Hayn MH, et al. Analysis of intracorporeal compared with extracorporeal urinary diversion after robot-assisted radical cystectomy: results from the International Robotic Cystectomy Consortium. Eur Urol 2014;65:340–7. http://dx.doi.org/10.1016/j.eururo.2013.09.042.

29. Jonsson MN, Adding LC, Hosseini A, et al. Robot-assisted radical cystectomy with intracorporeal urinary diversion in patients with transitional cell carcinoma of the bladder. Eur Urol 2011;60:1066–73. http://dx.doi.org/10.1016/j.eururo. 2011.07.035.

30. Gore JL, Yu HY, Setodji C, et al. Urinary diversion and morbidity after radical cystectomy for bladder cancer. Cancer 2010;116:331–9. http://dx.doi.org/10. 1002/cncr.24763.

31. Smith ND, Castle EP, Gonzalgo ML, et al. The RAZOR trial – randomized open versus robotic cystectomy -study design and trial update. BJU Int 2014. http:// dx.doi.org/10.1111/bju.12699.

32. Herr HW, Bochner BH, Dalbagni G, et al. Impact of the number of lymph nodes retrieved on outcome in patients with muscle invasive bladder cancer. J Urol 2002;167:1295–8.

33. Leissner J, Hohenfellner R, Thuroff JW, et al. Lymphadenectomy in patients with transitional cell carcinoma of the urinary bladder; significance for staging and prognosis. BJU Int 2000;85:817–23.

34. Wishnow KI, Johnson DE, Ro JY, et al. Incidence, extent and location of unsuspected pelvic lymph node metastasis in patients undergoing radical cystectomy for bladder cancer. J Urol 1987;137:408–10.

35. Skinner DG. Management of invasive bladder cancer: a meticulous pelvic node dissection can make a difference. J Urol 1982;128:34–6.
36. Herr HW, Faulkner JR, Grossman HB, et al. Surgical factors influence bladder cancer outcomes: a cooperative group report. J Clin Oncol 2004;22:2781–9. http://dx.doi.org/10.1200/JCO.2004.11.024.
37. Richards KA, Hemal AK, Kader AK, et al. Robot assisted laparoscopic pelvic lymphadenectomy at the time of radical cystectomy rivals that of open surgery: single institution report. Urology 2010;76:1400–4. http://dx.doi.org/10.1016/j. urology.2010.01.019.
38. Marshall SJ, Hayn MH, Stegemann AP, et al. Impact of surgeon and volume on extended lymphadenectomy at the time of robot-assisted radical cystectomy: results from the International Robotic Cystectomy Consortium (IRCC). BJU Int 2013;111:1075–80. http://dx.doi.org/10.1111/j.1464-410X. 2012.11583.x.
39. Bochner BH, Herr HW, Reuter VE. Impact of separate versus en bloc pelvic lymph node dissection on the number of lymph nodes retrieved in cystectomy specimens. J Urol 2001;166:2295–6.
40. Hollenbeck BK, Ye Z, Wong SL, et al. Hospital lymph node counts and survival after radical cystectomy. Cancer 2008;112:806–12. http://dx.doi.org/10.1002/ cncr.23234.
41. Wright JL, Lin DW, Porter MP. The association between extent of lymphadenectomy and survival among patients with lymph node metastases undergoing radical cystectomy. Cancer 2008;112:2401–8. http://dx.doi.org/10.1002/cncr. 23474.
42. Konety BR, Joslyn SA. Factors influencing aggressive therapy for bladder cancer: an analysis of data from the SEER program. J Urol 2003;170:1765–71. http://dx.doi.org/10.1097/01.ju.0000091620.86778.2e.
43. Steven K, Poulsen AL. Radical cystectomy and extended pelvic lymphadenectomy: survival of patients with lymph node metastasis above the bifurcation of the common iliac vessels treated with surgery only. J Urol 2007;178:1218–23. http://dx.doi.org/10.1016/j.juro.2007.05.160 [discussion: 1223–4].
44. Varadhan KK, Neal KR, Dejong CH, et al. The enhanced recovery after surgery (ERAS) pathway for patients undergoing major elective open colorectal surgery: a meta-analysis of randomized controlled trials. Clin Nutr 2010;29:434–40. http:// dx.doi.org/10.1016/j.clnu.2010.01.004.
45. Melnyk M, Casey RG, Black P, et al. Enhanced recovery after surgery (ERAS) protocols: time to change practice? Can Urol Assoc J 2011;5:342–8. http://dx. doi.org/10.5489/cuaj.11002.
46. Arumainayagam N, McGrath J, Jefferson KP, et al. Introduction of an enhanced recovery protocol for radical cystectomy. BJU Int 2008;101:698–701. http://dx. doi.org/10.1111/j.1464-410X.2007.07319.x.
47. Tabibi A, Simforoosh N, Basiri A, et al. Bowel preparation versus no preparation before ileal urinary diversion. Urology 2007;70:654–8. http://dx.doi.org/10.1016/j. urology.2007.06.1107.
48. Xu R, Zhao X, Zhong Z, et al. No advantage is gained by preoperative bowel preparation in radical cystectomy and ileal conduit: a randomized controlled trial of 86 patients. Int Urol Nephrol 2010;42:947–50. http://dx.doi.org/10.1007/ s11255-010-9732-9.
49. Daneshmand S, Ahmadi H, Schuckman AK, et al. Enhanced recovery protocol after radical cystectomy for bladder cancer. J Urol 2014. http://dx.doi.org/10. 1016/j.juro.2014.01.097.

50. Djaladat H, Daneshmand S. Enhanced recovery pathway following radical cystectomy. Curr Opin Urol 2014;24:135–9. http://dx.doi.org/10.1097/MOU.0000000000000027.

51. Awad S, Varadhan KK, Ljungqvist O, et al. A meta-analysis of randomised controlled trials on preoperative oral carbohydrate treatment in elective surgery. Clin Nutr 2013;32:34–44. http://dx.doi.org/10.1016/j.clnu.2012.10.011.

52. Wuethrich PY, Studer UE, Thalmann GN, et al. Intraoperative continuous norepinephrine infusion combined with restrictive deferred hydration significantly reduces the need for blood transfusion in patients undergoing open radical cystectomy: results of a prospective randomised trial. Eur Urol 2013. http://dx.doi.org/10.1016/j.eururo.2013.08.046.

53. Nelson R, Edwards S, Tse B. Prophylactic nasogastric decompression after abdominal surgery. Cochrane Database Syst Rev 2007:CD004929. http://dx.doi.org/10.1002/14651858.CD004929.pub3.

54. Cerantola Y, Valerio M, Persson B, et al. Guidelines for perioperative care after radical cystectomy for bladder cancer: enhanced recovery after surgery (ERAS((R))) society recommendations. Clin Nutr 2013;32:879–87. http://dx.doi.org/10.1016/j.clnu.2013.09.014.

55. Adamakis I, Tyritzis SI, Koutalellis G, et al. Early removal of nasogastric tube is beneficial for patients undergoing radical cystectomy with urinary diversion. Int Braz J Urol 2011;37:42–8.

56. Choi H, Kang SH, Yoon DK, et al. Chewing gum has a stimulatory effect on bowel motility in patients after open or robotic radical cystectomy for bladder cancer: a prospective randomized comparative study. Urology 2011;77:884–90. http://dx.doi.org/10.1016/j.urology.2010.06.042.

57. Zaghiyan K, Felder S, Ovsepyan G, et al. A prospective randomized controlled trial of sugared chewing gum on gastrointestinal recovery after major colorectal surgery in patients managed with early enteral feeding. Dis Colon Rectum 2013;56:328–35. http://dx.doi.org/10.1097/DCR.0b013e31827e4971.

58. Vora AA, Harbin A, Rayson R, et al. Alvimopan provides rapid gastrointestinal recovery without nasogastric tube decompression after radical cystectomy and urinary diversion. Can J Urol 2012;19:6293–8.

59. Lee CT, Chang SS, Kamat AM, et al. Alvimopan accelerates gastrointestinal recovery after radical cystectomy: a multicenter randomized placebo-controlled trial. Eur Urol 2014. http://dx.doi.org/10.1016/j.eururo.2014.02.036.

60. Birkmeyer JD, Siewers AE, Finlayson EV, et al. Hospital volume and surgical mortality in the United States. N Engl J Med 2002;346:1128–37. http://dx.doi.org/10.1056/NEJMsa012337.

61. Birkmeyer JD, Stukel TA, Siewers AE, et al. Surgeon volume and operative mortality in the United States. N Engl J Med 2003;349:2117–27. http://dx.doi.org/10.1056/NEJMsa035205.

62. Konety BR, Dhawan V, Allareddy V, et al. Impact of hospital and surgeon volume on in-hospital mortality from radical cystectomy: data from the Health Care Utilization Project. J Urol 2005;173:1695–700. http://dx.doi.org/10.1097/01.ju.0000154638.61621.03.

63. Gorin MA, Kates M, Mullins JK, et al. Impact of hospital volume on perioperative outcomes and costs of radical cystectomy: analysis of the Maryland Health Services Cost Review Commission database. Can J Urol 2014;21:7102–7.

64. Leow JJ, Reese S, Trinh QD, et al. The impact of surgeon volume on the morbidity and costs of radical cystectomy in the United States: a contemporary population-based analysis. BJU Int 2014. http://dx.doi.org/10.1111/bju.12749.

65. Sun M, Ravi P, Karakiewicz PI, et al. Is there a relationship between leapfrog volume thresholds and perioperative outcomes after radical cystectomy? Urol Oncol 2014;32:27.e7–13. http://dx.doi.org/10.1016/j.urolonc.2012.09.012.
66. Kulkarni GS, Urbach DR, Austin PC, et al. Higher surgeon and hospital volume improves long-term survival after radical cystectomy. Cancer 2013;119: 3546–54. http://dx.doi.org/10.1002/cncr.28235.
67. Trinh VQ, Trinh QD, Tian Z, et al. In-hospital mortality and failure-to-rescue rates after radical cystectomy. BJU Int 2013;112:E20–7. http://dx.doi.org/10.1111/bju. 12214.

Diagnosis and Management of Upper Tract Urothelial Carcinoma

Ilaria Lucca, MD[a,b,*,1], Jeffrey J. Leow, MBBS, MPH[c,d,1],
Shahrokh F. Shariat, MD[a,e,f,2], Steven L. Chang, MD, MS[c,d,2]

KEYWORDS

- Upper tract urothelial carcinoma • Kidney neoplasms • Ureteral neoplasms
- Urothelial carcinoma • Nephroureterectomy • Chemotherapy • Radiotherapy

KEY POINTS

- Upper tract urothelial carcinoma (UTUC) is a rare subset of urothelial cancers that portends a poor prognosis that has not improved in the past 2 decades.
- Numerous preoperative and postoperative prognostic factors have been identified to better predict survival outcomes and guide therapy.
- Treatment of low-risk noninvasive UTUC consists of conservative nephron-sparing surgery (eg, endoscopic treatments, segmental resection) and adjuvant topical therapies (eg, mitomycin C).
- Treatment of localized high-risk disease is most commonly open radical nephroureterectomy, although minimally invasive surgery is increasingly used, given equivalent oncologic and reduced surgical morbidity.

Continued

Funding Sources: Development fund of the CHUV-University Hospital (I. Lucca); Nil (J.J. Leow, S.F. Shariat, and S.L. Chang).
Conflict of Interest: Nil.
[a] Department of Urology, Comprehensive Cancer Center, Medical University of Vienna, Vienna General Hospital, Währinger Gürtel 18-20, Vienna A-1090, Austria; [b] Department of Urology, Centre Hospitalier Universitaire Vaudois, Rue du Bugnon 46, Lausanne 1011, Switzerland; [c] Department of Urology, Bladder Cancer Center, Dana-Farber/Brigham and Women's Cancer Center, Harvard Medical School, 450 Brookline Ave, Boston, MA 02215, USA; [d] Division of Urology, Center for Surgery and Public Health, Brigham and Women's Hospital, Harvard Medical School, 75 Francis Street, Boston, MA 02115, USA; [e] Department of Urology, University of Texas Southwestern Medical Center, 1801 Inwood Rd, Dallas, TX 75235, USA; [f] Department of Urology, Weill Cornell Medical College, New York-Presbyterian Hospital, Cornell University, 1300 York Avenue, New York, NY 10065, USA
[1] Act as equivalent co-first authors.
[2] Act as equivalent co-senior authors.
* Corresponding author. Department of Urology, Comprehensive Cancer Center, Medical University of Vienna, Vienna General Hospital, Währinger Gürtel 18-20, Vienna A-1090, Austria.
E-mail address: luccaila@gmail.com

Hematol Oncol Clin N Am 29 (2015) 271–288
http://dx.doi.org/10.1016/j.hoc.2014.10.003
0889-8588/15/$ – see front matter © 2015 Elsevier Inc. All rights reserved.

hemonc.theclinics.com

Continued

- Multimodal therapy, including neoadjuvant/adjuvant chemotherapy and combined chemoradiotherapy, may improve survival outcomes.
- Metastatic disease is commonly managed with systemic chemotherapy, with limited roles for salvage/adjuvant radiotherapy and surgery.

INTRODUCTION
Epidemiology

Urothelial cell carcinoma (UCC) is the fourth most common cancer worldwide, after prostate (or breast), lung, and colorectal cancer.[1] Among UCC, upper tract urothelial carcinoma (UTUC) is rare and accounts for 5% to 10% of all urothelial carcinomas with an annual incidence of 2 cases per 100,000 inhabitants in Western countries.[2] UTUC is more common in men than in women with a male-to-female ratio of 2:1 and the mean age at the diagnosis of 65 years old.[3] It is located twice more often in the renal pelvis than in the ureter and in about 20% of the cases a concomitant urothelial carcinoma of the bladder (UCB) is present.[4] UTUC tends to recur in the bladder or progress through the lymphatic and vascular systems to distant organs. To date, much of the decision-making in UTUC comes from knowledge acquired in UCB because of its relative rarity. Over the last 5 years, a large body of evidence has proven that UTUC and UCB have common features but differ as well in a significant degree.[5]

Risk Factors

Tobacco and occupational exposure are the main UTUC exogenous risk factors in most countries. The relative risk of developing UTUC in the case of tobacco exposure has been estimated to be 2.5 to 7, depending on the number of years of exposure and the number of cigarettes smoked per day.[6] Occupational exposure to certain aromatic amines has an estimated risk of 8.3.[7] However, exposure risk decreased since the 1960s because certain chemical substances, such as benzidine and β-naphthalene, have been banned from industrial production. The most exciting discovery in the last 10 years in UTUC has been the unraveling of aristolochic acid as an iatrogenic global risk factor for UTUC development.[8]

Balkan endemic nephropathy and Chinese herbs nephropathy, which are the same disease, are specifically related to UTUC.[9–11] They are characterized by a mutation of the p53 gene as a consequence of the exposure to aristolochic acid, a potent carcinogen derived from Aristolochia plants, which is used as an herbal ingredient or remedy.[12] A significant use of this plant has also been registered in Taiwan, where the incidence of UTUC is estimated to be approximately 20% to 25% of all urothelial cancers, the highest worldwide.[13] Unfortunately, clinical trials targeting these selected populations are lacking and further efforts are required to lower the exposure to this deadly substance, which is integral in many traditional Chinese and Indian pharmacopoeia.[14]

Rare cases of UTUC linked to hereditary nonpolyposis colorectal carcinoma (HNPCC, Lynch syndrome) have also been reported. UTUC patients younger than 60 years, with a personal history of an HNPCC-associated cancer, a first-degree relative younger than 50 years of age with HNPCC-associated cancer, or 2 first-degree relatives with HNPCC-associated cancer should be screened for hereditary cancers.[15,16]

Symptoms and Screening

UTUC are mainly silent in the first stages, diminishing the chance of an early diagnosis. Principal symptoms of UTUC are macrohematuria or microhematuria, followed by flank pain and lumbar mass. Systemic symptoms, such as fatigue, loss of weight, and fever, may suggest the presence of a metastatic disease when associated with UTUC.

Diagnosis

The diagnosis and evaluation of a patient with a suspected UTUC requires an accurate investigation, combining imaging and endoscopy, to better stage the patient and to carefully select for individualized therapy.[17]

Computed tomography (CT) urography is nowadays the first-line imaging examination used, because of a higher ability to identify small lesions with good anatomic characterization, compared with intravenous excretory urography and ultrasonography. The sensitivity and specificity of CT urography to detect UTUC are continuously improving and are estimated to be in the range of 67% to 100% and 93% to 99%, respectively.[18] Radiation exposure, allergic reactions, or nephropathy after contrast medium employment need to be considered before performing this examination. Magnetic resonance urography remains a valid alternative for some patients presenting with a contraindication to iodinated contrast material, with an estimated 74% rate of detection for lesions less than 2 cm.[19,20] Retrograde ureterorenopyelography through a ureteral catheter or during ureteroscopy (URS) remains an option to be considered to investigate UTUC, but it does not allow the prediction of tumor grade or stage.[21]

Positive urinary cytology may be the first sign of UTUC in the case of normal cystoscopy and after excluding carcinoma in situ (CIS) of the bladder and prostatic urethra.[18] Because cytology of UTUC is less sensitive compared with that of UCB cytology, it is recommended to perform it in situ before the contrast injection in case of retrograde ureteropyelography.[22]

Flexible URS associated with biopsy is an important diagnostic tool to evaluate patients with suspected UTUC. A reduction of misdiagnoses from 15.5% to 2.1% has been estimated when routine URS was performed ($P = .021$).[23] In addition to diagnosis, URS allows visual and pathologic evaluation of the tumor, thereby helping in clinical decision-making regarding treatment. It should be especially applied preoperatively in uncertain cases when radical surgery could be avoided or in the case of solitary kidney. Basket device biopsies seem to have a higher rate of successful diagnosis with a more precise definition of grade compared with other biopsy devices.[24] Complications associated with URS, such as urinary infection or iatrogenic lesion of the urinary upper tract, however, need to be taken into consideration.[25,26] Finally, despite the delay between diagnosis and radical surgery, diagnostic URS does not seem to significantly affect oncologic outcomes.[27] URS allows not only diagnosis, collection of information that imposes staging, and prognostication but also therapy in those patients benefitting from conservative therapy.[27]

PROGNOSTIC AND PREDICTIVE FACTORS

UTUC tends to have worse prognosis compared with UCB and the survival varies according to patient and tumor characteristics.[28] Five-year recurrence-free survival (RFS) and cancer-specific survival (CSS) are estimated to be 73% and 78%, respectively.[29] Identification of prognostic factors allows defining high-risk groups of patients, who should be treated with specific therapies. Therefore, nomograms and performance indices have been proposed as predictors of outcomes in patients with UTUC.[30–32]

Patient Characteristics

Female patients tend to have more advanced pathologic T stage and higher-grade tumor than male patients.[33] However, gender alone is no longer considered to be an independent prognostic factor of CSS. Also, ethnicity does not directly influence UTUC survival, even though some data show different tumor characteristics between Caucasians and Asians.[34] Older patients diagnosed with UTUC tend to have worse survival but many of them are still cured with radical surgical treatment, suggesting that age alone is not sufficient to influence clinical decision.[35]

Tumor Characteristics

Tumor stage and grade are the most powerful prognostic factors influencing UTUC outcome. The 5-year cancer-related survival in UTUC patients is higher than 90% for pTa/pT1/CIS tumors, less than 50% for pT2/pT3 tumors, and less than 10% for pT4 tumors.[18] The impact of positive lymph nodes, number of positive nodes, and extranodal extension are also well-established prognostic factors.[36,37] It has been estimated that the incidence of positive lymph nodes is approximately 0%, 5%, 24%, and 84% in patients with pTa/pT1/CIS, pT2, pT3, and pT4 UTUC, respectively.[38]

Tumor multifocality should be considered an independent prognostic factor of RFS and CSS in patients with organ-confined UTUC treated with radical nephroureterectomy (RNU).[39] In the case of a single lesion, ureteral location tends to have a worse oncologic outcome compared with renal pelvis or calice location.[40] As already shown in other types of cancers, lymphovascular invasion (LVI) is a strong independent prognostic factor for CSS and metastasis-free survival in UTUC patients, in particular when a lymph node dissection (LND) is not performed or in those without lymph node metastasis.[41] It has been estimated that LVI is present in approximately 20% of RNU samples, and its inclusion in the pathologic report is strongly recommended.[42] Finally, extensive tumor necrosis, tumor size 3 cm or greater, sessile tumor architecture, and hydronephrosis also negatively influence UTUC prognosis.[43–47]

Genetic and Biological Markers

Genetic and epigenetic biomarkers, based on tissue, urine, and blood, have achieved good sensitivities and specificities for UTUC diagnosis in pilot studies, but none has so far been validated. Their efficacy on large patient cohorts or for follow-up of UTUC patients to detect early recurrences still needs to be proven.

Interestingly, some studies have determined some specific genetic and epigenetic differences between UTUC and UCB.[48] The micro-RNA expression pattern seems to play a role in progressing and nonprogressing UTUC and a combination of new micro-RNAs may help to distinguish UTUC with a high probability of recurrence, improving patients' follow-up and CSS.[49] Among the oncofetal proteins, insulinlike growth factor messenger RNA binding proteins 3 and 5 have shown interesting results as independent factors associated with RFS, CCS, and all-cause mortality.[50,51] Few data are available on DNA methylation and UTUC detection and prognosis. GDF15, TMEFF2, VIM promoter methylation, GATA binding protein 3, KI-67, Bcl-xL, calreticulin, and annexin A2 and A3 are other valuable and promising diagnostic and prognostic biomarkers, but robust clinical data are still lacking.[52–55]

Increasing evidence suggests that host inflammatory response and procoagulant and fibrinolytic factors are stage-independent and grade-independent predictors of survival in patients with various solid tumors, including UTUC. Elevated preoperative neutrophil-lymphocyte ratio and erythrocyte sedimentation rate were independent risk factors of disease recurrence and cancer-specific mortality in UTUC patients treated with RNU.[56,57] Hemoglobin seems to be a promising marker as predictor of RFS and CSS in UTUC patients, being associated with aggressive tumor features, especially if a perioperative blood transfusion is required.[58,59] Finally, C-reactive protein, sodium, and albumin also may play a role for prognostication of UTUC patients treated with RNU.[60]

Taken together, these findings advocate testing of biomarkers in correlative clinical trials to validate their utility in UTUC management.

TREATMENT OF LOW-RISK CANCER (HIGH-GRADE TA, T1, AND CARCINOMA IN SITU)
Conservative Surgery

Although no randomized trials comparing UTUC conservative treatment with RNU are available nowadays, the nephron-sparing approach may be a valid alternative, especially in the case of renal insufficiency, solitary functional kidney, bilateral disease, or low-risk tumors.[18] Given the frequent bladder and ipsilateral upper tract recurrences, strict follow-up is required and, therefore, patient selection is crucial.[61] Despite a better protection of kidney function, endoscopic treatment of UTUC has a rate of local and bladder recurrence of approximately 25% and 15%, respectively.[62] Moreover, a change in grade and/or stage from the diagnostic biopsy to the endoscopic resection may occur in more than one-third of UTUC patients managed conservatively, with a considerable risk of undergrading and understaging.[63] The percutaneous approach in UTUC management could be considered for low-grade tumors in the lower caliceal system, even though only small case series have been reported and technical improvements in new flexible ureteroscopes are replacing this procedure.[64]

UTUC segmental resection has the main advantage of preserving renal function and conserving a good oncologic control, but should be reserved only for selected cases.[65] Complete distal ureterectomy and neocystostomy are a valid and oncologically safe alternative for large-volume noninvasive low-grade UTUC located in the distal ureter, which are not possible to manage endoscopically.[66] Ureteroureterostomy is a nonstandard option for proximal ureter or mid-ureter UTUC not completely resectable by the endoscopic approach in patients in whom kidney function preservation is imperative.[18] Segmental resection of the iliac and lumbar ureter and open resection of the renal pelvis tumor are hardly performed anymore because of the high risk of tumor spillages, complications, and recurrences, and the improved endoscopic tools.

Adjuvant Topical Agents

Despite a large experience on intravesical therapies in noninvasive UCB, only a few reports on the efficacy of instillation with chemotherapy or immunotherapy for UTUC treated with conservative intent have been published so far.[67] Instillation of topical agents is technically feasible anterogradely by means of a percutaneous nephrostomy or retrogradely through a single J or double JJ ureteric stent. To avoid complications, intracavitary pressure should be maintained low and absence of perforation or obstruction of the system needs to be proven. Although administration of bacillus Calmette-Guérin (BCG) or mitomycin C seems to be safe, its efficacy is still debated.

Patients with CIS UTUC treated with a curative intent by antegrade perfusions of BCG tend to have a better RFS, progression-free survival, and RNU-free survival compared with those treated with adjuvant intention after endoscopic resection of pTa/T1 tumors.[68] It is now becoming widely accepted that BCG is mainly indicated in CIS patients. Finally, it is difficult to obtain significant evidence on mitomycin C given that there are only a few studies available describing its use.[69,70] Another type of adjuvant therapy is single-dose intravesical mitomycin C after RNU,[71] and now, without evidence-based proof yet, after conservative endoscopic management of UTUC.

Follow-up of Bladder After Conservative Therapies

UTUC patients treated with conservative therapies need vigilant surveillance of the bladder and the ipsilateral upper tract. Currently, a combination of CT urography, ureteroscopy, cystoscopy, urinary cytology, and cytology in situ seems to be the most effective method. No consensus exists regarding the exact follow-up schedule, but at least routinely controls during the first 5 years are advisable.[18]

TREATMENT OF LOCALIZED HIGH-RISK (INVASIVE) CANCER
Radical Nephroureterectomy

The gold-standard treatment of localized high-risk UTUC is an RNU, which consists of en block removal of the kidney, renal pelvis, extramural and intramural ureter, ureteral orifice, and a cuff of bladder around the ureteral orifice. In patients with a neobladder or urinary diversion (eg, from bladder cancer progression), resection of the ureteral anastomosis and cuff of bowel should be performed instead. From an oncologic standpoint, it is imperative to (1) avoid entry into the urinary tract to prevent tumor spillage or seeding[72] and (2) completely excise the ureter distal to the tumor and bladder cuff because of a high risk of recurrence[73,74] arising in the remnant ureteral tissue translating into worse overall survival.[75,76]

Various surgical techniques for managing the distal ureter exist. The conventional approaches of bladder cuff removal via open surgery through the transvesical or extravesical approach appear similar in terms of oncologic outcomes.[77] The "pluck" technique was introduced by McDonald and colleagues[78] in 1952 but was not popularized until 1995 when this endoscopic approach to the distal ureter was found to have equivalent oncologic outcomes and reduced operative time.[79] These 3 competing methods of bladder cuff excision (transvesical, extravesical, and endoscopic) were recently evaluated by the UTUC Collaboration in a large study of 2681 patients, and no differences in terms of RFS, CSS, and overall survival were found.[77] However, patients who underwent the endoscopic approach were at significantly higher risk of intravesical recurrence compared with those who underwent the transvesical ($P = .02$) or extravesical approaches ($P = .02$), with no differences between the latter 2 groups. Regardless of technique chosen to manage the distal cuff, the underlying principle and consensus remains to avoid tumor spillage in the peritoneal cavity.[72,74–76]

Overall, oncologic outcomes after RNU remain relatively poor. The UTUC Collaboration reported results from 1363 patients treated with RNU at 12 academic centers and found that 5-year RFS and CSS probabilities were 69% and 73%, respectively. Furthermore, a study from MD Anderson Cancer Center showed that across the study period from 1986 to 2004, disease-specific survival rates were unchanged,[80] highlighting that current treatment paradigms may need to be augmented with multimodal therapy to improve outcomes.

Lymphadenectomy

Regional lymphadenectomy or LND allows for optimal staging of disease. Numerous retrospective studies have found a survival benefit in patients with greater or equal to a pT2 disease.[81,82] Because preoperative clinical staging is challenging, frequently inaccurate, some advocate performing LND for all patients undergoing RNU.[83–85] The template for LND depends on tumor location.[86] Based on a comprehensive mapping study, Kondo and colleagues[38] have proposed the following: for right-sided renal pelvic and midureter and upper-ureteral tumors, LND should include the hilar nodes, the paracaval, inter-aortocaval, and retrocaval lymph nodes, from the level of the renal hilus to the aortic bifurcation. For left-sided renal pelvic tumors and mid ureters and upper ureters, dissection should include para-aortic and hilar nodes from the renal hilus to the aortic bifurcation. The ipsilateral pelvic lymph nodes along the common, external, internal iliac, and obturator vessels should also be retrieved. A large multicenter retrospective study of 552 patients found that in the subgroup of patients with pN0 disease (n = 412), removal of at least 8 lymph nodes was a strong independent predictor of cancer-specific mortality (hazard ratio [HR]: 0.42, $P = .004$).[84] The benefits of LND lie in improved staging and local control as well as reduced risk of locoregional nodal relapse.[87] Therefore, although randomized trials are not available to clarify its role on overall survival, it is recommended when technically feasible.

Type of Surgical Approach

Most RNUs are performed via an open approach. A population-based study using the Nationwide Inpatient Sample between 1998 and 2009 found that 90.8% of patients with nonmetastatic UTUC underwent open RNU, whereas the rest underwent a minimally invasive approach.[88] As the urologic community gains experience with minimally invasive abdominal and pelvic surgery, the utilization of laparoscopic and robotic RNU is expected to increase correspondingly. Although peritoneal dissemination and port-site metastases are possible and have been reported,[89,90] these represent rare occurrences and have not deterred the adoption of the minimally invasive approach for RNU.[91]

The available data suggest comparable oncologic outcomes following either open or minimally invasive RNU. The only prospective randomized study examining this by Simone and colleagues[92] included 80 patients who underwent either open or laparoscopic RNU. The authors failed to identify a significant difference in 5-year CSS (open: 89.9% vs laparoscopic: 79.8%, $P = .2$).[92] A recent systematic review and meta-analysis of 21 nonrandomized studies with 1235 cases and 3093 controls examining oncologic outcomes of open versus laparoscopic RNU concluded that short-term to mid-term oncologic outcomes appear similar between open and laparoscopic RNU.[93–95] At this time, long-term results are sparse, especially for high-risk disease (eg, pT2, N+),[96] with oncologic equivalence between open and laparoscopic RNU reported in the longest median follow-up of 13.7 years.[97]

Laparoscopic RNU is associated with improved perioperative outcomes. The aforementioned randomized trial found shorter hospital length of stay and decreased blood loss among those receiving laparoscopic compared with open RNU.[92] A recent population-based study similarly reported that laparoscopic RNU was associated with fewer adverse intraoperative and postoperative outcomes compared with open RNU.[88] Robot-assisted laparoscopic RNU remains in its infancy, with only 10 studies reporting their initial experience, demonstrating feasibility and safety but lacking data at this time to confirm equivalent perioperative and long-term oncologic outcomes.[98]

Neoadjuvant and Adjuvant Chemotherapy

Compared with UCB,[99,100] there has been less robust evidence in terms of randomized clinical trials to clarify the role of perioperative chemotherapy in UTUC. Neoadjuvant chemotherapy is a promising and emerging approach for UTUC patients, particularly those with good renal function and histologic evidence of high-grade muscle-invasive disease. Pooled results from 2 retrospective studies found a 59% benefit in disease-specific survival (HR 0.41, P = .005).[101] Two prospective single-center phase 2 trials accrued patients with locally advanced urothelial cancers, including UTUC, and reported substantial pathologic downstaging (to inferior or equal to pT1N0) in up to 75% of patients.[102,103] Two ongoing trials evaluating the efficacy of neoadjuvant gemcitabine and cisplatin (NCT01663285, NCT01261728) are highly anticipated because positive results may shift the paradigm in the management of this disease.

There is a growing body of evidence supporting the use of adjuvant chemotherapy.[104–112] Adjuvant chemotherapy has strengths apparent to most: (1) accurate pathologic staging is available postoperatively; (2) any subclinical metastases can be eradicated to maximize the patient's overall and disease-specific survival. However, the downside is that a considerable proportion of patients will develop postoperative renal insufficiency potentially preventing the use of systemic therapies. Although cisplatin-based chemotherapy seems to be the most efficacious regimen to be administered from available evidence, it is also rather nephrotoxic, thereby limiting its utility. The latest meta-analysis investigating the role of adjuvant chemotherapy found that a pooled overall survival benefit (HR = 0.43, 95% CI: 0.21–0.89, P = .023), across 3 cisplatin-based studies, represents a 57% benefit in OS among those treated with adjuvant chemotherapy compared with those who received surgery alone.[101]

Radiotherapy

The aim of radiotherapy is to optimize local control of disease. This treatment targets the renal fossa, course of the ureter to the entire bladder, and the paracaval and para-aortic lymph nodes at risk of harboring micrometastatic or metastatic disease. Radiotherapy may be beneficial in delaying bladder tumor relapse and improving overall survival in both adjuvant[113,114] and salvage[115] settings. There may be prolonged overall and disease-free survival when administered concurrently with cisplatin-based chemotherapy[116] and a prescribed dose of 50 Gy or greater.[115] However, the systemic nature of UTUC is highlighted by the fact that 2 studies examining adjuvant radiotherapy have not found an OS benefit.[117,118]

TREATMENT OF METASTATIC CANCER

There is no clear survival benefit of an RNU in patients with metastatic (M1) disease. Instead, metastatic UTUC is typically managed with systemic chemotherapy. Currently, the same chemotherapeutic agents are used for bladder urothelial cancer; however, emerging evidence suggests these 2 diseases are different at the molecular level,[119–122] suggesting that future drug developments may be tailored specifically for UTUC.[5]

Chemotherapy

Extrapolating from the data for UCB,[123] platinum-based chemotherapy is the preferred treatment regimen for patients with metastatic UTUC.[124] MVAC (methotrexate, vinblastine, adriamycin, and cisplatin) yields modest survival advantage, although response rates are favorable with 72% overall response and 36% complete response rates[125]; however, optimal dosing is limited owing to associated toxicities, primarily mucocytis, and neutropenia.[126] As a result, gemcitabine with cisplatin is now preferred and considered first-line therapy, given better tolerability, similar response rates, time to progression, and survival rates in a disease that already portends poor prognosis in the metastatic setting.[127,128]

Options for patients who are poor candidates for first-line chemotherapy

A large proportion of patients with UTUC may be considered "unfit" for cisplatin-based regimens based on age (>75 years), decreased renal function (creatinine clearance <60 mL/min), or reduced performance status (Eastern Cooperative Oncology Group performance status ≥2).[126] For these patients, chemotherapy options are limited.

Carboplatin-based regimens may be offered and better tolerated[129]; however, the survival benefit is questionable. In a randomized trial comparing a carboplatin-based regimen (methotrexate, carboplatin, vinblastine) with a cisplatin-based regimen (MVAC) for the treatment of advanced urothelial carcinoma, investigators found a statistically significant difference in median disease-related survival time favoring MVAC (16 months; range, 6 to 22+) versus the carboplatin-based regimen (9 months; range, 6 to 14+) ($P = .03$),[130] underscoring the efficacy of cisplatin in the treatment of urothelial carcinomas.

Another strategy increasingly used by oncologists to overcome the toxicity of typical cisplatin-based regimens is to increase the dose of chemotherapy with hematologic growth factor supporting the use of granulocyte colony stimulating factor (ie, high-dose intensity or dose-dense chemotherapy). This regimen has been met with good success with a randomized phase 3 trial demonstrating progression-free survival benefit in advanced urothelial carcinoma.[131] Dose-dense therapy is being increasingly investigated by centers of excellence particularly for bladder urothelial cancer and may be a promising alternative to gemcitabine-cisplatin for UTUC. In fact, it is already being investigated in the neoadjuvant setting, for bladder[132,133] and high-grade UTUCs.[134] Another corollary is the administration of gemcitabine with cisplatin every 2 weeks in a split-dose fashion; this strategy yielded partial response in 39% of patients with median progression-free and overall survival of 3.5 and 8.5 months, respectively.[127]

Radiotherapy

Compared with adjuvant radiotherapy, salvage radiotherapy has dismal overall survival and progression-free survival rates.[115] Therefore, the role of radiotherapy among patients with metastatic UTUC is limited to palliation. Although palliative radiotherapy is an established treatment in the management of symptoms caused by many forms of cancer,[135] there are limited data exploring this option for patients with advanced UTUC. Drawing from the experience of palliative radiotherapy in patients with advanced bladder urothelial carcinoma,[136,137] radiotherapy can address intractable hemorrhage and pain associated with metastatic UTUC. Novel approaches, potentially involving chemotherapy, may be helpful in expanding the applicability of radiotherapy in managing patients with metastatic UTUC.

Surgery

Information on the role of surgery among patients with metastatic UTUC is lacking. In this setting, a nephrectomy may palliate symptoms including pain and bleeding from the involved kidney akin to palliative radiotherapy. Inferring from data for bladder cancer, there may also be a survival benefit for select patients who undergo salvage surgery to resect limited metastatic disease[138,139] or consolidation surgery in those who respond well to chemotherapy.[140,141] Additional studies are needed to better delineate the utility of surgery for patients with metastatic UTUC.

SUMMARY

Although UTUC is a relatively uncommon disease, it typically has an aggressive natural history. The overall prognosis for UTUC is relatively poor and has not substantially improved over the past 2 decades. However, continued research has led to the discovery of risk factors, such as the environmental carcinogen, aristolochic acid, improving the understanding of this disease and potentially improving the prevention and early detection of UTUC. Although RNU remains the gold-standard treatment of localized invasive UTUC, the use of nephron-sparing options for select patients as well as minimally invasive RNU has decreased morbidity and will likely play an increasingly important role in the care of patients with UTUC. There has been little improvement in the prognosis of this disease over the past 2 decades, highlighting the necessity for better multimodality therapeutic options incorporating the latest advances in chemotherapy and radiotherapy to achieve improved outcomes for our patients with UTUC.

REFERENCES

1. Siegel R, Ma J, Zou Z, et al. Cancer statistics, 2014. CA Cancer J Clin 2014; 64(1):9–29.
2. Raman JD, Messer J, Sielatycki JA, et al. Incidence and survival of patients with carcinoma of the ureter and renal pelvis in the USA, 1973-2005. BJU Int 2011; 107(7):1059–64.
3. Munoz JJ, Ellison LM. Upper tract urothelial neoplasms: incidence and survival during the last 2 decades. J Urol 2000;164(5):1523–5.
4. Cosentino M, Palou J, Gaya JM, et al. Upper urinary tract urothelial cell carcinoma: location as a predictive factor for concomitant bladder carcinoma. World J Urol 2013;31(1):141–5.
5. Green DA, Rink M, Xylinas E, et al. Urothelial carcinoma of the bladder and the upper tract: disparate twins. J Urol 2013;189(4):1214–21.
6. Colin P, Koenig P, Ouzzane A, et al. Environmental factors involved in carcinogenesis of urothelial cell carcinomas of the upper urinary tract. BJU Int 2009; 104(10):1436–40.
7. Shinka T, Miyai M, Sawada Y, et al. Factors affecting the occurrence of urothelial tumors in dye workers exposed to aromatic amines. Int J Urol 1995;2(4):243–8.
8. Grollman AP. Aristolochic acid nephropathy: Harbinger of a global iatrogenic disease. Environ Mol Mutagen 2013;54(1):1–7.
9. Patel N, Arya M, Muneer A, et al. Molecular aspects of upper tract urothelial carcinoma. Urol Oncol 2014;32(1):28.e11–20.
10. Fang D, Zhang L, Li X, et al. Risk factors and treatment outcomes of new contralateral upper urinary urothelial carcinoma after nephroureterectomy: the experiences of a large Chinese center. J Cancer Res Clin Oncol 2014; 140(3):477–85.
11. Gokmen MR, Cosyns JP, Arlt VM, et al. The epidemiology, diagnosis, and management of aristolochic acid nephropathy: a narrative review. Ann Intern Med 2013;158(6):469–77.
12. Hollstein M, Moriya M, Grollman AP, et al. Analysis of TP53 mutation spectra reveals the fingerprint of the potent environmental carcinogen, aristolochic acid. Mutat Res 2013;753(1):41–9.
13. Chen CH, Dickman KG, Moriya M, et al. Aristolochic acid-associated urothelial cancer in Taiwan. Proc Natl Acad Sci U S A 2012;109(21):8241–6.
14. Matin SF, Shariat SF, Milowsky MI, et al. Highlights from the first symposium on upper tract urothelial carcinoma. Urol Oncol 2014;32(3):309–16.
15. Roupret M, Yates DR, Comperat E, et al. Upper urinary tract urothelial cell carcinomas and other urological malignancies involved in the hereditary

nonpolyposis colorectal cancer (lynch syndrome) tumor spectrum. Eur Urol 2008;54(6):1226–36.

16. Audenet F, Colin P, Yates DR, et al. A proportion of hereditary upper urinary tract urothelial carcinomas are misclassified as sporadic according to a multi-institutional database analysis: proposal of patient-specific risk identification tool. BJU Int 2012;110(11 Pt B):E583–9.

17. Kaag M, Trost L, Thompson RH, et al. Preoperative predictors of renal function decline following radical nephroureterectomy for upper tract urothelial carcinoma. BJU Int 2014;114(5):674–9.

18. Roupret M, Babjuk M, Comperat E, et al. European guidelines on upper tract urothelial carcinomas: 2013 update. Eur Urol 2013;63(6):1059–71.

19. Takahashi N, Kawashima A, Glockner JF, et al. Small (<2-cm) upper-tract urothelial carcinoma: evaluation with gadolinium-enhanced three-dimensional spoiled gradient-recalled echo MR urography. Radiology 2008;247(2):451–7.

20. Takahashi N, Kawashima A, Glockner JF, et al. MR urography for suspected upper tract urothelial carcinoma. Eur Radiol 2009;19(4):912–23.

21. Williams SK, Denton KJ, Minervini A, et al. Correlation of upper-tract cytology, retrograde pyelography, ureteroscopic appearance, and ureteroscopic biopsy with histologic examination of upper-tract transitional cell carcinoma. J Endourol 2008;22(1):71–6.

22. Messer J, Shariat SF, Brien JC, et al. Urinary cytology has a poor performance for predicting invasive or high-grade upper-tract urothelial carcinoma. BJU Int 2011;108(5):701–5.

23. Tsivian A, Tsivian M, Stanevsky Y, et al. Routine diagnostic ureteroscopy for suspected upper tract transitional-cell carcinoma. J Endourol 2014;28(8): 922–5.

24. Kleinmann N, Healy KA, Hubosky SG, et al. Ureteroscopic biopsy of upper tract urothelial carcinoma: comparison of basket and forceps. J Endourol 2013; 27(12):1450–4.

25. Taie K, Jasemi M, Khazaeli D, et al. Prevalence and management of complications of ureteroscopy: a seven-year experience with introduction of a new maneuver to prevent ureteral avulsion. Urol J 2012;9(1):356–60.

26. Grabe M. Controversies in antibiotic prophylaxis in urology. Int J Antimicrob Agents 2004;23(Suppl 1):S17–23.

27. Nison L, Roupret M, Bozzini G, et al. The oncologic impact of a delay between diagnosis and radical nephroureterectomy due to diagnostic ureteroscopy in upper urinary tract urothelial carcinomas: results from a large collaborative database. World J Urol 2013;31(1):69–76.

28. Gandaglia G, Bianchi M, Trinh QD, et al. Survival after nephroureterectomy for upper tract urothelial carcinoma: a population-based competing-risks analysis. Int J Urol 2014;21(3):249–56.

29. Ehdaie B, Shariat SF, Savage C, et al. Postoperative nomogram for disease recurrence and cancer-specific death for upper tract urothelial carcinoma: comparison to American Joint Committee on Cancer staging classification. Urol J 2014;11(2):1435–41.

30. Seisen T, Colin P, Hupertan V, et al. Postoperative nomogram to predict cancer-specific survival after radical nephroureterectomy in patients with localised and/or locally advanced upper tract urothelial carcinoma without metastasis. BJU Int 2014;114(5):733–40.

31. Roupret M, Hupertan V, Seisen T, et al. Prediction of cancer specific survival after radical nephroureterectomy for upper tract urothelial carcinoma: development of

an optimized postoperative nomogram using decision curve analysis. J Urol 2013; 189(5):1662–9.

32. Aziz A, Fritsche HM, Gakis G, et al. Comparative analysis of comorbidity and performance indices for prediction of oncological outcomes in patients with upper tract urothelial carcinoma who were treated with radical nephroureterectomy. Urol Oncol 2014. [Epub ahead of print].

33. Lughezzani G, Briganti A, Karakiewicz PI, et al. Predictive and prognostic models in radical prostatectomy candidates: a critical analysis of the literature. Eur Urol 2010;58(5):687–700.

34. Matsumoto K, Novara G, Gupta A, et al. Racial differences in the outcome of patients with urothelial carcinoma of the upper urinary tract: an international study. BJU Int 2011;108(8 Pt 2):E304–9.

35. Shariat SF, Godoy G, Lotan Y, et al. Advanced patient age is associated with inferior cancer-specific survival after radical nephroureterectomy. BJU Int 2010;105(12):1672–7.

36. Xylinas E, Rink M, Margulis V, et al. Prediction of true nodal status in patients with pathological lymph node negative upper tract urothelial carcinoma at radical nephroureterectomy. J Urol 2013;189(2):468–73.

37. Roscigno M, Brausi M, Heidenreich A, et al. Lymphadenectomy at the time of nephroureterectomy for upper tract urothelial cancer. Eur Urol 2011;60(4):776–83.

38. Kondo T, Nakazawa H, Ito F, et al. Primary site and incidence of lymph node metastases in urothelial carcinoma of upper urinary tract. Urology 2007;69(2): 265–9.

39. Chromecki TF, Cha EK, Fajkovic H, et al. The impact of tumor multifocality on outcomes in patients treated with radical nephroureterectomy. Eur Urol 2012; 61(2):245–53.

40. Hurel S, Roupret M, Seisen T, et al. Influence of preoperative factors on the oncologic outcome for upper urinary tract urothelial carcinoma after radical nephroureterectomy. World J Urol 2014. [Epub ahead of print].

41. Ku JH, Byun SS, Jeong H, et al. Lymphovascular invasion as a prognostic factor in the upper urinary tract urothelial carcinoma: a systematic review and meta-analysis. Eur J Cancer 2013;49(12):2665–80.

42. Novara G, Matsumoto K, Kassouf W, et al. Prognostic role of lymphovascular invasion in patients with urothelial carcinoma of the upper urinary tract: an international validation study. Eur Urol 2010;57(6):1064–71.

43. Ishioka J, Saito K, Kijima T, et al. Risk stratification for bladder recurrence of upper urinary tract urothelial carcinoma after radical nephroureterectomy. BJU Int 2014. [Epub ahead of print].

44. Espiritu PN, Sverrisson EF, Sexton WJ, et al. Effect of tumor size on recurrence-free survival of upper tract urothelial carcinoma following surgical resection. Urol Oncol 2014;32(5):619–24.

45. Cha EK, Shariat SF, Kormaksson M, et al. Predicting clinical outcomes after radical nephroureterectomy for upper tract urothelial carcinoma. Eur Urol 2012;61(4):818–25.

46. Zigeuner R, Shariat SF, Margulis V, et al. Tumour necrosis is an indicator of aggressive biology in patients with urothelial carcinoma of the upper urinary tract. Eur Urol 2010;57(4):575–81.

47. Bozzini G, Nison L, Colin P, et al. Influence of preoperative hydronephrosis on the outcome of urothelial carcinoma of the upper urinary tract after nephroureterectomy: the results from a multi-institutional French cohort. World J Urol 2013;31(1):83–91.

48. Yates DR, Catto JW. Distinct patterns and behaviour of urothelial carcinoma with respect to anatomical location: how molecular biomarkers can augment clinico-pathological predictors in upper urinary tract tumours. World J Urol 2013;31(1):21–9.

49. Izquierdo L, Ingelmo-Torres M, Mallofre C, et al. Prognostic value of microRNA expression pattern in upper tract urothelial carcinoma. BJU Int 2014;113(5): 813–21.

50. Lee DJ, Xylinas E, Rieken M, et al. Insulin-like growth factor messenger RNA-binding protein 3 expression helps prognostication in patients with upper tract urothelial carcinoma. Eur Urol 2014;66(2):379–85.

51. Liang PI, Wang YH, Wu TF, et al. IGFBP-5 overexpression as a poor prognostic factor in patients with urothelial carcinomas of upper urinary tracts and urinary bladder. J Clin Pathol 2013;66(7):573–82.

52. Yoshimine S, Kikuchi E, Kosaka T, et al. Prognostic significance of Bcl-xL expression and efficacy of Bcl-xL targeting therapy in urothelial carcinoma. Br J Cancer 2013;108(11):2312–20.

53. Lu CM, Lin JJ, Huang HH, et al. A panel of tumor markers, calreticulin, annexin A2, and annexin A3 in upper tract urothelial carcinoma identified by proteomic and immunological analysis. BMC Cancer 2014;14:363.

54. Gonzalez-Roibon N, Albadine R, Sharma R, et al. The role of GATA binding protein 3 in the differential diagnosis of collecting duct and upper tract urothelial carcinomas. Hum Pathol 2013;44(12):2651–7.

55. Monteiro-Reis S, Leca L, Almeida M, et al. Accurate detection of upper tract urothelial carcinoma in tissue and urine by means of quantitative GDF15, TMEFF2 and VIM promoter methylation. Eur J Cancer 2014;50(1):226–33.

56. Tanaka N, Kikuchi E, Kanao K, et al. A multi-institutional validation of the prognostic value of the neutrophil-to-lymphocyte ratio for upper tract urothelial carcinoma treated with radical nephroureterectomy. Ann Surg Oncol 2014; 21(12):4041–8.

57. Sung HH, Jeon HG, Jeong BC, et al. Clinical significance of prognosis of the neutrophil-lymphocyte ratio and erythrocyte sedimentation rate in patients undergoing radical nephroureterectomy for upper urinary tract urothelial carci-noma. BJU Int 2014. [Epub ahead of print].

58. Rink M, Sharifi N, Fritsche HM, et al. Impact of preoperative anemia on oncologic outcomes of upper tract urothelial carcinoma treated with radical nephroureterectomy. J Urol 2014;191(2):316–22.

59. Rieken M, Schubert T, Xylinas E, et al. Association of perioperative blood trans-fusion with oncologic outcomes after radical nephroureterectomy for upper tract urothelial carcinoma. Eur J Surg Oncol 2014. [Epub ahead of print].

60. Fujita K, Uemura M, Yamamoto Y, et al. Preoperative risk stratification for cancer-specific survival of patients with upper urinary tract urothelial carci-noma treated by nephroureterectomy. Int J Clin Oncol 2014. [Epub ahead of print].

61. Polcari AJ, Hugen CM, Turk TM. Endoscopic management of upper tract urothe-lial carcinoma. Can J Urol 2009;16(6):4887–94.

62. Fajkovic H, Klatte T, Nagele U, et al. Results and outcomes after endoscopic treatment of upper urinary tract carcinoma: the Austrian experience. World J Urol 2013;31(1):37–44.

63. Smith AK, Stephenson AJ, Lane BR, et al. Inadequacy of biopsy for diagnosis of upper tract urothelial carcinoma: implications for conservative management. Urology 2011;78(1):82–6.

64. Cutress ML, Stewart GD, Zakikhani P, et al. Ureteroscopic and percutaneous management of upper tract urothelial carcinoma (UTUC): systematic review. BJU Int 2012;110(5):614–28.
65. Smith P, Mandel J, Raman JD. Conservative nephron-sparing treatment of upper-tract tumors. Curr Urol Rep 2013;14(2):102–8.
66. Dalpiaz O, Ehrlich G, Quehenberger F, et al. Distal ureterectomy is a safe surgical option in patients with urothelial carcinoma of the distal ureter. Urol Oncol 2014;32(1):34.e1–8.
67. Bachir BG, Kassouf W. Efficacy of instillations with chemotherapy or immunotherapy following endoscopic resection for upper tract urothelial carcinoma. Expert Rev Anticancer Ther 2012;12(1):63–75.
68. Giannarini G, Kessler TM, Birkhauser FD, et al. Antegrade perfusion with bacillus Calmette-Guerin in patients with non-muscle-invasive urothelial carcinoma of the upper urinary tract: who may benefit? Eur Urol 2011;60(5):955–60.
69. Carmignani L, Bianchi R, Cozzi G, et al. Intracavitary immunotherapy and chemotherapy for upper urinary tract cancer: current evidence. Rev Urol 2013;15(4):145–53.
70. Aboumarzouk OM, Somani B, Ahmad S, et al. Mitomycin C instillation following ureterorenoscopic laser ablation of upper urinary tract carcinoma. Urol Ann 2013;5(3):184–9.
71. O'Brien T, Ray E, Singh R, et al. Prevention of bladder tumours after nephroureterectomy for primary upper urinary tract urothelial carcinoma: a prospective, multicentre, randomised clinical trial of a single postoperative intravesical dose of mitomycin C (the ODMIT-C Trial). Eur Urol 2011;60(4):703–10.
72. Margulis V, Shariat SF, Matin SF, et al. Outcomes of radical nephroureterectomy: a series from the Upper Tract Urothelial Carcinoma Collaboration. Cancer 2009; 115(6):1224–33.
73. Romero FR, Schaeffer EM, Muntener M, et al. Oncologic outcomes of extravesical stapling of distal ureter in laparoscopic nephroureterectomy. J Endourol 2007;21(9):1025–7.
74. Macejko AM, Pazona JF, Loeb S, et al. Management of distal ureter in laparoscopic nephroureterectomy–a comprehensive review of techniques. Urology 2008;72(5):974–81.
75. Lughezzani G, Sun M, Perrotte P, et al. Should bladder cuff excision remain the standard of care at nephroureterectomy in patients with urothelial carcinoma of the renal pelvis? A population-based study. Eur Urol 2010;57(6): 956–62.
76. Phe V, Cussenot O, Bitker MO, et al. Does the surgical technique for management of the distal ureter influence the outcome after nephroureterectomy? BJU Int 2011;108(1):130–8.
77. Xylinas E, Rink M, Cha EK, et al. Impact of distal ureter management on oncologic outcomes following radical nephroureterectomy for upper tract urothelial carcinoma. Eur Urol 2014;65(1):210–7.
78. H.P. McDonald, W.E. Upchurch, C.E. Sturdevant Nephro-ureterectomy: a new technique. J Urol, 67 (1952), pp. 804–809.
79. Walton TJ, Novara G, Matsumoto K, et al. Oncological outcomes after laparoscopic and open radical nephroureterectomy: results from an international cohort. BJU Int 2011;108(3):406–12.
80. Brown GA, Busby JE, Wood CG, et al. Nephroureterectomy for treating upper urinary tract transitional cell carcinoma: time to change the treatment paradigm? BJU Int 2006;98(6):1176–80.

81. Brausi MA, Gavioli M, De Luca G, et al. Retroperitoneal lymph node dissection (RPLD) in conjunction with nephroureterectomy in the treatment of infiltrative transitional cell carcinoma (TCC) of the upper urinary tract: impact on survival. Eur Urol 2007;52(5):1414–8.

82. Kondo T, Nakazawa H, Ito F, et al. Impact of the extent of regional lymphadenectomy on the survival of patients with urothelial carcinoma of the upper urinary tract. J Urol 2007;178(4 Pt 1):1212–7 [discussion: 1217].

83. Roscigno M, Shariat SF, Freschi M, et al. Assessment of the minimum number of lymph nodes needed to detect lymph node invasion at radical nephroureterectomy in patients with upper tract urothelial cancer. Urology 2009;74(5):1070–4.

84. Roscigno M, Shariat SF, Margulis V, et al. The extent of lymphadenectomy seems to be associated with better survival in patients with nonmetastatic upper-tract urothelial carcinoma: how many lymph nodes should be removed? Eur Urol 2009;56(3):512–8.

85. Roscigno M, Shariat SF, Margulis V, et al. Impact of lymph node dissection on cancer specific survival in patients with upper tract urothelial carcinoma treated with radical nephroureterectomy. J Urol 2009;181(6):2482–9.

86. Kondo T, Hashimoto Y, Kobayashi H, et al. Template-based lymphadenectomy in urothelial carcinoma of the upper urinary tract: impact on patient survival. Int J Urol 2010;17(10):848–54.

87. Weight CJ, Gettman MT. The emerging role of lymphadenectomy in upper tract urothelial carcinoma. Urol Clin North Am 2011;38(4):429–37, vi.

88. Hanna N, Sun M, Trinh QD, et al. Propensity-score-matched comparison of perioperative outcomes between open and laparoscopic nephroureterectomy: a national series. Eur Urol 2012;61(4):715–21.

89. Ong AM, Bhayani SB, Pavlovich CP. Trocar site recurrence after laparoscopic nephroureterectomy. J Urol 2003;170(4 Pt 1):1301.

90. Roupret M, Smyth G, Irani J, et al. Oncological risk of laparoscopic surgery in urothelial carcinomas. World J Urol 2009;27(1):81–8.

91. Greco F, Fornara P. Words of wisdom. Re: laparoscopic versus open nephroureterectomy: perioperative and oncologic outcomes from a randomised prospective study. Eur Urol 2010;57(6):1117–8.

92. Simone G, Papalia R, Guaglianone S, et al. Laparoscopic versus open nephroureterectomy: perioperative and oncologic outcomes from a randomised prospective study. Eur Urol 2009;56(3):520–6.

93. Ni S, Tao W, Chen Q, et al. Laparoscopic versus open nephroureterectomy for the treatment of upper urinary tract urothelial carcinoma: a systematic review and cumulative analysis of comparative studies. Eur Urol 2012;61(6):1142–53.

94. Capitanio U, Shariat SF, Isbarn H, et al. Comparison of oncologic outcomes for open and laparoscopic nephroureterectomy: a multi-institutional analysis of 1249 cases. Eur Urol 2009;56(1):1–9.

95. Favaretto RL, Shariat SF, Chade DC, et al. Comparison between laparoscopic and open radical nephroureterectomy in a contemporary group of patients: are recurrence and disease-specific survival associated with surgical technique? Eur Urol 2010;58(5):645–51.

96. Rassweiler JJ, Schulze M, Marrero R, et al. Laparoscopic nephroureterectomy for upper urinary tract transitional cell carcinoma: is it better than open surgery? Eur Urol 2004;46(6):690–7.

97. Stewart GD, Humphries KJ, Cutress ML, et al. Long-term comparative outcomes of open versus laparoscopic nephroureterectomy for upper urinary tract

urothelial-cell carcinoma after a median follow-up of 13 years. J Endourol 2011; 25(8):1329–35.

98. Lim SK, Shin TY, Rha KH. Current status of robot assisted laparoscopic radical nephroureterectomy for management of upper tract urothelial carcinoma. Curr Urol Rep 2013;14(2):138–46.

99. Leow JJ, Martin-Doyle W, Rajagopal PS, et al. Adjuvant chemotherapy for invasive bladder cancer: a 2013 updated systematic review and meta-analysis of randomized trials. Eur Urol 2014;66(1):42–54.

100. Sternberg CN, Bellmunt J, Sonpavde G, et al. ICUD-EAU International Consultation on Bladder Cancer 2012: chemotherapy for urothelial carcinoma-neoadjuvant and adjuvant settings. Eur Urol 2013;63(1):58–66.

101. Leow JJ, Martin-Doyle W, Fay AP, et al. A systematic review and meta-analysis of adjuvant and neoadjuvant chemotherapy for upper tract urothelial carcinoma. Eur Urol 2014;66(3):529–41.

102. Siefker-Radtke AO, Dinney CP, Shen Y, et al. A phase 2 clinical trial of sequential neoadjuvant chemotherapy with ifosfamide, doxorubicin, and gemcitabine followed by cisplatin, gemcitabine, and ifosfamide in locally advanced urothelial cancer: final results. Cancer 2013;119(3):540–7.

103. Siefker-Radtke A, Kamat A, Corn P, et al. Neoadjuvant chemotherapy with DDMVAC and bevacizumab in high-risk urothelial cancer: results from a phase II trial at the M. D. Anderson Cancer Center. J Clin Oncol 2012;30(Suppl 5) [abstract: 261].

104. Hellenthal NJ, Shariat SF, Margulis V, et al. Adjuvant chemotherapy for high risk upper tract urothelial carcinoma: results from the Upper Tract Urothelial Carcinoma Collaboration. J Urol 2009;182(3):900–6.

105. Kawashima A, Nakai Y, Nakayama M, et al. The result of adjuvant chemotherapy for localized pT3 upper urinary tract carcinoma in a multi-institutional study. World J Urol 2012;30(5):701–6.

106. Kim TS, Oh JH, Rhew HY. The efficacy of adjuvant chemotherapy for locally advanced upper tract urothelial cell carcinoma. J Cancer 2013;4(8):686–90.

107. Kwak C, Lee SE, Jeong IG, et al. Adjuvant systemic chemotherapy in the treatment of patients with invasive transitional cell carcinoma of the upper urinary tract. Urology 2006;68(1):53–7.

108. Lee SE, Byun SS, Park YH, et al. Adjuvant chemotherapy in the management of pT3N0M0 transitional cell carcinoma of the upper urinary tract. Urol Int 2006; 77(1):22–6.

109. Soga N, Arima K, Sugimura Y. Adjuvant methotrexate, vinblastine, adriamycin, and cisplatin chemotherapy has potential to prevent recurrence of bladder tumors after surgical removal of upper urinary tract transitional cell carcinoma. Int J Urol 2008;15(9):800–3.

110. Suzuki S, Shinohara N, Harabayashi T, et al. Impact of adjuvant systemic chemotherapy on postoperative survival in patients with high-risk urothelial cancer. Int J Urol 2004;11(7):456–60.

111. Vassilakopoulou M, de la Motte Rouge T, Colin P, et al. Outcomes after adjuvant chemotherapy in the treatment of high-risk urothelial carcinoma of the upper urinary tract (UUT-UC): results from a large multicenter collaborative study. Cancer 2011;117(24):5500–8.

112. Yafi FA, Tanguay S, Rendon R, et al. Adjuvant chemotherapy for upper-tract urothelial carcinoma treated with nephroureterectomy: assessment of adequate renal function and influence on outcome. Urol Oncol 2014;32(1): 31.e17–24.

113. Hall MC, Womack JS, Roehrborn CG, et al. Advanced transitional cell carcinoma of the upper urinary tract: patterns of failure, survival and impact of postoperative adjuvant radiotherapy. J Urol 1998;160(3 Pt 1):703–6.

114. Chen B, Zeng ZC, Wang GM, et al. Radiotherapy may improve overall survival of patients with T3/T4 transitional cell carcinoma of the renal pelvis or ureter and delay bladder tumour relapse. BMC Cancer 2011;11:297.

115. Fan KH, Chen YC, Leung WM, et al. Adjuvant and salvage radiotherapy for urothelial cell carcinoma of the upper urinary tract: experience in a single institution. Chang Gung Med J 2012;35(3):247–54.

116. Czito B, Zietman A, Kaufman D, et al. Adjuvant radiotherapy with and without concurrent chemotherapy for locally advanced transitional cell carcinoma of the renal pelvis and ureter. J Urol 2004;172(4 Pt 1):1271–5.

117. Cozad SC, Smalley SR, Austenfeld M, et al. Adjuvant radiotherapy in high stage transitional cell carcinoma of the renal pelvis and ureter. Int J Radiat Oncol Biol Phys 1992;24(4):743–5.

118. Maulard-Durdux C, Dufour B, Hennequin C, et al. Postoperative radiation therapy in 26 patients with invasive transitional cell carcinoma of the upper urinary tract: no impact on survival? J Urol 1996;155(1):115–7.

119. Cuckow PM, Nyirady P, Winyard PJ. Normal and abnormal development of the urogenital tract. Prenat Diagn 2001;21(11):908–16.

120. Riedel I, Liang FX, Deng FM, et al. Urothelial umbrella cells of human ureter are heterogeneous with respect to their uroplakin composition: different degrees of urothelial maturity in ureter and bladder? Eur J Cell Biol 2005;84(2–3):393–405.

121. Hudson AE, Feng WC, Delostrinos CF, et al. Spreading of embryologically distinct urothelial cells is inhibited by SPARC. J Cell Physiol 2005;202(2):453–63.

122. Catto JW, Azzouzi AR, Rehman I, et al. Promoter hypermethylation is associated with tumor location, stage, and subsequent progression in transitional cell carcinoma. J Clin Oncol 2005;23(13):2903–10.

123. Carballido EM, Rosenberg JE. Optimal treatment for metastatic bladder cancer. Curr Oncol Rep 2014;16(9):404.

124. Audenet F, Yates DR, Cussenot O, et al. The role of chemotherapy in the treatment of urothelial cell carcinoma of the upper urinary tract (UUT-UCC). Urol Oncol 2013;31(4):407–13.

125. Sternberg CN, Yagoda A, Scher HI, et al. M-VAC (methotrexate, vinblastine, doxorubicin and cisplatin) for advanced transitional cell carcinoma of the urothelium. J Urol 1988;139(3):461–9.

126. Galsky MD, Hahn NM, Rosenberg J, et al. Treatment of patients with metastatic urothelial cancer "unfit" for Cisplatin-based chemotherapy. J Clin Oncol 2011; 29(17):2432–8.

127. Morales-Barrera R, Bellmunt J, Suarez C, et al. Cisplatin and gemcitabine administered every two weeks in patients with locally advanced or metastatic urothelial carcinoma and impaired renal function. Eur J Cancer 2012;48(12): 1816–21.

128. von der Maase H, Hansen SW, Roberts JT, et al. Gemcitabine and cisplatin versus methotrexate, vinblastine, doxorubicin, and cisplatin in advanced or metastatic bladder cancer: results of a large, randomized, multinational, multicenter, phase III study. J Clin Oncol 2000;18(17):3068–77.

129. Dogliotti L, Carteni G, Siena S, et al. Gemcitabine plus cisplatin versus gemcitabine plus carboplatin as first-line chemotherapy in advanced transitional cell carcinoma of the urothelium: results of a randomized phase 2 trial. Eur Urol 2007;52(1):134–41.

130. Bellmunt J, Ribas A, Eres N, et al. Carboplatin-based versus cisplatin-based chemotherapy in the treatment of surgically incurable advanced bladder carcinoma. Cancer 1997;80(10):1966–72.

131. Sternberg CN, de Mulder PH, Schornagel JH, et al. Randomized phase III trial of high-dose-intensity methotrexate, vinblastine, doxorubicin, and cisplatin (MVAC) chemotherapy and recombinant human granulocyte colony-stimulating factor versus classic MVAC in advanced urothelial tract tumors: European Organization for Research and Treatment of Cancer Protocol no. 30924. J Clin Oncol 2001;19(10):2638–46.

132. Choueiri TK, Jacobus S, Bellmunt J, et al. Neoadjuvant dose-dense methotrexate, vinblastine, doxorubicin, and cisplatin with pegfilgrastim support in muscle-invasive urothelial cancer: pathologic, radiologic, and biomarker correlates. J Clin Oncol 2014;32(18):1889–94.

133. Plimack ER, Hoffman-Censits JH, Viterbo R, et al. Accelerated methotrexate, vinblastine, doxorubicin, and cisplatin is safe, effective, and efficient neoadjuvant treatment for muscle-invasive bladder cancer: results of a multicenter phase II study with molecular correlates of response and toxicity. J Clin Oncol 2014;32(18):1895–901.

134. Hoffman-Censits JH, Trabulsi EJ, Chen DY, et al. Neoadjuvant accelerated methotrexate, vinblastine, doxorubicin, and cisplatin (AMVAC) in patients with high-grade upper-tract urothelial carcinoma. J Clin Oncol 2014;32(S4) [abstract: 326].

135. Konski A, Feigenberg S, Chow E. Palliative radiation therapy. Semin Oncol 2005; 32(2):156–64.

136. Duchesne GM, Bolger JJ, Griffiths GO, et al. A randomized trial of hypofractionated schedules of palliative radiotherapy in the management of bladder carcinoma: results of medical research council trial BA09. Int J Radiat Oncol Biol Phys 2000;47(2):379–88.

137. McLaren DB, Morrey D, Mason MD. Hypofractionated radiotherapy for muscle invasive bladder cancer in the elderly. Radiother Oncol 1997;43(2):171–4.

138. Cowles RS, Johnson DE, McMurtrey MJ. Long-term results following thoracotomy for metastatic bladder cancer. Urology 1982;20(4):390–2.

139. Abe T, Shinohara N, Harabayashi T, et al. Impact of multimodal treatment on survival in patients with metastatic urothelial cancer. Eur Urol 2007;52(4): 1106–13.

140. Dodd PM, McCaffrey JA, Herr H, et al. Outcome of postchemotherapy surgery after treatment with methotrexate, vinblastine, doxorubicin, and cisplatin in patients with unresectable or metastatic transitional cell carcinoma. J Clin Oncol 1999;17(8):2546–52.

141. Herr HW, Donat SM, Bajorin DF. Post-chemotherapy surgery in patients with unresectable or regionally metastatic bladder cancer. J Urol 2001;165(3):811–4.

Bladder Preservation Strategies

Ashesh B. Jani, MD, MSEE[a],*, Jason A. Efstathiou, MD, DPhil[b],
William U. Shipley, MD, FACR[b]

KEYWORDS

- Bladder cancer • Cystectomy • Chemotherapy • Radiotherapy • Organ preservation

KEY POINTS

- Organ preservation by concurrent chemoradiotherapy following an aggressive transurethral resection (TUR) of muscle-invasive bladder cancer (MIBC) is an established treatment of selected patients with bladder cancer as an alternative to cystectomy with or without chemotherapy.
- Established patient and disease factors must be considered when deciding to offer patients with bladder cancer organ-preserving chemoradiotherapy, and attention must also be paid to the treatment regimen and the radiation technique.
- Ongoing biomarker studies of the TUR of bladder tumor (TURBT) specimen suggest that subsets of patients may respond favorably to an organ-preservation approach using radiation or chemoradiotherapy regimens, but prospective studies are needed to validate these observations.
- Concurrent chemoradiotherapy following a complete TURBT for organ preservation is now being studied prospectively for patients with non-MIBC who are refractory to intravesical therapy.

INTRODUCTION

Bladder cancer has a significant incidence and mortality, with approximately 75,000 new cases and 15,000 deaths in the United States in 2013.[1] Management of muscle-invasive bladder cancer (MIBC) has evolved significantly over the past few decades. Cystectomy remains the standard treatment, but organ-preservation approaches combining concurrent chemotherapy and radiation following an aggressive transurethral resection of bladder tumor (TURBT) have emerged as appropriate alternatives in selected patients.[2–11] Although preoperative radiotherapy followed by cystectomy was found to initially improve local control, this approach was later abandoned.[12,13]

The authors have nothing to disclose.
[a] Department of Radiation Oncology, Emory University, 1365 Clifton Road, Northeast, Suite A1300, Atlanta, GA 30322, USA; [b] Department of Radiation Oncology, Massachusetts General Hospital, Harvard Medical School, 100 Blossom Street, Cox 3, Boston, MA 02114, USA
* Corresponding author.
E-mail address: abjani@emory.edu

Postoperative nonconformal radiotherapy was associated with significant toxicity when earlier radiotherapy techniques were used, but postoperative radiation using intensity-modulated radiotherapy (IMRT) is now again under study.[14–17] Although the addition of radiotherapy with surgery (in either the preoperative or postoperative study) is not currently standard, the addition of neoadjuvant (and probably adjuvant) chemotherapy with surgery has been demonstrated to improve survival. The combination of surgery and chemotherapy is now the optimal standard in patients suitable for cisplatin-based multidrug therapy from the standpoint of cancer control outcomes, with a 5-year overall survival of approximately 70% for muscle-invasive disease.[18–21]

The morbidity of surgery must be weighed into consideration, particularly because of the extensiveness of the surgery and associated recovery.[6–11] In this context, a trimodality therapeutic organ-preservation approach (TURBT plus concurrent chemotherapy and radiation) was developed in order to attempt to achieve a high cancer control rate while preserving good bladder function and a good quality of life. Organ-preservation approaches are now commonly used in other areas of cancer treatment whereby extensive surgeries were once standard: lumpectomy plus radiotherapy in place of modified radical mastectomy for breast cancer, chemoradiotherapy in place of abdominoperineal resection for anal cancer, chemoradiotherapy and limb-sparing surgery in place of amputation for sarcomas, and chemoradiotherapy in place of extensive surgery for head and neck cancers. In all of these disease sites, an organ-preservation technique (with the more extensive surgery reserved for salvage therapy), achieved similar rates of local control and overall survival as up-front extensive surgery.

It is with this same general goal that bladder preservation strategies were developed. Although radiotherapy alone in general has poorer cancer control outcomes in comparison with cystectomy, the addition of chemotherapy to radiotherapy produced results commensurate with cystectomy series.[2,22–33] Recently, cooperative group trials (Radiation Therapy Oncology Group [RTOG] 0233 and BC2001) report 5-year cystectomy-free survival rates of more than 60% for selected patients with muscle-invasive disease without any demonstrated compromise to the overall survival in comparison with up-front cystectomy series.[30,31]

PATIENT EVALUATION OVERVIEW

Risk factors for bladder cancer are smoking, chronic physical irritation (such as bladder stones, *schistosoma haematobium*, or indwelling catheter), and chronic chemical irritation (such as phenacetin, cyclophosphamide, and occupational factors in the dye, rubber, and paint industries).[34] Urothelial carcinoma (formerly called transitional cell carcinoma) is the most common histologic variant (representing more than 90% of bladder cancer cases in North America), and further discussion in the current article is restricted to urothelial carcinoma. Diagnostic workup initially begins with a thorough physical examination with particular attention to a bimanual examination to determine the extent of pelvic involvement. A cystoscopic/TURBT examination is critical, with biopsies taken from all visualized areas of abnormalities and often random normal areas (including prostatic urethra biopsies, as indicated). The size, number, and morphology of each lesion should be documented as well as a tumor map. It may be important to evaluate by imaging the upper urinary tract for synchronous lesions, although these are rare. The laboratory workup consists of a urinalysis, cytology, and basic chemistry/blood counts. The radiological workup consists of computed tomography (CT) or MRI of the pelvis and abdomen and a chest radiograph or CT; a bone scan is typically obtained for muscle-invasive lesions, particularly if the alkaline phosphatase is elevated. The reader is referred to the American Joint Committee on Cancer's manual for staging.[35] Discussion in this article is primarily related to muscle-invasive, node-negative, nonmetastatic disease (cT2-T4, cN0, M0) after the aforementioned workup.

PHARMACOLOGIC TREATMENT OPTIONS

A variety of drugs from several different classes have been found to have single-agent activity against metastatic bladder cancer, including (alphabetically) carbogen, cisplatin, doxorubicin, 5-fluorouracil (5FU), gemcitabine, ifosfamide, methotrexate, mitomycin C, nicotinamide, paclitaxel, and vinblastine.[24–33,36,37] Consistent with approaches at other disease sites, several multi-agent regimens have been designed to overcome single-agent resistance as well as to have nonoverlapping toxicity; these regimens have been used in the neoadjuvant, adjuvant, and concomitant settings with surgery and radiotherapy and are summarized in **Table 1**.

NONPHARMACOLOGIC TREATMENT OPTIONS
Surgical Treatment Options

A range of surgical options is available, ranging from minor office procedures to major operating room procedures requiring weeks of recovery time.[7–11] The TURBT is the standard of care for non-MIBC (N-MIBC) and typically serves a diagnostic role for MIBC. A partial cystectomy, which involves extraperitoneal cystostomy and wide local excision, is indicated for a solitary, well-defined tumor with no evidence of carcinoma in situ in a mobile portion of the bladder and for which no ureteral implant is needed; only approximately 5% of patients with muscle-invasive disease are candidates for partial cystectomy. The next most aggressive procedure is the simple cystectomy, in which the plane of dissection is the bladder wall; this procedure involves the removal of the bladder plus various amounts of ureters/urethra and is a palliative procedure only; the standard curative surgery for muscle-invasive disease is the radical cystectomy.[7–11]

In men, radical cystectomy involves the removal of the bladder, prostate, seminal vesicles, proximal vas deferens, distal ureters, proximal urethra, and the margin of

Table 1
List of active chemotherapy agents and commonly used multi-agent regimens in bladder cancer

Major Drugs with Single-Agent Activity	Neoadjuvant or Adjuvant Regimens (with Surgery or Radiotherapy)	Concomitant Agents/ Regimens with Radiotherapy
Carbogen	MVAC	Cisplatin
Cisplatin	MCV (also called CMV)	5FU & cisplatin
Doxorubicin	ITF	Paclitaxel & cisplatin
5FU	Gemcitabine & cisplatin	Gemcitabine (low dose)
Gemcitabine	Gemcitabine & paclitaxel	5FU & mitomycin C
Ifosfamide		Carbogen & nicotinamide
Methotrexate		
Mitomycin C		
Nicotinamide		
Paclitaxel		
Vinblastine		

Abbreviations: ITF, ifosfamide, paclitaxel, and cisplatin; MCAV, methotrexate, vinblastine, doxorubicin, and cisplatin; MCV, methotrexate, cisplatin, and vinblastine.

the adipose and peritoneum and includes a pelvic lymph-node dissection. In women, the procedure involves the removal of the bladder, urethra, uterus, oviducts, ovaries, anterior vaginal wall, distal ureters, and the surrounding adipose tissue/fascia and also involves a pelvic lymph-node dissection; note that in women, the radical cystectomy is synonymous with an anterior exenteration. Urinary diversions fall into 2 major categories: incontinent and continent. Incontinent diversions, in which there is no internal reservoir, are typically conduit diversions, the most common of which is the ileal conduit. Continent diversions typically involve diverting the ureters into a resected segment of ileum or ileocecum that is then either fixed to the abdominal wall with an external stoma created or anastomosed to the urethra in men or the sigmoid colon in women. The continent diversion can either require self-catheterization or can function similar to that of a normal bladder.[7–11]

Radiotherapy Treatment Options

External beam radiotherapy (EBRT) alone, as described earlier, typically has lower cancer control rates than radical cystectomy for a given stage; its use as a sole treatment is typically reserved for those who are poor surgical candidates, poor organ-preservation chemoradiotherapy candidates, have metastatic disease with a symptomatic bladder issues, or have unresectable locally advanced disease.[22] Interstitial brachytherapy can be used for selected patients either alone or in combination with EBRT, both in the context of primary treatment with radiotherapy or as adjuvant treatment in conjunction with partial cystectomy.[23] Further discussion herein is restricted to EBRT as the radiotherapy modality.

COMBINATION THERAPIES
Surgery Plus Radiotherapy

Preoperative or neoadjuvant irradiation was explored in several randomized trials, with several different fractionation schemes evaluated.[12,13] Although a local control benefit was demonstrated and a dose response was suggested in several studies, the practice has largely been abandoned.

Postoperative/adjuvant radiotherapy was investigated in an RTOG/Jefferson study (conducted during an era of older treatment techniques) with toxicity found to be prohibitively high.[14,15] Postoperative radiotherapy remains an active area of investigation (in the context of modern treatment techniques) with several ongoing single-institution phase II studies as well as a randomized phase II protocol being developed by the NRG cooperative group/National Cancer Institute clinical trial network in patients with pT3/4 and/or pN+ disease.[7,16]

Surgery Plus Chemotherapy

Neoadjuvant chemotherapy with surgery has several theoretic advantages: early therapy for potential micrometastases, drug delivery not being compromised by an altered surgical bed, and improved tumor resectability. Neoadjuvant chemotherapy has been found in randomized trials to improve disease-free survival and overall survival over surgery alone.[18,19]

Adjuvant chemotherapy also has several theoretic advantages: not delaying the definitive local therapy and knowledge of pathologic staging (and consequent application for adverse disease features, such as positive nodal status, extravesical tumor extension, and/or lymphovascular invasion). With respect to adjuvant chemotherapy, although earlier meta-analyses did not suggest a benefit to this strategy, a more recent meta-analysis suggests a disease-free survival and overall survival advantage with adjuvant cisplatin-based chemotherapy after surgery; this remains an area of active investigation.[20,21]

Chemotherapy Plus Radiotherapy

Chemotherapy in combination with radiotherapy has 2 goals. First, as the case when combined with surgery, one goal is to eradicate distant micrometastases and to improve distant control. The other goal is radiosensitization. The overall objective is to achieve local control and distant control while achieving organ preservation and, thus, reserving an extensive surgical procedure for salvage therapy.

The general flow path as practiced in the US cooperative group setting consists of (1) complete TURBT; (2) induction chemoradiotherapy; (3) response assessment with cystoscopy/biopsy; (4) if a complete response is achieved, consolidation chemoradiotherapy; (5) further response assessment with cystoscopy/biopsy; and (6) continued surveillance.[24–30,32] The aforementioned treatment describes a split-course regimen; one alternative is to omit the midtreatment course response assessment (item 3 previously mentioned) and deliver the chemoradiotherapy in a single course.[31] With either regimen (full course or split course), salvage cystectomy is curative for many poorly responding patients or those who recur with an invasive tumor. **Fig. 1** shows the aforementioned flow path; note that this flow path does not show a step for neoadjuvant

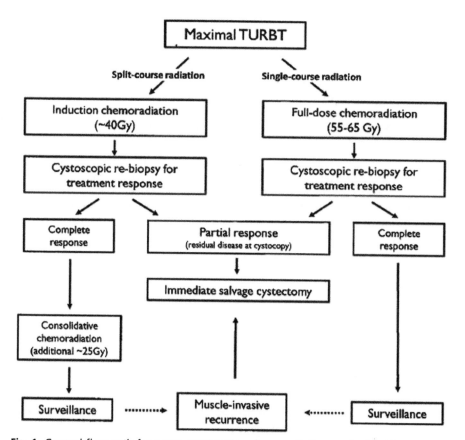

Fig. 1. General flow path for organ-preservation chemoradiotherapy for bladder cancer.

chemotherapy that had been used in some earlier regimens (and may warrant further investigation).[24–26]

Patient selection for organ preservation is important. A host of disease and patient factors were found to be unfavorable or can be considered relative contraindications; these are summarized in **Table 2**. The ideal patient is the one with good urinary function, is healthy enough to tolerate radio-sensitizing chemotherapy concurrent with radiotherapy, and is one for whom radical cystectomy is a salvage option in the event the desired response is not achieved at any response assessment on the flow path in **Fig. 1**. The ideal setting is one in which care is carefully coordinated by the urologist, medical oncologist, radiation oncologist, pathologist, and radiologist in order to adhere to what is an intrinsically complex treatment algorithm.

TREATMENT COMPLICATIONS

The individual chemotherapy agents, the different surgical approaches, and the radiotherapy all have their separate individual toxicities. The main side effects of the chemotherapy component of the bladder preservation regimen of course depend on the agents used but are most commonly hematosuppression, nausea, and neuropathy.[21,24–32] The principal toxicities of the radiotherapy component are gastrointestinal (GI) and genitourinary (GU); overall RTOG grade 3 or higher GI and GU toxicity have been found to be approximately 4% (range 0%–7%) and 5% (range 0%–8%), respectively.[24–33]

EVALUATION OF OUTCOME AND LONG-TERM RECOMMENDATIONS

A range of multicenter studies conducted by cooperative groups over the last few decades has examined the outcomes of bladder preservation chemoradiotherapy. These studies have sequentially asked the questions of the role neoadjuvant chemotherapy, the tolerability of hyper-fractionation, and the comparison of successful regimens. A brief summary of this experience is provided next:

1. RTOG 88–02: single-arm phase II study examining neoadjuvant methotrexate, cisplatin, and vinblastine (MCV) followed by cisplatin with once-daily radiotherapy[25]; demonstrated feasibility of organ-preservation approach
2. RTOG 89–03: randomized phase III trial comparing neoadjuvant MCV versus no MCV followed by cisplatin with once-daily radiotherapy chemotherapy; did not demonstrate significant benefit to neoadjuvant chemotherapy[26]

Table 2	
Disease and patient factors not favoring organ-preservation chemoradiotherapy	
Disease Factors	**Patient Factors**
Tumor-related hydronephrosis	Unsuitable for radio-sensitizing chemotherapy
Diffuse involvement of bladder mucosa with Tis plus MIBC	Urinary incontinence/poor bladder function
Tumor located in a diverticulum making it not resectable by TURBT or able to be well followed cystoscopically	Small bladder capacity
Clinical T4 disease with prostatic stromal invasion	Inflammatory bowel disease
Positive lymph nodes by both imaging and biopsy	Adhesions from prior pelvic surgery
Nonurothelial carcinoma histology	

3. RTOG 95–06: a single-arm phase I/II study looking at 5FU/cisplatin and twice-daily radiotherapy[27]; demonstrated feasibility/tolerability of chemotherapy and twice-daily radiotherapy
4. RTOG 97–06: single-arm phase I/II study examining cisplatin concomitant with twice-daily radiotherapy, followed by adjuvant MCV[28]; established feasibility of adjuvant chemotherapy following organ-preservation chemoradiotherapy
5. RTOG 99–06: single-arm phase I/II trial examining concomitant paclitaxel/cisplatin and twice-daily radiotherapy, followed by adjuvant gemcitabine/cisplatin[29]; modification of previous strategy with incorporation of paclitaxel during concomitant phase and gemcitabine during adjuvant phase
6. RTOG 02–33: randomized phase II trial comparing either paclitaxel/cisplatin or 5FU/cisplatin concomitant with twice-daily radiotherapy, followed by adjuvant gemcitabine/(cisplatin or paclitaxel)[30]; high rates of completion, complete response, and bladder preservation found in both induction regimens
7. BC 2001: randomized trial (with 2 × 2 design) permitting optional neoadjuvant chemotherapy and simultaneously examining (1) no chemotherapy versus 5FU/mitomycin concomitant with once-daily radiotherapy and (2) whole-bladder radiotherapy or modified-volume radiotherapy[31]; locoregional control over radiotherapy alone significantly improved with addition of chemotherapy, and reducing the volume of bladder receiving full radiotherapy dose reduces late toxicity without detriment to tumor control
8. RTOG 07–12: randomized phase II trial of gemcitabine concomitant with once-daily radiotherapy versus 5FU/cisplatin concomitant with twice-daily radiotherapy, in either case followed by adjuvant gemcitabine/(cisplatin or paclitaxel)[32]; results not yet available

A summary of this experience is provided in **Table 3**. Note that **Table 3** also includes the results of a pooled analysis of the first 6 RTOG studies (trials 1 through 8 discussed earlier).[4] Note the progressive improvement over the course of the studies in both cystectomy-free survival and overall survival. Nomograms have recently been developed (which consider factors such as clinical T stage, presence of hydronephrosis, completeness of TURBT, age, sex, and tumor grade) to assist in the individualized patient discussion of outcomes with organ-preservation chemoradiotherapy.[38]

FUTURE DIRECTIONS
Molecular Markers

Identification of suitable candidates for organ-preservation chemoradiotherapy, beyond the standard patient and disease factors listed in **Table 2**, is a process of ongoing study; biomarkers may serve this role. Her-2 expression has been found to correlate with survival.[39] Recently, MRE11, which is a protein involved in DNA repair, has been investigated in 2 studies as a predictive biomarker in which overexpression was associated with improved disease-specific survival in patients receiving radiation or chemoradiation but not in those undergoing radical surgery.[40,41] MRE11 will be investigated in the prospective setting to attempt to validate if high MRE 11 expression is a useful biomarker to assist in individualizing the treatment decision for bladder cancer.

Nonmuscle Invasive Bladder Cancer

Standard treatment of N-MIBC is complete TURBT and intravesical therapy, typically bacillus Calmette-Guérin with or without interferon. Local recurrence rates are quite high (nearly half), and standard treatment is cystectomy in these cases. Two recent

Table 3
Summary of major bladder organ-preservation chemoradiotherapy studies

Study	N	Neoadjuvant Chemo	Induction Chemo-XRT	Consolidation Chemo-XRT	Adjuvant Chemo	CR Rate (%)	CFS	OS
RTOG 88-02[25]	91	MCV	Cisplatin + once-daily XRT	Cisplatin + once-daily XRT	None	75	4 y: 44%	4 y: 62%
RTOG 89-03[26]	61	MCV	Cisplatin + once-daily XRT	Cisplatin + once-daily XRT	None	59	5 y: 38%	5 y: 48%
	62	None	Cisplatin + once-daily XRT	Cisplatin + once-daily XRT	None		5 y: 40%	5 y: 49%
RTOG 95-06[27]	34	None	Cisplatin + 5FU + twice-daily XRT	Cisplatin + 5FU + twice-daily XRT	None	67	3 y: 66%	3 y: 83%
RTOG 97-06[28]	47	None	Cisplatin + twice-daily XRT	Cisplatin + once-daily XRT	MCV	74	3 y: 48%	3 y: 61%
RTOG 99-06[29]	81	None	Paclitaxel + cisplatin + twice-daily XRT	Paclitaxel + cisplatin + once-daily XRT	Gem + CP	81	5 y: 47%	5 y: 56%
RTOG 02-33[30]	46	None	Paclitaxel + cisplatin + twice-daily XRT	Paclitaxel + cisplatin + twice-daily XRT	Gem + (CP or paclitaxel)	87	5 y: 67%	5 y: 71%
	47	None	Cisplatin + 5FU + twice-daily XRT	Cisplatin + 5FU + twice-daily XRT	Gem + (CP or paclitaxel)	79	5 y: 71%	5 y: 75%
Pooled results of above[4]	468	See above for RTOG 88-02 through RTOG 02-33				69	5 y: 56% 10 y: 55% DSS 5 y: 71% 10 y: 65%	5 y: 57% 10 y: 36%
BC 2001[31]	182	Optional (31% received)	5FU + Mitomycin + once-daily XRT		None	67	2 y: 88%	5 y: 48%
	178	Optional (34% received)	None		None	66	2 y: 83%	5 y: 35%
RTOG 07-12[32]	32	None	Cisplatin + 5FU + twice-daily XRT	Cisplatin + 5FU + twice-daily XRT	Gem + (CP or paclitaxel)	Not available		
	32	None	[a]Low-dose Gem + once-daily XRT	Low-dose Gem + once-daily XRT	Gem + (CP or paclitaxel)	Not available		

Abbreviations: CFS, cystectomy-free survival (ie, both bladder intact and disease-specific survival); CP, cisplatin; DSS, disease-specific survival; Gem, gemcitabine; OS, overall survival; XRT, radiotherapy.
[a] Low-dose gemcitabine: 27 mg/m^2 twice weekly.

studies have shown high rates of complete response and recurrence-free survival with the use of organ-preservation chemoradiotherapy in this population, whereby cystectomy would be the next step in standard management, and have demonstrated disease-specific survival of 70%.[42,43] These experiences inspired the development of an ongoing RTOG phase II study of concomitant chemoradiotherapy (once-daily radiotherapy and concomitant chemotherapy consisting of either cisplatin or 5FU/mitomycin C).[44]

Radiotherapy Technique

As described earlier, recently radiotherapy in both the intact-bladder setting and in the postcystectomy setting has been found to have acceptable GI and GU morbidity. Newer radiotherapy techniques, such as IMRT and image-guided radiotherapy, may be associated with further reduction in toxicity over earlier techniques.[45-47]

REFERENCES

1. Siegel R, Naishadham D, Jemal A. Cancer statistics, 2013. CA Cancer J Clin 2013;63(1):11–30.
2. Efstathiou JA, Spiegel DY, Shipley WU, et al. Long-term outcomes of selective bladder preservation by combined-modality therapy for invasive bladder cancer: the MGH experience. Eur Urol 2012;61(4):705–11.
3. Chen RC, Shipley WU, Efstathiou JA, et al. Trimodality bladder preservation therapy for muscle-invasive bladder cancer. J Natl Compr Canc Netw 2013; 11(8):952–60.
4. Mak RH, Hunt D, Shipley WU, et al. Long-term outcomes in patients with muscle-invasive bladder cancer after bladder-preserving combined-modality therapy: a pooled analysis of RTOG 8802, 8903, 9706, 9906, and 0233. J Clin Oncol, in press.
5. Gakis G, Efstathiou JA, Lerner SP, et al. ICUD-EAU International Consultation on Bladder Cancer 2012: radical cystectomy and bladder preservation for muscle-invasive urothelial carcinoma of the bladder. Eur Urol 2013;63:45–57.
6. Clark PE, Agarwal N, Biagioli MC, et al, National Comprehensive Cancer Network (NCCN). Bladder cancer. J Natl Compr Canc Netw 2013;11(4):446–75.
7. Madersbacher S, Hochreiter W, Burkhard F, et al. Radical cystectomy for bladder cancer today–a homogeneous series without neoadjuvant therapy. J Clin Oncol 2003;21(4):690–6.
8. Stein JP, Lieskovsky G, Cote R, et al. Radical cystectomy in the treatment of invasive bladder cancer: long-term results in 1,054 patients. J Clin Oncol 2001;19(3):666–75.
9. Hautmann RE, Gshwend JE, de Petriconi RC, et al. Cystectomy for transitional cell carcinoma of the bladder: results of a surgery only series in the neobladder era. J Urol 2006;176(2):486–92.
10. Dhar NB, Klein EA, Reuther AM, et al. Outcome after radical cystectomy with limited or extended pelvic lymph node dissection. J Urol 2008;179(3):873–8.
11. Donat SM, Shabsigh A, Savage C, et al. Potential impact of postoperative early complications on the timing of adjuvant chemotherapy in patients undergoing radical cystectomy: a high-volume tertiary cancer center experience. Eur Urol 2009;55(1):177–85.
12. Batata MA, Chu FC, Hilaris BS, et al. Radiation therapy before cystectomy in the management of patients with bladder cancer. Clin Radiol 1982;33(1):109–14.
13. Cole CJ, Pollack A, Zagars GK, et al. Local control of muscle-invasive bladder cancer: preoperative radiotherapy and cystectomy versus cystectomy alone. Int J Radiat Oncol Biol Phys 1995;32(2):331–40.

14. Mohiuddin M, Kramer S, Newall J, et al. Combined preoperative and postoperative radiation for bladder cancer. Results of RTOG/Jefferson Study. Cancer 1985; 55(5):963–6.

15. Reisinger SA, Mohiuddin M, Mulholland SG. Combined pre- and postoperative adjuvant radiation therapy for bladder cancer–a ten year experience. Int J Radiat Oncol Biol Phys 1992;24(3):463–8.

16. Zaghloul MS, Nouh A, Nazmy M, et al. Long-term results of primary adenocarcinoma of the urinary bladder: a report on 192 patients. Urol Oncol 2006;24(1): 13–20.

17. NRG-GU 001. Available at: www.nrgoncology.org. (protocol pending). Accessed August 14, 2014.

18. Grossman HB, Natale RB, Tangen CM, et al. Neoadjuvant chemotherapy plus cystectomy compared with cystectomy alone for locally advanced bladder cancer. N Engl J Med 2003;349(9):859–66.

19. Plimack ER, Hoffman-Censits JH, Viterbo R, et al. Accelerated methotrexate, vinblastine, doxorubicin, and cisplatin is safe, effective, and efficient neoadjuvant treatment for muscle-invasive bladder cancer: results of a multicenter phase II study with molecular correlates of response and toxicity. J Clin Oncol 2014; 32(18):1895–901.

20. Advanced Bladder Cancer (ABC) Meta-analysis Collaboration. Adjuvant chemotherapy in invasive bladder cancer: a systematic review and meta-analysis of individual patient data. Eur Urol 2005;48(2):189–99.

21. Leow JJ, Martin-Doyle W, Rajagopal PS, et al. Adjuvant chemotherapy for invasive bladder cancer: a 2013 updated systematic review and meta-analysis of randomized trials. Eur Urol 2014;66(1):42–54.

22. Efstathiou JA, Coen JJ, Zietman AL, et al. Bladder Cancer. In: Gunderson LL, Tepper JE, editors. Clinical Radiation Oncology. 3rd edition. Churchill Livingstone Saunders/Elsevier; 2011.

23. van der Werf-Messing BH, van Putten WL. Carcinoma of the urinary bladder category T2,3NXM0 treated by 40 Gy external irradiation followed by cesium137 implant at reduced dose (50%). Int J Radiat Oncol Biol Phys 1989;16(2):369–71.

24. Shipley WU, Prout GR Jr, Einstein AB Jr, et al. Treatment of invasive bladder cancer by cisplatin and irradiation in patients unsuited for surgery: a high success rate in clinical stage T2 tumors in a National Bladder Cancer Group trial. JAMA 1987;258:931–5.

25. Tester W, Caplan R, Heaney J, et al. Neoadjuvant combined modality program with selective organ preservation for invasive bladder cancer: results of Radiation Therapy Oncology Group phase II trial 8802. J Clin Oncol 1996;14(1):119–26.

26. Shipley WU, Winter KA, Kaufman DS, et al. Phase III trial of neoadjuvant chemotherapy in patients with invasive bladder cancer treated with selective bladder preservation by combined radiation therapy and chemotherapy: initial results of Radiation Therapy Oncology Group 89-03. J Clin Oncol 1998;16(11):3576–83.

27. Kaufman DS, Winter KA, Shipley WU, et al. The initial results in muscle-invading bladder cancer of RTOG 95-06: phase I/II trial of transurethral surgery plus radiation therapy with concurrent cisplatin and 5-fluorouracil followed by selective bladder preservation or cystectomy depending on the initial response. Oncologist 2000;5(6):471–6.

28. Hagan MP, Winter KA, Kaufman DS, et al. RTOG 97-06: initial report of a phase I-II trial of selective bladder conservation using TURBT, twice-daily accelerated irradiation sensitized with cisplatin, and adjuvant MCV combination chemotherapy. Int J Radiat Oncol Biol Phys 2003;57(3):665–72.

29. Kaufman DS, Winter KA, Shipley WU, et al. Phase I-II RTOG study (99-06) of patients with muscle-invasive bladder cancer undergoing transurethral surgery, paclitaxel, cisplatin, and twice-daily radiotherapy followed by selective bladder preservation or radical cystectomy and adjuvant chemotherapy. Urology 2009; 73(4):833–7.

30. Mitin T, Hunt D, Shipley WU, et al. Transurethral surgery and twice-daily radiation plus paclitaxel-cisplatin or fluorouracil-cisplatin with selective bladder preservation and adjuvant chemotherapy for patients with muscle invasive bladder cancer (RTOG 0233): a randomised multicentre phase 2 trial. Lancet Oncol 2013;14(9): 863–72.

31. James ND, Hussain SA, Hall E, et al, BC2001 Investigators. Radiotherapy with or without chemotherapy in muscle-invasive bladder cancer. N Engl J Med 2012; 366(16):1477–88.

32. RTOG 0712: a phase II randomized study for patients with muscle-invasive bladder cancer evaluating transurethral surgery and concomitant chemoradiation by either BID irradiation plus 5-fluorouracil and cisplatin or QD irradiation plus gemcitabine followed by selective bladder preservation and gemcitabine/ cisplatin adjuvant chemotherapy. Available at: www.rtog.org. Accessed August 14, 2014.

33. Efstathiou JA, Bae K, Shipley WU, et al. Late pelvic toxicity after bladder-sparing therapy in patients with invasive bladder cancer: RTOG 89-03, 95-06, 97-06, 99-06. J Clin Oncol 2009;27(25):4055–61.

34. Frank SJ, Zelesky MJ. Bladder cancer. In: Leibel SA, Phillips TL, editors. Textbook of radiation oncology. Philadelphia: WB Saunders; 1998. p. 725–39.

35. American Joint Committee on Cancer. AJCC cancer staging manual. In: Urinary bladder. 7th edition. New York: Springer; 2010. p. 497–506.

36. Gartrell BA, Sonpavde G. Emerging drugs for urothelial carcinoma. Expert Opin Emerg Drugs 2013;18(4):477–94.

37. Hoskin PJ, Rojas AM, Bentzen SM, et al. Radiotherapy with concurrent carbogen and nicotinamide in bladder carcinoma. J Clin Oncol 2010;28(33): 4912–8.

38. Coen JJ, Paly JJ, Niemierko A, et al. Nomograms predicting response to therapy and outcomes after bladder-preserving trimodality therapy for muscle-invasive bladder cancer. Int J Radiat Oncol Biol Phys 2013;86(2):311–6.

39. Chakravarti A, Winter K, Wu CL, et al. Expression of the epidermal growth factor receptor and Her-2 are predictors of favorable outcome and reduced complete response rates, respectively, in patients with muscle-invading bladder cancers treated by concurrent radiation and cisplatin-based chemotherapy: a report from the Radiation Therapy Oncology Group. Int J Radiat Oncol Biol Phys 2005;62(2):309–17.

40. Choudhury A, Nelson LD, Teo MT, et al. MRE11 expression is predictive of cause-specific survival following radical radiotherapy for muscle-invasive bladder cancer. Cancer Res 2010;70(18):7017–26.

41. Laurberg JR, Brems-Eskildsen AS, Nordentoft I, et al. Expression of TIP60 (tat-interactive protein) and MRE11 (meiotic recombination 11 homolog) predict treatment-specific outcome of localised invasive bladder cancer. BJU Int 2012; 110(11 Pt C):E1228–36.

42. Wo JY, Shipley WU, Dahl DM, et al. The results of concurrent chemo-radiotherapy for recurrence after treatment with bacillus Calmette-Guérin for non-muscle-invasive bladder cancer: is immediate cystectomy always necessary? BJU Int 2009;104(2):179–83.

43. Weiss C, Wolze C, Engehausen DG, et al. Radiochemotherapy after transurethral resection for high-risk T1 bladder cancer: an alternative to intravesical therapy or early cystectomy? J Clin Oncol 2006;24(15):2318–24.

44. RTOG 0926. A phase II protocol for patients with stage T1 bladder cancer to evaluate selective bladder preserving treatment by radiation therapy concurrent with radiosensitizing chemotherapy following a thorough transurethral surgical re-staging. Available at: www.rtog.org. Accessed August 14, 2014.

45. Søndergaard J, Høyer M, Petersen JB, et al. The normal tissue sparing obtained with simultaneous treatment of pelvic lymph nodes and bladder using intensity-modulated radiotherapy. Acta Oncol 2009;48(2):238–44.

46. McBain CA, Logue JP. Radiation therapy for muscle-invasive bladder cancer: treatment planning and delivery in the 21st century. Semin Radiat Oncol 2005; 15(1):42–8.

47. Søndergaard J, Holmberg M, Jakobsen AR, et al. A comparison of morbidity following conformal versus intensity-modulated radiotherapy for urinary bladder cancer. Acta Oncol 2014;1:1–8.

Perioperative Therapy for Muscle Invasive Bladder Cancer

Jeffrey J. Leow, MBBS, MPH[a,b,*,1], André P. Fay, MD[a,1], Stephanie A. Mullane, BS[a], Joaquim Bellmunt, MD, PhD[a,c]

KEYWORDS

- Urinary bladder neoplasms • Neoadjuvant therapy • Adjuvant therapy
- Chemotherapy • Radiotherapy • Radical cystectomy • Chemotherapy

KEY POINTS

- Bladder cancer has a high incidence of local and distant recurrence, which may be the result of micrometastatic disease at the time of localized treatment.
- Eradicating deposits of micrometastases from bladder cancer is best achieved via perioperative systemic neoadjuvant or adjuvant therapy.
- Postcystectomy nomograms and risk stratification help to identify patients who may benefit from adjuvant therapy.
- Use of platinum-based combination chemotherapy in the neoadjuvant setting improves survival. Adjuvant chemotherapy is also beneficial, although the evidence is less robust.
- Investigation of molecular pathways underlying bladder cancer has led to the discovery of genomic alterations, which may lead to the development of patient-specific therapies.

INTRODUCTION

Urothelial carcinoma (UC) of the bladder is the fourth most commonly diagnosed malignancy in the United States. About 20% to 30% of patients present with muscle invasive ($\geq$T2) bladder cancer (MIBC).[1] Initial treatment for most of these patients consists of localized therapy, including surgery or radiation; however, the risk of recurrence after localized therapy exceeds 50%,[2] and the 5-year mortality rate ranges from 33% to

Funding Sources: Nil.
Conflict of Interest: Nil.
[a] Bladder Cancer Center, Dana-Farber/Brigham and Women's Cancer Center, Harvard Medical School, 450 Brookline Avenue, Boston, MA 02215, USA; [b] Department of Urology, Tan Tock Seng Hospital, Singapore; [c] University Hospital del Mar-IMIM, Barcelona, Spain
[1] These authors contributed equally to this work.
* Corresponding author. Bladder Cancer Center, Dana-Farber/Brigham and Women's Cancer Center, Harvard Medical School, Boston, MA.
E-mail address: jeffrey.leow@mail.harvard.edu

Hematol Oncol Clin N Am 29 (2015) 301–318
http://dx.doi.org/10.1016/j.hoc.2014.11.002
0889-8588/15/$ – see front matter © 2015 Elsevier Inc. All rights reserved.

hemonc.theclinics.com

73%.[3] It is thought that the high incidence of local and distant recurrence is due to micrometastatic disease at the time of localized treatment. Therefore, perioperative systemic therapy is often used in the form of neoadjuvant or adjuvant therapy, with the goal of eradicating deposits of micrometastases.

Based on level I evidence (meta-analysis of randomized trials), the current gold standard for the treatment of MIBC is neoadjuvant cisplatin-based chemotherapy, followed by surgery, which shows an increased overall survival benefit of 5%.[4] Despite this evidence, recent studies have reported that this therapeutic strategy is still not widely used.[5]

Adjuvant treatment has increased survival in patients with different malignancies such as breast and colon cancer.[6,7] In MIBC, the role of adjuvant chemotherapy has been investigated throughout the last 3 decades, but the benefit still remains controversial. Most clinical trials evaluating the impact of adjuvant chemotherapy on MIBC have important methodological limitations, including small sample size, early termination owing to poor accrual, few events (deaths), and different chemotherapy regimens, leading to unequivocal results and few studies reporting a survival benefit.

This article discusses advantages and disadvantages of each therapeutic strategy, highlighting the most important studies supporting their use.

STRATIFICATION OF RISK AND PROGNOSTIC VARIABLES

Whereas there is strong evidence for the use of neoadjuvant chemotherapy in MIBC, there has been little information on the risk stratification of this group in the prelocalized treatment setting. In the meta-analysis of neoadjuvant trials performed in 2005, there was no specific risk stratification involving age, gender, clinical T or N stage, or performance status.[4]

The most widely used risk stratification in the precystectomy setting is staging. However, there is a large difference between clinical and pathologic staging at radical cystectomy (RC), with up to 54% of patients being upstaged[8] and 18% being downstaged at the time of surgery.[9] A nomogram designed to help predict pT3 or pT4 at RC was found to confer only a modest (4%) improvement over clinical staging alone.[10] Qureshi and colleagues[11] constructed an artificial neural network with 2 difference categories (Ta/T1 and T2–T4), using variables including genomic alterations, smoking status, gender, carcinoma in situ (CIS), metaplasia, architecture, and location of the tumor. This model predicted progression-free survival (PFS) and 1-year cancer-specific survival (CSS) at 80% and 82% accuracy, respectively. Catto and colleagues'[12] neuro–fuzzy models predicted recurrence-free survival (RFS) of Ta-T4 cases with 88% to 95% accuracy. The prediction model included p53, mismatch repair proteins, stage, grade, age, smoking status, and previous cancer. Although all of these models could be used to help identify patients who need neoadjuvant therapy, it has not proved to be better than clinical staging alone.

There have been multiple postcystectomy nomograms and risk stratifications that help identify patients who may benefit from adjuvant therapy.[13–18] Most prediction models include pathologic features from RC, including lymphovascular invasion (LVI), grade, and lymph node involvement, yet there is still only a minimal increase in accuracy of survival or recurrence compared with staging alone.

Karakiewicz and colleagues[13] created probability nomograms including age, T stage, N stage, grade, LVI, CIS, adjuvant radiotherapy, adjuvant chemotherapy, and neoadjuvant chemotherapy, which predict 2-, 5-, and 8-year RFS with 78% accuracy. Shariat and colleagues[14,15] had a similar probability nomogram, using the same categories as Karakiewicz, which predicted 2-, 5-, and 8-year overall survival (OS) and bladder CSS at 79% and 73% accuracy, respectively. Additional nomograms created by the groups of Bassi and Bochner[16,17] have been found to be able to predict 5-year RFS and 5-year OS at 75% and 76% accuracy, respectively.

One of the best markers for survival is a complete pathologic response (pT0). There is approximately a 15% complete response (CR) from transurethral resection alone, whereas there is about a 35% to 45% CR after neoadjuvant chemotherapy.[18] In the Southwest Oncology Group (SWOG) neoadjuvant trial, 85% of patients with pT0 were alive after 5 years of follow-up.[19]

Biomarkers to help predict response to therapy could possibly increase the CR rate. A 20-gene expression profile has been shown to predict advanced or metastatic UC; however, this requires further prospective validation before incorporating it into routine clinical practice.[20] The COXEN (CO eXpression ExtapolatioN) model has shown promise in the preclinical setting at predicting which cell lines will respond to gemcitabine/cisplatin or MVAC (methotrexate, vinblastine, doxorubicin, cisplatin) therapy. This model is currently being tested in a prospective clinical trial.[21] Recently, Van Allen and colleagues[22] found that mutations in ERCC2, a DNA damage repair protein, correlate with CR in patients receiving cisplatin-based combination neoadjuvant chemotherapy. There is a need to validate these markers and investigate additional novel prediction models in both precystectomy and postcystectomy settings.

NEOADJUVANT STRATEGIES FOR MUSCLE INVASIVE BLADDER CANCER
Advantages

Neoadjuvant chemotherapy has several advantages. The 2 main advantages are the ability to eradicate micrometastases early, and the potential to downstage chemotherapy sensitive tumors.[23] Approximately 38% of patients who are able to receive cisplatin combination chemotherapy have a pathologic CR, compared with the pathologic CR rate of 6% to 15% for patients who did not receive cisplatin-based combination neoadjuvant chemotherapy.[2,19,20] Pathologic CR has been shown to strongly predict outcomes, and is used as an important end point for patient prognosis.[23]

Disadvantages

There are some potential disadvantages to neoadjuvant chemotherapy. Because there are no validated ways to predict response to neoadjuvant chemotherapy, patients with chemoresistant bladder tumors who undergo neoadjuvant chemotherapy are inevitably delayed from receipt of a potentially curative surgical therapeutic option (ie, RC). This delay and its association with survival outcomes remain unclear. In addition, there is some concern that neoadjuvant chemotherapy may subsequently increase the risk of complications during RC, although this has recently been contended in population-based studies.[24,25]

Evidence Summary

Chemotherapy
Randomized clinical trials Multiple clinical trials have demonstrated the benefit of neoadjuvant chemotherapy (**Table 1**). The Nordic I trial included 311 patients with T1-T4NxM0 who were randomized to receive 2 cycles of cisplatin and doxorubicin versus no neoadjuvant treatment before RC. All patients received 20 Gy of irradiation before RC. There was no statistically significant difference in OS or CSS at 5 years. However, in a subgroup analysis of patients with pT3-T4 disease, a 15% survival benefit was seen in patients receiving chemotherapy.[26] In the Nordic II trial, 309 patients were randomized to receive 3 cycles of neoadjuvant cisplatin and methotrexate or to RC alone. Again, no overall significant difference in 5-year survival was seen

Table 1
Randomized trials for neoadjuvant therapy

Series	Study Population	Year	No. of Patients	Chemotherapy	Follow-up[a] (mo) (Range)	Overall Survival[b] (%)	Overall Survival HR (95% CI)	Significant (Yes/No)
Cortesi[74]	T2–T4, N0, M0	(Unpublished)	171	Cisplatin Methotrexate Epirubicin Vinblastine	—	52.4 vs 57.7	—	No
Wallace[75]	T2–T4, Nx, M0	1991	255[c]	Cisplatin	—	71.1 vs 65.8	1.13 (0.80–1.57)	No
Coppin[76]	T2–T4b	1996	102	Cisplatin	78	16 vs 13, $P = .34$	0.75 (90% CI 0.50–1.12)	No
Abol-Enein[77]	T2–T4a, Nx, M0	1997	196	Cisplatin Methotrexate Vinblastine	—	—	—	—
Martinez-Pineiro[78]	T2–T4a, Nx–N2, M0	1995	122	Cisplatin	78.2 (48–101)	35.5 vs 37.3	—	No
Italian Bladder Study (GISTV)[79]	T2–T4a	1996	206	Methotrexate Vinblastine Adriamycin Cisplatin	—	—	—	No
International Collaboration of Trialists[30]	T2–T4a, N0–x, M0	2011	976	Cisplatin Methotrexate Vinblastine	120	36 vs 30, $P = .037$	0.84 (0.72–0.99)	Yes

Study	Stage	Year	No. of patients	Regimen	Follow-up (mo)	Survival (%)	HR (95% CI)	Significant
Malmstrom[80] **Bassi**	T3–T4, N0 Any T, N+	1996	325	Cisplatin Doxorubicin	60	59 vs 51, $P = .1$	—	No
Bassi (GUONE)[81]	T2–T4b, N0-x, M0	2002	153	Cisplatin Methotrexate Vinblastine	—	52 vs 57.6	—	No
Sherif (Nordic II)[27]	T2–T4a, Nx, M0	2002	317	Cisplatin and methotrexate Cisplatin and adriamycin	56.4	56 vs 48	0.80 (0.64–0.99)	Yes
Grossman (SWOG Intergroup)[19]	T2–T4a	2003	317	Methotrexate Vinblastine Adriamycin Cisplatin	104	57 vs 43, $P = .06$	1.33 (1.00–1.76)	Yes

Abbreviations: CI, confidence interval; HR, hazard ratio.

[a] Mean or median follow-up time (in months) as reported by each study during time of publication. Types of range reported include minimum to maximum, interquartile range, and 95% confidence intervals.

[b] Based on number of events out of total number of patients in treatment (neoadjuvant) versus control arm (local treatment: radical cystectomy or radiotherapy).

[c] All 255 patients underwent neoadjuvant chemotherapy, but the control arm received local treatment in the form of radiotherapy in 2 different regimens: (1) 159 patients received 45–50 Gy in 22 fractions and (2) 96 patients received 65 Gy in 22 fractions + 10–15 Gy.

between the treatment groups (53%, neoadjuvant plus RC vs 46%, RC only).[27] One limitation to both Nordic trials is that they both used unconventional regimens that are uncommonly used in current practice (doxorubicin/cisplatin and methotrexate/cisplatin, respectively). However, a combined analysis of the 2 Nordic trials revealed an OS favoring neoadjuvant chemotherapy (5-year survival 56% vs 48%; $P = .049$), highlighting the efficacy of cisplatin-based neoadjuvant chemotherapy.[28]

The largest neoadjuvant prospective trial, published in 1999, included 976 patients (T2-T4N0) who were randomized to receive 3 cycles with the combination chemotherapy regimen of cisplatin, methotrexate, and vinblastine (CMV) or no systemic therapy. Patients were then treated with 1 of the following local therapies: (1) radiation therapy (RT), (2) a combination of low-dose radiotherapy and RC, or (3) RC alone.[29] Although the trial did not initially demonstrate statistical significance in survival, a long-term update, presented in 2002, demonstrated a 10-year OS benefit credited to neoadjuvant chemotherapy (36% vs 30%; hazard ratio [HR] 0.84).[30] The type of localized treatment did not change the survival outcomes. Pathologic CR was attained in 32.5% of patients receiving neoadjuvant therapy, versus 12.3% with RC alone.[30]

The SWOG performed a prospective, randomized controlled trial of 317 patients with T2-T4aN0M0 UC comparing 3 cycles of neoadjuvant MVAC chemotherapy preceding RC with RC alone. Although the trial did not show a statistically significant advantage for neoadjuvant therapy with 5-year OS (57% vs 43%; $P = .06$) or median survival (77 vs 46 mo), the trial is still considered to demonstrate level I superiority of neoadjuvant therapy because the original goal of statistically significant difference, defined as a one-sided $P<.05$, was attained. Patients receiving neoadjuvant therapy had a CR rate of 38%, compared with 15% with RC alone. Most patients (81%–82%) were able to proceed to cystectomy after receiving neoadjuvant chemotherapy. Toxicities of chemotherapy were manageable, with no toxic deaths, grade 4 neutropenia seen in 33%, and grade 3 gastrointestinal toxicities seen in 17%. No increase in postoperative complications was observed.[20]

Finally, single-agent platinum did not yield significantly better outcomes. No single platinum-based combination regimen combined with any local therapy (RC alone, radiotherapy alone, or radiotherapy in combination with RC) has demonstrated superiority over only localized therapy. Cisplatin tends to be the platinum agent used in most patients (>90%), with carboplatin used only in 6% to 7% of patients, owing to carboplatin being shown to be significantly inferior to cisplatin-based treatment.[31]

Nonrandomized prospective and retrospective studies The 2 main neoadjuvant chemotherapy regimens, gemcitabine-cisplatin (GC) and MVAC, have only been compared in retrospective studies. Current data suggest similar rates of pathologic CR and survival outcomes with both regimens (relative risk of CR 0.97, 95% confidence interval [CI] 0.60–1.56; $P = .9$).[32]

Dose-dense MVAC is being used more frequently in the neoadjuvant setting. A phase II study explored the efficacy and safety of this regimen with pegfilgrastim support in patients with muscle-invasive UC. Neoadjuvant chemotherapy resulted in significant pathologic and radiologic downstaging (49% achieved CR defined as ≤ pT1N0M0) with a favorable toxicity profile.[33] One advantage of this strategy is the short time to complete the 4 cycles of therapy, thus not delaying surgical treatment in patients who are not sensitive to systemic chemotherapy. Dose-dense therapy is being increasingly investigated by centers of excellence, particularly for bladder UC, and may also be a promising alternative to GC for high-grade upper tract urothelial carcinoma (UTUC).[34]

Meta-analysis The pooling of data from the aforementioned randomized clinical trials using meta-analysis statistical techniques has allowed us to advance our understanding regarding the true utility of neoadjuvant chemotherapy in bladder cancer, in addition to statistically increasing the total number of patients in both arms. The latest published meta-analysis of 11 randomized trials was performed by the Advanced Bladder Cancer Meta-Analysis Collaboration, and included 3005 patients. There was a significant survival benefit (HR 0.86, 95% CI 0.77–0.95; P = .003) among those who received neoadjuvant cisplatin-based chemotherapy, compared with those who did not; this translated into a 5% absolute increase in 5-year OS and a 9% absolute increase in 5-year disease-free survival (DFS) in comparison with RC alone.[4] Given this demonstrated survival benefit, in 2012 the National Comprehensive Cancer Network Guidelines recommend the use of neoadjuvant platinum-based combination chemotherapy for cT2 and strongly recommend it for cT3 node-negative disease,[35] similar to guidelines from the European Association of Urology[36] and European Society of Medical Oncology.[37]

At present, there is no effective regimen for patients with poor performance status and/or renal inefficiencies. There has been a meta-analysis comparing carboplatin-based with cisplatin-based chemotherapy regimens, with cisplatin-based therapies showing clear superiority (relative risk 3.54; P = .005).[31]

Radiation therapy

UC is relatively radiosensitive, and in the neoadjuvant setting RT may be able to prevent intraoperative seeding of tumor cells in the operative field and to sterilize microscopic extension in the perivesical tissues. There exists only one randomized trial demonstrating the superiority of preoperative radiotherapy over cystectomy alone in 2-year OS in patients with T3 bladder cancer.[38,39] Studies performed in the 1980s investigated the role of preoperative radiotherapy in either T2 or all stages of bladder cancer, and no marked benefits were found. One of the more recent studies was a phase III trial in the United States, which had a total of 140 patients who were randomized to receive 2000 Gy of pelvic irradiation followed by RC within 1 week, or RC alone. The 5-year survival rates were 43% (95% CI 30%–56%) and 53% (95% CI 41%–65%), respectively (P = .23).[40] Since then, research into this treatment modality has stagnated. In the contemporary management of bladder cancer, the role of RT in the neoadjuvant setting seems limited. With recent advances in the use of more targeted radiotherapies such as intensity-modulated RT, which has been shown in some studies to significantly reduce the volume of normal tissues affected while treating a variety of abdominopelvic tumors, neoadjuvant radiotherapy may resurface as a potential investigative option for patients with bladder cancer.[41,42]

ADJUVANT STRATEGIES FOR MUSCLE INVASIVE BLADDER CANCER
Advantages

The major advantage of administering adjuvant treatment is the appropriate patient selection according to the risk of recurrence. The adequate pathologic staging reduces the risk of overtreatment and allows for the selection of patients most likely to benefit from systemic therapy.[43] A large retrospective cohort evaluated discrepancies in clinical and pathologic staging in patients who underwent RC for MIBC. Clinical understaging was identified in approximately 50% of the patients, and pathologic downstaging occurred in 18%.[9]

Adjuvant chemotherapy does not delay local treatment for patients with chemoresistant tumors. Moreover, when neoadjuvant was compared with adjuvant chemotherapy, there were no differences in perioperative morbidity.[44] Therefore, adjuvant therapy certainly has its place in contemporary management.

Disadvantages

The major disadvantage to adjuvant treatment is delaying the treatment of micrometastatic disease. In addition, response to treatment measured by pathologic downstaging may provide important prognostic information.[45] With adjuvant chemotherapy, the only way to assess the benefit of this treatment is the absence of disease progression during long-term follow-up.

Another potential disadvantage is the possibility of postsurgical complications that may preclude patients from receiving adjuvant cisplatin-based chemotherapy. Donat and colleagues[46] have found at their high-volume tertiary center that nearly one-third (30%) of patients develop complications after RC of Clavien grade 2 or higher. Although surgical morbidity at their center may reflect the more complicated case mix they encounter, this highlights the importance of considering contributors to postoperative morbidity, as this may delay the administration of adjuvant chemotherapy.

Summary of Evidence

Chemotherapy

Randomized clinical trials Several randomized clinical trials attempted to define the role of adjuvant treatment in MIBC (**Table 2**). In 1994, Studer and colleagues[47] reported the results of a study designed to evaluate the role of adjuvant cisplatin monotherapy after RC. Seventy-seven patients with nonmetastatic MIBC were stratified based on nodal status (stage pN0 vs pN1–N2) and were randomly assigned to observation or adjuvant chemotherapy. In this study, no differences in OS were observed between the 2 groups in patients with all disease stages. Similarly, patients who had pN1-N2 did not benefit from the adjuvant treatment.[47]

Skinner and colleagues[48] randomized 91 patients with T3/T4 or positive lymph node MIBC to receive adjuvant cisplatin, doxorubicin, and cyclophosphamide or to observation after RC. In this study, median OS was 4.3 years for patients who received chemotherapy versus 2.4 years in the observation group ($P = .0062$). Of note, these results could be explained by several methodological biases.[48]

A German phase III clinical trial showed a benefit in OS and PFS with adjuvant chemotherapy (MVAC or MVEC [methotrexate, vinblastine, epirubicin, cisplatin]). This study was prematurely closed because of suggested striking benefits of adjuvant chemotherapy, so only a small number of patients was included in the final analysis. Of note, patients assigned to the observation arm did not receive any further treatment at the time of recurrence. By contrast, another German study showed that patients treated with adjuvant MVEC versus observation did not show significant differences in OS.[49]

Another clinical trial compared 2 neoadjuvant cycles followed by 3 adjuvant cycles after RC versus 5 adjuvant cycles of MVAC. This study enrolled 140 patients and suggested that neoadjuvant chemotherapy may be more feasible than adjuvant chemotherapy, although no difference in survival outcome was demonstrated.[44]

Recently, trials using cisplatin/gemcitabine-based regimens in the adjuvant setting were performed, based on results of this regimen in the metastatic setting. The prospective Italian trial of 194 patients was underpowered to demonstrate a survival difference in patients receiving 4 cycles of adjuvant GC (HR 1.29).[50] The Spanish Oncology Genitourinary Group trial randomized 340 patients with high-risk disease (T3–T4 or lymph node positive) to receive 4 cycles of paclitaxel, gemcitabine, and cisplatin (PCG) versus observation. Adjuvant PCG resulted in a significant increase in OS compared with no chemotherapy (60% vs 31%, HR 0.44).[51] Of note, both trials were prematurely closed, and the power of these analyses limits the conclusion regarding the efficacy of this strategy.

A biomarker-driven clinical trial, based on altered p53 levels, randomized patients with organ-confined disease (pT1 or pT2, N0M0) to 3 cycles of MVAC versus observation. No statistically significant difference in clinical outcome was identified based on p53 status.[52]

Most recently, the results of the European Organization for Research and Treatment of Cancer (EORTC) intergroup randomized phase III clinical trial was presented. The study's initial plan was to enroll a total of 1344 patients with MIBC to receive 4 cycles of adjuvant chemotherapy according to physician choice (GC, MVAC, or dose-dense MVAC) versus 6 cycles of deferred therapy at the time of recurrence. The trial was prematurely closed after enrollment of 284 patients with pT3-T4 and/or lymph node–positive and M0 disease. Adjuvant chemotherapy resulted in a statistically significant difference in PFS: 46.8% in the adjuvant treatment arm versus 29.5% in patients in the deferred arm. However, the median OS (primary end point) was 53.6% for patients who received immediate treatment versus 47.7% for patients in the deferred chemotherapy group (HR 0.78, 95% CI 0.56–1.10; $P = .13$).[53]

Nonrandomized prospective and retrospective studies Logothesis and colleagues[54] are among the first to report the impact of adjuvant chemotherapy in patients with MIBC. In this study, 71 patients presenting with pT3b, pT4, N1, or vascular/lymphatic invasion were treated with cisplatin, cyclophosphamide, and adriamycin. The 5-year survival rate for patients treated with this strategy was 70%, compared with 37% for those patients who were part of a historical control treated with surgery alone. Similar results in terms of long-term survival were reported from another study in which adjuvant CMV (n = 23) was compared with the same drugs plus doxorubicin (n = 12).[55] These studies supported the rationale for randomized investigation of this therapeutic strategy.

A large retrospective study evaluated 932 patients from 11 centers who received adjuvant chemotherapy after RC, and found that adjuvant chemotherapy was independently associated with longer OS (HR 0.83, 95% CI 0.72–0.97; $P = .017$). As expected, the benefit was higher in patients who presented both pT3 stage and lymph node–positive disease (HR 0.75, 95% CI 0.62–0.90; $P = .002$).[56]

Meta-analysis As the results from the prospective randomized clinical trials were not definitive and have several methodological limitations, meta-analyses have been conducted to help interpret the available data. The Advanced Bladder Cancer Meta-Analysis Collaboration conducted a meta-analysis with individual patient data from 491 patients enrolled in 6 studies. In this analysis, patients who were treated with adjuvant chemotherapy had a relative reduction in the risk of death of 25%.[57]

Recently, a study-level meta-analysis of 9 randomized trials including 945 patients was published.[58] In this updated analysis, patients receiving adjuvant treatment with cisplatin-based regimens had a DFS benefit (HR 0.66, 95% CI 0.45–0.91, $P = .014$) and OS benefit (HR 0.78, 95% CI 0.61–0.99; $P = .044$) compared with those who underwent RC alone. Moreover, lymph node–positive patients seem to have greater benefit with this strategy. Interpretation of these results should be taken cautiously, as individual patient data were not analyzed.[59–61] Therefore, the next study to look out for will be an updated individual patient data meta-analysis including the latest EORTC intergroup study, as the pooled HR is likely to demonstrate OS benefit for adjuvant chemotherapy. Such findings may influence clinical practice substantially.

Radiation therapy

RT has no well-established role in the adjuvant setting. Although the rationale of decreasing local recurrences may lead to subsequently lower rates of distant disease,

Table 2
Randomized trials for adjuvant therapy

Series	Year	Study Population	No. of Patients Total	Treatment Arm (Chemotherapy Regimen)	Control Arm (Locoregional Treatment)	Follow-Up (mo) (Range)[a]	Overall Survival (%)	Overall Survival HR (95% CI)	Significance (Yes/No)
Freiha[82]	1996	T3–T4, Any N	55	Cisplatin and methotrexate Vinblastine	Radical cystectomy	62 (24–96)	63 vs 36	0.74 (0.36–1.53)	No
Otto[83]	2001	T3/N1–N22	108	Methotrexate Vinblastine Epirubicin Cisplatin	Radical cystectomy	44	50.9 vs 54.7	0.82 (0.48–1.38)	No
Skinner[48]	1991	T3–T4, N0	102	Patients 1–17: 16 cisplatin-based, in combinations with doxorubicin, cyclophosphamide, 5-fluorouracil, vinblastine, or bleomycin Patients 18–91: Cisplatin, doxorubicin, cyclophosphamide	Radical cystectomy	—	51.6 vs 28.8	0.75 (0.48–1.19)	Yes

(the rows for "Skinner[48]" also list: Any T, N+)

Lehmann[84]	2006	Any T, N+ T3–T4, Any N	49	MVAC or MVEC (1 patient received carboplatin instead of cisplatin)	Radical cystectomy	120	17.4 vs 26.9	1.75 (0.95–3.23)	No
Studer[47]	1994	Any T, Any N	91	Cisplatin	Radical cystectomy	69 (36–96)	57 vs 54	1.02 (0.57–1.84)	No
Stadler[52]	2011	T1–T2, N0 p53+	114	Methotrexate Vinblastine Doxorubicin Cisplatin	Radical cystectomy	64.8 (61.2–70.8)	20.7 vs 16.1	1.11 (0.45–2.72)	No
Italian trial[50]	2012	T2 (grade 3) T3–T4, N0–N2	194	Gemcitabine Cisplatin	Radical cystectomy	35 (15–57)	46.6 vs 39.9	1.29 (0.84–1.99)	No
Spanish trial[51]	2010	T3–T4, N0 Any T, N+	142	Paclitaxel Gemcitabine Cisplatin	Radical cystectomy	29.8 (1–95)	60 vs 31	0.38 (0.22–0.65)	Yes
EORTC Intergroup Trial[53]	2014	T3–T4, N0 Any T, N+	284	Gemcitabine, cisplatin or MVAC or High-dose MVAC	Radical cystectomy	83.6 (-) vs 86.5 (-)	53.6 vs 47.7	0.78 (0.56–1.08)	No

Abbreviations: EORTC, European Organization for Research and Treatment of Cancer; MVAC, methotrexate, vinblastine, doxorubicin, cisplatin; MVEC, methotrexate, vinblastine, epirubicin, cisplatin.

[a] Mean or median follow-up time (in months) as reported by each study during time of publication. Types of range reported include minimum to maximum, interquartile range, and 95% confidence intervals.

the use of RT after an RC has resulted in suboptimal results and has been associated with higher toxicity levels.

A small randomized trial showed that adjuvant radiotherapy may improve both local control and DFS in comparison with surgery alone.[62] In addition, a retrospective study reported similar results.[63] Results of a phase III randomized clinical trial were reported in 2006 at the American Society of Clinical Oncology Annual Meeting, whereby no statistical differences were observed in DFS rates in high-risk patients with bladder cancer who received adjuvant chemoradiation with cisplatin plus gemcitabine versus radiation alone.[64]

Regarding the limitations of these studies, further evaluation and a better characterization of patients who may benefit from this therapy are warranted. Similarly to the neoadjuvant setting, modern RT techniques may have a role in improving the toxicity profile and adding clinical benefit.

MOLECULAR BIOLOGY AND TARGETED THERAPIES

Our understanding of the molecular pathways underlying bladder cancer has benefited from recent advances in technologies such as high-throughput transcript profiling, microarrays, metabolomics, and proteomics. Intense research efforts in this area have borne fruit through the discovery of numerous molecular markers. These markers may be useful for screening, early diagnosis, and surveillance in addition to staging and prognosis.[65] Leading the effort is The Cancer Genome Atlas project (TCGA), which has identified potential therapeutic targets in 69% of UC tumors, including pathways suitable for further investigation.[66] It has been estimated that at least 60% of genomic alterations could be treated by drugs that are already available or under clinical testing.[67] Some potential new targets for treatment intervention have been described for UC, including the most recurrent reported mutations in the receptor tyrosine kinases (*RTK*)-*RAS-RAF*, phosphoinositide 3-kinase (*PI3K*)/*AKT*/mammalian target of rapamycin pathways (mTOR), and regulators of G1-S cell cycle progression such as TP53 and RB1.[67]

Other potential therapeutic targets lie in the mutation and/or gene amplifications present in a large proportion of urothelial tumors, including *FGFR3* mutations,[68] *PTEN* deletions, and *FGFR1*, *CCND1*, and *MDM2* amplifications.[66] More than half of UC have also been found to contain aberrations of the chromatin remodeling genes (*UTX*, *MLL-MLL3*, *CREBBP-EP300*, *NCOR1*, *ARID1A*, and *CHD6*) and, more recently, *STAG2* mutations.[67,69] Nevertheless, it must be cautioned that the functional effect of mutations in these genes encoding epigenomic regulatory proteins remains relatively unknown. It may be possible that identifying these driving genomic alterations, even if occurring in only a small subset of patients with bladder cancer, may lead to the development of patient-specific therapies. For example, recently described mutations in *TSC1* were useful in helping investigators examine the response to mTOR inhibitors such as everolimus, or in the *PIK3CA* gene, mutated in up to 26% of cases, which may predict sensitivity to *PIK3CA*/mTOR inhibitors.[70–73] Cancer immunotherapy also represents an exciting avenue for research, with the Food and Drug Administration recently granting "Breakthrough Therapy Designation" for MPDL3280A (anti-PDL1) in bladder cancer.

ONGOING CLINICAL TRIALS

Several clinical investigations have also been performed to address some open questions in the neoadjuvant and adjuvant treatment scenarios. A phase III trial clinical trial of GC versus high-dose intensity MVAC, with regimen selection decisions driven by genomic profile, will help to define the optimal chemotherapy regimen in the perioperative setting for patients with locally advanced UC (NCT01812369). In addition, the role of taxanes in the neoadjuvant setting is being evaluated in a phase I study consisting of administering 4 cycles of cabazitaxel and cisplatin before RC. The study's primary end point is response rate (NCT01616875). In the adjuvant setting, a German phase III study was designed to evaluate gemcitabine alone versus nontreatment in the control arm in a subset of patients who are not suitable for cisplatin-based chemotherapy (NCT00146276). This study, like the previous studies in the adjuvant setting, was closed because of poor accrual, but can still be valuable. Another study is evaluating the impact of an immunotherapeutic agent recMAGE-A3 + AS-15 in patients with MIBC who were surgically treated and are positive for the antigen MAGE-A3 (MAGNOLIA) (NCT01435356). Finally, a randomized phase II study is evaluating DN24-02 (a Her2 targeting autologous antigen-presenting cell-based vaccine) as adjuvant therapy in subjects with high-risk HER2+ UC.

SUMMARY AND FUTURE DIRECTIONS

MIBC is an aggressive disease associated with poor survival rates. Although RC alone may result in cure for a subset of patients, the higher rates of relapse suggest that early administration of systemic therapy may improve clinical outcomes. Therefore, contemporary management of patients with MIBC involves the combination of surgery, systemic chemotherapy, and chemoradiation in select patients who are candidates for bladder preservation.

Neoadjuvant treatment with cisplatin-based combination regimens is an established standard of care and has improved long-term survival in MIBC. However, owing to the low rates of adoption of neoadjuvant chemotherapy, clinicians will still face the decision of whether to administer adjuvant chemotherapy to high-risk patients who have not received neoadjuvant chemotherapy. In the absence of definitive evidence justifying the recommendation of adjuvant chemotherapy, administering systemic therapy after an RC in high-risk patients is still an option if clinical trials are not available.

In the genomic era, the biology underlying MIBC has been elucidated. The TCGA has characterized genes and molecular pathways involved in cancer development and tumor progression, providing insights to improve the therapeutic arsenal. In addition, these results may add to the development of biomarkers to select patients for the available or new therapies. Of importance is that immunotherapy strategies have produced encouraging results in patients with advanced disease. However, how this new knowledge will affect the perioperative treatment in MIBC is still undefined, and efforts should be undertaken to integrate molecular aspects in innovative clinical trial designs in this setting.

REFERENCES

1. Siegel R, Naishadham D, Jemal A. Cancer statistics, 2013. CA Cancer J Clin 2013;63:11–30.
2. Stein JP, Lieskovsky G, Cote R, et al. Radical cystectomy in the treatment of invasive bladder cancer: long-term results in 1,054 patients. J Clin Oncol 2001;19: 666–75.
3. Herr HW, Dotan Z, Donat SM, et al. Defining optimal therapy for muscle invasive bladder cancer. J Urol 2007;177:437–43.
4. Vale CL. Neoadjuvant chemotherapy in invasive bladder cancer: update of a systematic review and meta-analysis of individual patient data. Eur Urol 2005;48: 202–6.

5. Reardon ZD, Patel SG, Zaid HB, et al. Trends in the use of perioperative chemotherapy for localized and locally advanced muscle-invasive bladder cancer: a sign of changing tides. Eur Urol 2014. http://dx.doi.org/10.1016/j.eururo.2014.01.009.

6. Early Breast Cancer Trialists' Collaborative Group, Peto R, Davies C, et al. Comparisons between different polychemotherapy regimens for early breast cancer: meta-analyses of long-term outcome among 100,000 women in 123 randomised trials. Lancet 2012;379:432–44.

7. Labianca R, Nordlinger B, Beretta GD, et al. Early colon cancer: ESMO Clinical Practice Guidelines for diagnosis, treatment and follow-up. Ann Oncol 2013; 24(Suppl 6):vi64–72.

8. Mitra AP, Datar RH, Cote RJ. Molecular pathways in invasive bladder cancer: new insights into mechanisms, progression, and target identification. J Clin Oncol 2006;24:5552–64.

9. Svatek RS, Shariat SF, Novara G, et al. Discrepancy between clinical and pathological stage: external validation of the impact on prognosis in an international radical cystectomy cohort. BJU Int 2011;107:898–904.

10. Karakiewicz PI, Shariat SF, Palapattu GS, et al. Precystectomy nomogram for prediction of advanced bladder cancer stage. Eur Urol 2006;50:1254–60 [discussion: 1261–2].

11. Qureshi KN, Naguib RN, Hamdy FC, et al. Neural network analysis of clinicopathological and molecular markers in bladder cancer. J Urol 2000;163: 630–3.

12. Catto JW, Linkens DA, Abbod MF, et al. Artificial intelligence in predicting bladder cancer outcome: a comparison of neuro-fuzzy modeling and artificial neural networks. Clin Cancer Res 2003;9(11):4172–7.

13. Karakiewicz PI, Shariat SF, Palapattu GS, et al. Nomogram for predicting disease recurrence after radical cystectomy for transitional cell carcinoma of the bladder. J Urol 2006;176:1354–61 [discussion: 1361–2].

14. Shariat SF, Margulis V, Lotan Y, et al. Nomograms for bladder cancer. Eur Urol 2008;54:41–53.

15. Shariat SF, Karakiewicz PI, Palapattu GS, et al. Nomograms provide improved accuracy for predicting survival after radical cystectomy. Clin Cancer Res 2006;12:6663–76.

16. Bassi P, Sacco E, De Marco V, et al. Prognostic accuracy of an artificial neural network in patients undergoing radical cystectomy for bladder cancer: a comparison with logistic regression analysis. BJU Int 2007;99:1007–12.

17. International Bladder Cancer Nomogram Consortium, Bochner BH, Kattan MW, Vora KC. Postoperative nomogram predicting risk of recurrence after radical cystectomy for bladder cancer. J Clin Oncol 2006;24:3967–72.

18. Tollefson MK, Boorjian SA, Farmer SA, et al. Downstaging to non-invasive urothelial carcinoma is associated with improved outcome following radical cystectomy for patients with cT2 disease. World J Urol 2012;30:795–9.

19. Grossman HB, Natale RB, Tangen CM, et al. Neoadjuvant chemotherapy plus cystectomy compared with cystectomy alone for locally advanced bladder cancer. N Engl J Med 2003;349:859–66.

20. Dancik G, Aisner D, Theodorescu DA. 20 gene model for predicting nodal involvement in bladder cancer patients with muscle invasive tumors. PLoS Curr 2011;3:RRN1248.

21. Smith SC, Baras AS, Lee JK, et al. The COXEN principle: translating signatures of in vitro chemosensitivity into tools for clinical outcome prediction and drug discovery in cancer. Cancer Res 2010;70(5):1753–8.

22. Van Allen EM, Mouw KW, Kim P, et al. Somatic ERCC2 mutations correlate with cisplatin sensitivity in muscle-invasive urothelial carcinoma. Cancer Discov 2014; 4:1140–53.
23. Rosenblatt R, Sherif A, Rintala E, et al. Pathologic downstaging is a surrogate marker for efficacy and increased survival following neoadjuvant chemotherapy and radical cystectomy for muscle-invasive urothelial bladder cancer. Eur Urol 2012;61:1229–38.
24. Johnson DC, Nielsen ME, Matthews J, et al. Neoadjuvant chemotherapy for bladder cancer does not increase risk of perioperative morbidity. BJU Int 2014; 114:221–8.
25. Gandaglia G, Popa I, Abdollah F, et al. The effect of neoadjuvant chemotherapy on perioperative outcomes in patients who have bladder cancer treated with radical cystectomy: a population-based study. Eur Urol 2014. http://dx.doi.org/10.1016/j.eururo.2014.01.014.
26. Hellsten S, Rintala E, Wahlqvist R, et al. Nordic prospective trials of radical cystectomy and neoadjuvant chemotherapy. The Nordic Cooperative Bladder Cancer Study Group. Eur Urol 1998;33(Suppl 4):35–8.
27. Sherif A, Rintala E, Mestad O, et al. Neoadjuvant cisplatin-methotrexate chemotherapy for invasive bladder cancer—Nordic Cystectomy Trial 2. Scand J Urol Nephrol 2002;36:419–25.
28. Sherif A, Holmberg L, Rintala E, et al. Neoadjuvant cisplatinum based combination chemotherapy in patients with invasive bladder cancer: a combined analysis of two Nordic studies. Eur Urol 2004;45:297–303.
29. Neoadjuvant cisplatin, methotrexate, and vinblastine chemotherapy for muscle-invasive bladder cancer: a randomised controlled trial. International collaboration of trialists. Lancet 1999;354:533–40.
30. International Collaboration of Trialists, Medical Research Council Advanced Bladder Cancer Working Party (now the National Cancer Research Institute Bladder Cancer Clinical Studies Group), European Organisation for Research and Treatment of Cancer Genito-Urinary Tract Cancer Group, et al. International phase III trial assessing neoadjuvant cisplatin, methotrexate, and vinblastine chemotherapy for muscle-invasive bladder cancer: long-term results of the BA06 30894 trial. J Clin Oncol 2011;29:2171–7.
31. Galsky MD, Chen GJ, Oh WK, et al. Comparative effectiveness of cisplatin-based and carboplatin-based chemotherapy for treatment of advanced urothelial carcinoma. Ann Oncol 2012;23:406–10.
32. Yeshchina O, Badalato GM, Wosnitzer MS, et al. Relative efficacy of perioperative gemcitabine and cisplatin versus methotrexate, vinblastine, adriamycin, and cisplatin in the management of locally advanced urothelial carcinoma of the bladder. Urology 2012;79:384.
33. Choueiri TK, Jacobus S, Bellmunt J, et al. Neoadjuvant dose-dense methotrexate, vinblastine, doxorubicin, and cisplatin with pegfilgrastim support in muscle-invasive urothelial cancer: pathologic, radiologic, and biomarker correlates. J Clin Oncol 2014;32:1889–94.
34. Apolo AB, Kim JW, Bochner BH, et al. Examining the management of muscle-invasive bladder cancer by medical oncologists in the United States. Urol Oncol 2014;32:637–44.
35. Clark PE, Agarwal N, Biagioli MC, et al. Bladder cancer. J Natl Compr Canc Netw 2013;11(4):446–75.
36. Witjes JA, Comperat E, Cowan NC, et al. EAU guidelines on muscle-invasive and metastatic bladder cancer: summary of the 2013 guidelines. Eur Urol 2014;65:778–92.

37. Bellmunt J, Orsola A, Leow JJ, et al. Bladder cancer: ESMO practice guidelines for diagnosis, treatment and follow-up. Ann Oncol 2014. http://dx.doi.org/10.1093/annonc/mdu223.

38. Zaghloul MS. Adjuvant and neoadjuvant radiotherapy for bladder cancer: revisited. Future Oncol 2010;6:1177–91.

39. Caldwell WL. Preoperative irradiation of patients with T3 carcinoma in bilharzial bladder. Int J Radiat Oncol Biol Phys 1979;5:1007–8.

40. Smith JA, Crawford ED, Paradelo JC, et al. Treatment of advanced bladder cancer with combined preoperative irradiation and radical cystectomy versus radical cystectomy alone: a phase III intergroup study. J Urol 1997;157:805–7 [discussion: 807–8].

41. Murthy V, Zaghloul MS. Adjuvant radiotherapy in bladder cancer: time to take a fresh look? Urol Oncol 2007;25:353–4.

42. Troiano M, Corsa P, Raguso A, et al. Radiation therapy in urinary cancer: state of the art and perspective. Radiol Med 2009;114:70–82.

43. Sternberg CN, Bellmunt J, Sonpavde G, et al. ICUD-EAU International Consultation on Bladder Cancer 2012: chemotherapy for urothelial carcinoma-neoadjuvant and adjuvant settings. Eur Urol 2013;63:58–66.

44. Millikan R, Dinney C, Swanson D, et al. Integrated therapy for locally advanced bladder cancer: final report of a randomized trial of cystectomy plus adjuvant M-VAC versus cystectomy with both preoperative and postoperative M-VAC. J Clin Oncol 2001;19:4005–13.

45. Schultz PK, Herr HW, Zhang ZF, et al. Neoadjuvant chemotherapy for invasive bladder cancer: prognostic factors for survival of patients treated with M-VAC with 5-year follow-up. J Clin Oncol 1994;12:1394–401.

46. Donat SM, Shabsigh A, Savage C, et al. Potential impact of postoperative early complications on the timing of adjuvant chemotherapy in patients undergoing radical cystectomy: a high-volume tertiary cancer center experience. Eur Urol 2009;55:177–85.

47. Studer UE, Bacchi M, Biedermann C, et al. Adjuvant cisplatin chemotherapy following cystectomy for bladder cancer: results of a prospective randomized trial. J Urol 1994;152:81–4.

48. Skinner DG, Daniels JR, Russell CA, et al. The role of adjuvant chemotherapy following cystectomy for invasive bladder cancer: a prospective comparative trial. J Urol 1991;145(3):459–64.

49. Stockle M, Meyenburg W, Wellek S, et al. Adjuvant polychemotherapy of nonorgan-confined bladder cancer after radical cystectomy revisited: long-term results of a controlled prospective study and further clinical experience. J Urol 1995;153:47–52.

50. Cognetti F, Ruggeri EM, Felici A, et al. Adjuvant chemotherapy with cisplatin and gemcitabine versus chemotherapy at relapse in patients with muscle-invasive bladder cancer submitted to radical cystectomy: an Italian, multicenter, randomized phase III trial. Ann Oncol 2012;23:695–700.

51. Paz-Ares L, Solsona E, Esteban E, et al. Randomized phase III trial comparing adjuvant paclitaxel/gemcitabine/cisplatin (PGC) to observation in patients with resected invasive bladder cancer: Results of the Spanish Oncology Genitourinary Group (SOGUG) 99/01 study. J Clin Oncol 28:18s, 2010 (suppl; abstr LBA4518) Available at: http://meetinglibrary.asco.org/content/51401-74.

52. Stadler WM, Lerner SP, Groshen S, et al. Phase III study of molecularly targeted adjuvant therapy in locally advanced urothelial cancer of the bladder based on p53 status. J Clin Oncol 2011;29:3443–9.

53. Sternberg CN, Skoneczna I, Kerst JM, et al. Final results of EORTC intergroup randomized phase III trial comparing immediate versus deferred chemotherapy after radical cystectomy in patients with pT3T4 and/or N+ M0 transitional cell carcinoma (TCC) of the bladder. J Clin Oncol 2014;32(Suppl 5):4500. Available at: http://meetinglibrary.asco.org/content/130351-144.
54. Logothetis CJ, Dexeus FH, Chong C, et al. Cisplatin, cyclophosphamide and doxorubicin chemotherapy for unresectable urothelial tumors: the M.D. Anderson experience. J Urol 1989;141:33–7.
55. Michael M, Tannock IF, Czaykowski PM, et al. Adjuvant chemotherapy for high-risk urothelial transitional cell carcinoma: the Princess Margaret Hospital experience. Br J Urol 1998;82:366–72.
56. Svatek RS, Shariat SF, Lasky RE, et al. The effectiveness of off-protocol adjuvant chemotherapy for patients with urothelial carcinoma of the urinary bladder. Clin Cancer Res 2010;16:4461–7.
57. Advanced Bladder Cancer (ABC) Meta-analysis Collaboration. Adjuvant chemotherapy in invasive bladder cancer: a systematic review and meta-analysis of individual patient data Advanced Bladder Cancer (ABC) Meta-analysis Collaboration. Eur Urol 2005;48:189–99 [discussion: 199–201].
58. Leow JJ, Martin-Doyle W, Rajagopal PS, et al. Adjuvant chemotherapy for invasive bladder cancer: a 2013 updated systematic review and meta-analysis of randomized trials. Eur Urol 2014;66:42–54.
59. Raghavan D, Bawtinhimer A, Mahoney J, et al. Adjuvant chemotherapy for bladder cancer—why does level 1 evidence not support it? Ann Oncol 2014; 25:1930–4.
60. Leow JJ, Chang SL, Bellmunt J. Reply from authors re: Cora N. Sternberg, Richard Sylvester. Thoughts on a Systematic Review and Meta-analysis of Adjuvant Chemotherapy in Muscle-invasive Bladder Cancer. Eur Urol 2014;66:55–6. Eur Urol 2014;66:57–8.
61. Sternberg CN, Sylvester R. Thoughts on a systematic review and meta-analysis of adjuvant chemotherapy in muscle-invasive bladder cancer. Eur Urol 2014;66: 55–6.
62. Zaghloul MS, Awwad HK, Akoush HH, et al. Postoperative radiotherapy of carcinoma in bilharzial bladder: improved disease free survival through improving local control. Int J Radiat Oncol Biol Phys 1992;23:511–7.
63. Reisinger SA, Mohiuddin M, Mulholland SG. Combined pre- and postoperative adjuvant radiation therapy for bladder cancer–a ten year experience. Int J Radiat Oncol Biol Phys 1992;24:463–8.
64. James ND, Hussain SA, Hall E, et al. Results of a phase III randomized trial of synchronous chemoradiotherapy (CRT) compared to radiotherapy (RT) alone in muscle-invasive bladder cancer (MIBC) (BC2001 CRUK/01/004). J Clin Oncol 28:15s, 2010 (suppl; abstr 4517). Available at: http://meetinglibrary.asco.org/content/40892-74.
65. Kamat AM, Hegarty PK, Gee JR, et al. ICUD-EAU International Consultation on Bladder Cancer 2012: screening, diagnosis, and molecular markers. Eur Urol 2013;63:4–15.
66. Cancer Genome Atlas Research Network. Comprehensive molecular characterization of urothelial bladder carcinoma. Nature 2014. http://dx.doi.org/10.1038/nature12965.
67. Iyer G, Al-Ahmadie H, Schultz N, et al. Prevalence and co-occurrence of actionable genomic alterations in high-grade bladder cancer. J Clin Oncol 2013;31: 3133–40.

68. Al-Ahmadie HA, Iyer G, Janakiraman M, et al. Somatic mutation of fibroblast growth factor receptor-3 (FGFR3) defines a distinct morphological subtype of high-grade urothelial carcinoma. J Pathol 2011;224:270–9.

69. Gui Y, Guo G, Huang Y, et al. Frequent mutations of chromatin remodeling genes in transitional cell carcinoma of the bladder. Nat Genet 2011;43:875–8.

70. Iyer G, Hanrahan AJ, Milowsky MI, et al. Genome sequencing identifies a basis for everolimus sensitivity. Science 2012;338:221.

71. Houédé N, Pourquier P. Targeting the genetic alterations of the PI3K-AKT-mTOR pathway: its potential use in the treatment of bladder cancers. Pharmacol Ther 2014. http://dx.doi.org/10.1016/j.pharmthera.2014.06.004.

72. Nadal R, Bellmunt J. New treatments for bladder cancer: when will we make progress? Curr Treat Options Oncol 2014;15:99–114.

73. Wagle N, Grabiner BC, Van Allen EM, et al. Response and acquired resistance to everolimus in anaplastic thyroid cancer. N Engl J Med 2014;371:1426–33.

74. Cortesi E. Neoadjuvant treatment for locally advanced bladder cancer: a randomized prospective clinical trial. Proc Am Soc Clin Oncol 1995;14:Abstr 623.

75. Wallace DMA, et al. Neo-adjuvant (pre-emptive) cisplatin therapy in invasive transitional cell carcinoma of the Bladder. British journal of urology 1991;67(6): 608–15.

76. Coppin CM, et al. Improved local control of invasive bladder cancer by concurrent cisplatin and preoperative or definitive radiation. The National Cancer Institute of Canada Clinical Trials Group. Journal of clinical oncology 1996;14(11): 2901–7.

77. Abol-Enein H, El-Mekresh M, El-Baz M, et al. Neo-adjuvant chemotherapy in the treatment of invasive transitional bladder cancer. A controlled, prospective randomized study [abstract]. Br J Urol 1997;79 Suppl 4:43.

78. Martinez-Piñeiro JA, Martin MG, Arocena F, et al. Neoadjuvant cisplatin chemotherapy before radical cystectomy in invasive transitional cell carcinoma of the bladder: a prospective randomized phase III study. J Urol 1995;153:964–73.

79. GISTV (Italian Bladder Cancer Study Group). Neoadjuvant treatment for locally advanced bladder cancer: a randomized prospective clinical trial. J Chemother 1996;8:345–6.

80. Malström P-U, Rintala E, Walhqvist R, et al. Five-year follow up of a prospective trial of radical cystectomy and neoadjuvant chemotherapy: Nordic cystectomy trial I. J Urol 1996;155:1903–6.

81. Bassi P, Pagano F, Pappagallo G, et al. Neo-adjuvant M-VAC of invasive bladder cancer: The G.U.O.N.E. multicenter phase III trial. Eur Urol 1998;33(Suppl 1):142.

82. Freiha F, Reese J, Torti FM. A randomized trial of radical cystectomy versus radical cystectomy plus cisplatin, vinblastine and methotrexate chemotherapy for muscle invasive bladder cancer. J Urol 1996;155(2):495–9, discussion 499–500.

83. Otto T, Börgermann C, Krege S, et al. Adjuvant chemotherapy in locally advanced bladder cancer (pT3/pT4a, pN1-2, M0): a phase III study. Eur Urol 2001;39(147 suppl 5):577. Abstract.

84. Lehmann J, Franzaring L, Thüroff J, et al. Complete long-term survival data from a trial of adjuvant chemotherapy vs control after radical cystectomy for locally advanced bladder cancer. BJU international 2006;97(1):42–7.

First-Line Treatment and Prognostic Factors of Metastatic Bladder Cancer for Platinum-Eligible Patients

Wassim Abida, MD, PhD*, Dean F. Bajorin, MD,
Jonathan E. Rosenberg, MD

KEYWORDS

- Urothelial carcinoma, metastatic • Platinum chemotherapy • Prognostic factors

KEY POINTS

- Metastatic urothelial carcinoma occurs primarily in an elderly population.
- The median overall survival of patients with metastatic urothelial carcinoma is approximately 15 months.
- Cisplatin-containing regimens are standard first-line therapy in eligible patients.
- In patients unfit to receive cisplatin, carboplatin-containing regimens are appropriate alternatives.
- Prognostic models incorporating clinical risk factors have been validated; molecular prognostic models are under investigation.

INTRODUCTION

Carcinoma of the bladder is a common malignancy in the United States, with an estimated incidence of 74,690 cases in 2014, and a median age at diagnosis of 73 years.[1] Approximately 20% to 25% of all patients develop metastatic disease, resulting in an estimated 15,580 deaths in 2014.

Greater than 90% of urothelial carcinomas (UCs) occur in the bladder, with a smaller number occurring in the ureter, renal pelvis, and urethra. Given the preponderance of disease originating in the bladder, treatments derived from studies of metastatic bladder cancer are extended to patients with UC originating in other sites.

Metastatic UC is generally incurable, with a median survival of approximately 14 to 15 months with modern chemotherapy regimens.[2] The most effective first-line

Disclosures: None (W. Abida). Consultant to Novartis (D.F. Bajorin). Consultant to Oncogenex and Janssen (J.E. Rosenberg).
Genitourinary Oncology Service, Department of Medicine, Memorial Sloan Kettering Cancer Center, 1275 York Avenue, New York, NY 10065, USA
* Corresponding author.
E-mail address: abidam@mskcc.org

regimens for this disease are cisplatin-based, with carboplatin-based regimens used as an alternative for unfit patients. This article focuses on prognostic and predictive factors for metastatic UC, and reviews the current status of first-line treatment of patients who are eligible for platinum-based therapy.

FIRST-LINE TREATMENT OF METASTATIC DISEASE
Combination Cisplatin-Containing Chemotherapy is Standard First-Line Treatment

Cisplatin has been used for the treatment of epithelial malignancies since the 1970s, with initial reports describing response rates ranging from 30% to 70% for advanced UC treated with cisplatin-containing regimens.[3–5] These response rates were higher than observed with other chemotherapeutic agents at the time, establishing cisplatin as a preferred first-line agent in this disease. One study comparing cisplatin, methotrexate, and vinblastine (CMV) versus methotrexate and vinblastine revealed increased overall survival (OS) in the CMV arm, confirming the advantage of platinum-containing regimens in the first-line setting.[6]

Methotrexate, vinblastine, adriamycin, and cisplatin: standard first-line therapy

A landmark randomized study compared single-agent cisplatin with combination methotrexate, vinblastine, adriamycin, and cisplatin (MVAC) in 269 patients with advanced UC.[7,8] MVAC was superior with respect to overall response rate (RR) (39% vs 12%), progression-free survival (PFS) (10.0 vs 4.3 months), and median OS (12.5 vs 8.2 months). MVAC was also compared with cisplatin, cyclophosphamide, and doxorubicin (CISCA), and was shown to be superior.[9] These studies established the superiority of MVAC over other cisplatin-containing regimens. However, the toxicity of MVAC was significant, with increased rates of myelosuppression, neutropenic fever, and mucositis[7] limiting the use of this regimen in a primarily elderly population with frequent comorbidities.

Gemcitabine and cisplatin: an appropriate alternative to methotrexate, vinblastine, adriamycin, and cisplatin

In an effort to improve on the response and toxicity of MVAC, cisplatin-containing doublets incorporating other chemotherapeutic agents have been tested.[10] One regimen, gemcitabine and cisplatin (GC), showed promising results in single-arm phase II studies.[11–13] Based on these findings, this regimen was advanced to a phase III trial comparing it with MVAC in 405 patients with stage IV UC.[2,14] Both arms had similar RRs (46%–49%) and OS (13.8–14.8 months), with improved toxicity profile in the GC arm. Although this study was designed to show superiority of GC and was underpowered to prove equivalency, the similar disease outcomes and favorable toxicity profile of GC have established this regimen as an appropriate first-line treatment for patients with metastatic UC.

Building on the GC backbone, a phase III randomized study compared paclitaxel, cisplatin, and gemcitabine (PCG) with GC in patients with advanced and metastatic UC.[15] Although RRs were higher in the PCG arm, the study failed to show a statistically significant OS benefit.

Alternative dosing regimens

The advent of growth factor support (granulocyte colony-stimulating factor [G-CSF]) has allowed for the investigation of dose-dense chemotherapy regimens, with the goal of reducing myelosuppression and improving response. A key randomized study compared standard MVAC administered in 4-week cycles and high-dose intensity MVAC (HD-MVAC) administered in 2-week cycles with G-CSF.[16,17] Although no statistically significant difference in OS was seen, RRs and PFS were higher and toxicity rates were lower in the HD-MVAC arm. As a result, HD-MVAC, also called *dose-dense MVAC* (ddMVAC), is now considered an option in the first-line setting.[18] ddMVAC was also compared with a dose-dense GC regimen, wherein treatment was administered in 2-week cycles with G-CSF support.[19] This study was limited by premature closure, precluding firm conclusions.

GC was traditionally given in 4-week cycles, with gemcitabine administered on days 1, 8, and 15, resulting in significant rates of hematologic toxicity and treatment delay.[14] Two studies, one in non–small cell lung cancer and the other in metastatic UC, compared 4-week dosing versus a 3-week schedule in which gemcitabine was administered on days 1 and 8.[20,21] Both found similar RRs, with a better toxicity profile in the 3-week dosing arm, concluding that 3-week dosing of GC is an appropriate alternative. Additionally, in an effort to reduce cisplatin toxicity, several phase II trials investigated GC with split-dose cisplatin, wherein the drug is administered at 35 to 45 mg/m^2 on days 1 and 8 instead of the full dose of 70 mg/m^2 on day 1.[22–24] All concluded that the split-dose regimen is active and well tolerated. Although no clear evidence shows that split-dose cisplatin is equivalent to full-dose, the studies described earlier suggest that split-dose cisplatin may be a reasonable alternative with less toxicity for selected patients.

Other Platinum Agents in Patients Unfit to Receive Cisplatin

The evidence described previously strongly supports the use of cisplatin in the first-line treatment of patients with metastatic UC. However, cisplatin toxicity limits its use, particularly in patients with a glomerular filtration rate of less than 60 mL/min and those with baseline neuropathy. To this end, regimens incorporating other platinum drugs have been investigated. Several early-phase studies examined gemcitabine and oxaliplatin in patients unfit to receive cisplatin,[25,26] suggesting that it is an active and tolerable combination in this population, but the regimen has not been tested in larger studies.

Carboplatin combination regimens have been investigated more extensively. However, multiple studies, although underpowered, established the superiority of cisplatin over carboplatin-containing regimens. One such study compared MVAC with methotrexate, carboplatin, and vinblastine (M-CAVI), revealing higher RRs and survival in the MVAC arm.[27] Another randomized study comparing MVAC with carboplatin and paclitaxel closed early because of poor accrual, but seemed to favor the MVAC arm.[28] A third underpowered study comparing GC with gemcitabine and carboplatin also seemed to favor the cisplatin arm.[29]

Despite the apparent superiority of cisplatin to carboplatin, many patients are considered unfit to receive cisplatin because of poor performance status or comorbidities. An expert consensus statement was released in 2011 with the goal of defining unfit patients (**Table 1**).[30] For those patients, carboplatin-containing regimens may be appropriate because of the toxicity profile. A randomized study compared two carboplatin-containing regimens, M-CAVI and gemcitabine/carboplatin, in unfit patients.[31] Although median survival was comparable, toxicity was significantly lower with gemcitabine/carboplatin, establishing it as an appropriate first-line regimen in this patient population. A triplet regimen consisting of gemcitabine, carboplatin, and paclitaxel was also tested in a phase II trial, revealing a favorable response rate of 68% and median survival of 14.7 months.[32]

Targeted Therapies in the First-Line Treatment of Metastatic Disease

The effectiveness of platinum-containing chemotherapy regimens in the first-line treatment of metastatic UC has been established. Current efforts are directed at

Table 1
Consensus criteria for patients unfit to receive cisplatin-based therapy

Category	Proposed Severity for 'Unfit' Classification (1 Category Must Be Met)
Performance status	WHO or ECOG grade 2 or KPS of 60%–70%
Renal function	<60 mL/min (calculated or measured)
Hearing	CTCAE v4 grade ≥2 audiometric hearing loss
Neuropathy	CTCAE v4 grade ≥2 peripheral neuropathy
Cardiac function	New York Heart Association class III heart failure

Abbreviations: CTCAE, Common Terminology Criteria for Adverse Events; ECOG, Eastern Cooperative Oncology Group; KPS, Karnofsky performance status; WHO, World Health Organization.

Adapted from Galsky MD, Hahn NM, Rosenberg J, et al. A consensus definition of patients with metastatic urothelial carcinoma who are unfit for cisplatin-based chemotherapy. Lancet Oncol 2011;12:212; with permission.

investigating the added benefit of targeted therapies in this setting.[33] Targeting angiogenesis with bevacizumab has shown promise in early-phase studies. One phase II study treated 43 patients with GC and bevacizumab, showing an overall RR of 72% and median survival of 19.1 months,[34] leading to an ongoing phase III trial. Another study treated 51 patients unfit to receive cisplatin with combination gemcitabine, carboplatin, and bevacizumab.[35] This study reported an RR of 49% and median OS of 13.9 months, but did not strictly meet its PFS end point.

Given the success of immune checkpoint blockade in other epithelial malignancies,[36] significant interest has been shown in investigating the role of immunomodulatory agents in metastatic UC. An ongoing phase II trial is testing the safety and efficacy of the cytotoxic T-lymphocyte–associated protein 4 (CTLA-4) blocking agent ipilimumab in combination with GC in the first-line setting.

Treatment of Variant Urothelial and Nonurothelial Histologies

More than 90% of cancers of the urinary tract are of urothelial histology, although urothelial histologic variants, including squamous and glandular differentiated tumors, are increasingly being recognized.[37,38] No prospective studies have specifically addressed the treatment of urothelial variants, and these tumors are treated similarly to those of pure urothelial histology.

Pure nonurothelial urinary tract cancers are rare and poorly studied. Retrospective studies have reported variable responses with platinum-containing regimens.[39,40] One prospective trial enrolled 20 patients with advanced and metastatic adenocarcinoma, squamous cell, small cell, sarcomatoid, or poorly differentiated carcinoma of the urinary tract, and treated them with combination ifosfamide, paclitaxel, and cisplatin.[41] This regimen was noted to be active in the overall population, with a 35% response rate, albeit with inconclusive outcomes in the small histologic subsets. Pure small cell carcinoma of the bladder has been treated with a variety of platinum-containing regimens extrapolated from small cell lung cancer.[42,43]

PROGNOSTIC AND PREDICTIVE FACTORS
Clinical Prognostic Factors

Drawing on a database of 203 patients treated with MVAC, Bajorin and colleagues[44] developed a prognostic model whereby Karnofsky performance status (KPS) of less than 80% and the presence of bone or visceral metastases present independent risk factors for poor prognosis in unresectable and metastatic disease. This model was subsequently validated in independent series.[2,45,46] Recently a prognostic nomogram was developed by Galsky and colleagues,[47] incorporating baseline performance status, number of visceral metastatic sites, white blood cell count, and response to first-line treatment as independent variables predicting survival after completion of first-line therapy.

Molecular Predictive Factors

Significant interest has been shown in identifying molecular factors that accurately predict survival and response to therapy in metastatic UC. However, currently no molecular markers are in standard clinical use in this disease.

Alterations in several genes involved in DNA damage response and repair have been correlated with response to platinum-based therapy. Multiple studies reported an association between high expression of *ERCC1* and poor response to platinum-based therapy in metastatic UC and other malignancies.[48,49] However, other studies found no significant correlation,[50,51] and a recent report described inconsistent results with antibodies commonly used to score *ERCC1* expression.[52] Mutation in another repair gene, *ERCC2*, was recently reported to correlate with platinum response in a retrospective study of patients undergoing neoadjuvant therapy for muscle-invasive bladder cancer,[53] although further validation is needed in metastatic disease. The prognostic role of *BRCA1* expression has also been investigated, but no clear association between mRNA expression and survival was observed in a retrospective study.[48]

Microarray technology has allowed for the identification of gene signatures associated with UC molecular subtypes and platinum response.[54–58] Using this technology, Takata and colleagues[56,57] identified a 14-gene signature that correlates with tumor response to neoadjuvant MVAC. Another group developed an algorithm called COXEN (CO-eXpression gENe analysis) that correlates gene expression with drug response of bladder cancer cell lines,[55] and validated this model in a group of patients treated with neoadjuvant chemotherapy.[58] These algorithms have yet to be validated in metastatic disease. Of significant promise is the large amount of genomic data being generated through international and institutional efforts, including the Cancer Genome Atlas project.[59] Tumor molecular characteristics, correlated retrospectively with clinical outcomes, can guide the way for the identification of prognostic and predictive markers and for the selection of targeted therapies.[60]

Histology and Disease Prognosis

The small numbers of variant and pure nonurothelial histologies have limited investigation of their prognostic role.[37] Although the data are not conclusive, retrospective analyses suggest that nonurothelial histologies result in worse response to chemotherapy and survival compared with UC in metastatic disease.[8,61,62]

SUMMARY

Metastatic UC is an aggressive disease; patients have a median survival of approximately 15 months when treated with modern chemotherapy regimens. Several randomized trials, summarized in **Table 2**, have established GC and MVAC as the preferred first-line regimens in eligible patients. Although cisplatin has been shown to be superior to carboplatin-containing regimens, carboplatin doublets and triplets are reasonable alternatives for unfit patients. Current investigative approaches include the addition of targeted therapies to first-line platinum combination regimens. With regard to prognosis, two models using clinical risk factors have been shown to predict survival in patients treated with first-line platinum-containing therapy. Although

Table 2
Summary of practice-changing randomized trials in advanced urothelial carcinoma

Study	Patients Enrolled	Response Rate (%)	Median Survival (mo)	Conclusion
Cisplatin vs MVAC[7,8]	Cisplatin: 120	12	8.2	MVAC is superior
	MVAC: 126	39	12.5	
GC vs MVAC[2,14]	GC: 203	49	14.0	Regimens appear equivalent with less toxicity for GC
	MVAC: 202	46	15.2	
MVAC vs ddMVAC[16,17]	MVAC: 129	50	14.9	RR and PFS are superior, toxicity is lower with ddMVAC
	ddMVAC: 134	64	15.1	
MVAC vs M-CAVI[27]	MVAC: 24	52	16.0	Underpowered, but appears to favor MVAC
	M-CAVI: 23	39	9.0	

molecular characteristics have not yet found standard clinical use in determining prognosis in metastatic UC, intensive molecular profiling efforts are paving the way for molecular subtyping, improved prognostication, and patient stratification for clinical trials testing targeted therapies in the first-line setting and beyond.

REFERENCES

1. National Cancer Institute Surveillance, Epidemiology, and End Results Program. Cancer Stat Fact Sheets. http://seer.cancer.gov/statfacts/html/urinb.html. Accessed on 8/1/2014.
2. von der Maase H, Sengelov L, Roberts JT, et al. Long-term survival results of a randomized trial comparing gemcitabine plus cisplatin, with methotrexate, vinblastine, doxorubicin, plus cisplatin in patients with bladder cancer. J Clin Oncol 2005;23:4602–8.
3. Sternberg CN, Yagoda A, Scher HI, et al. Preliminary results of M-VAC (methotrexate, vinblastine, doxorubicin and cisplatin) for transitional cell carcinoma of the urothelium. J Urol 1985;133:403–7.
4. Sternberg JJ, Bracken RB, Handel PB, et al. Combination chemotherapy (CISCA) for advanced urinary tract carcinoma. A preliminary report. JAMA 1977;238: 2282–7.
5. Yagoda A. Future implications of phase 2 chemotherapy trials in ninety-five patients with measurable advanced bladder cancer. Cancer Res 1977;37:2775–80.
6. Mead GM, Russell M, Clark P, et al. A randomized trial comparing methotrexate and vinblastine (MV) with cisplatin, methotrexate and vinblastine (CMV) in advanced transitional cell carcinoma: results and a report on prognostic factors in a Medical Research Council study. MRC Advanced Bladder Cancer Working Party. Br J Cancer 1998;78:1067–75.
7. Loehrer PJ Sr, Einhorn LH, Elson PJ, et al. A randomized comparison of cisplatin alone or in combination with methotrexate, vinblastine, and doxorubicin in patients with metastatic urothelial carcinoma: a cooperative group study. J Clin Oncol 1992;10:1066–73.
8. Saxman SB, Propert KJ, Einhorn LH, et al. Long-term follow-up of a phase III intergroup study of cisplatin alone or in combination with methotrexate, vinblastine, and doxorubicin in patients with metastatic urothelial carcinoma: a cooperative group study. J Clin Oncol 1997;15:2564–9.

9. Logothetis CJ, Dexeus FH, Finn L, et al. A prospective randomized trial comparing MVAC and CISCA chemotherapy for patients with metastatic urothelial tumors. J Clin Oncol 1990;8:1050–5.

10. Bellmunt J, Albiol S. New chemotherapy combinations for advanced bladder cancer. Curr Opin Urol 2001;11:517–22.

11. Kaufman D, Raghavan D, Carducci M, et al. Phase II trial of gemcitabine plus cisplatin in patients with metastatic urothelial cancer. J Clin Oncol 2000;18:1921–7.

12. Moore MJ, Winquist EW, Murray N, et al. Gemcitabine plus cisplatin, an active regimen in advanced urothelial cancer: a phase II trial of the National Cancer Institute of Canada Clinical Trials Group. J Clin Oncol 1999;17:2876–81.

13. von der Maase H, Andersen L, Crino L, et al. Weekly gemcitabine and cisplatin combination therapy in patients with transitional cell carcinoma of the urothelium: a phase II clinical trial. Ann Oncol 1999;10:1461–5.

14. von der Maase H, Hansen SW, Roberts JT, et al. Gemcitabine and cisplatin versus methotrexate, vinblastine, doxorubicin, and cisplatin in advanced or metastatic bladder cancer: results of a large, randomized, multinational, multicenter, phase III study. J Clin Oncol 2000;18:3068–77.

15. Bellmunt J, von der Maase H, Mead GM, et al. Randomized phase III study comparing paclitaxel/cisplatin/gemcitabine and gemcitabine/cisplatin in patients with locally advanced or metastatic urothelial cancer without prior systemic therapy: EORTC Intergroup Study 30987. J Clin Oncol 2012;30:1107–13.

16. Sternberg CN, de Mulder P, Schornagel JH, et al. Seven year update of an EORTC phase III trial of high-dose intensity M-VAC chemotherapy and G-CSF versus classic M-VAC in advanced urothelial tract tumours. Eur J Cancer 2006;42:50–4.

17. Sternberg CN, de Mulder PH, Schornagel JH, et al. Randomized phase III trial of high-dose-intensity methotrexate, vinblastine, doxorubicin, and cisplatin (MVAC) chemotherapy and recombinant human granulocyte colony-stimulating factor versus classic MVAC in advanced urothelial tract tumors: European Organization for Research and Treatment of Cancer Protocol no. 30924. J Clin Oncol 2001;19:2638–46.

18. Clark PE, Agarwal N, Biagioli MC, et al. Bladder cancer. J Natl Compr Canc Netw 2013;11:446–75.

19. Bamias A, Dafni U, Karadimou A, et al. Prospective, open-label, randomized, phase III study of two dose-dense regimens MVAC versus gemcitabine/cisplatin in patients with inoperable, metastatic or relapsed urothelial cancer: a Hellenic Cooperative Oncology Group study (HE 16/03). Ann Oncol 2013;24:1011–7.

20. Als AB, Sengelov L, Von Der Maase H. Gemcitabine and cisplatin in locally advanced and metastatic bladder cancer; 3- or 4-week schedule? Acta Oncol 2008;47:110–9.

21. Soto Parra H, Cavina R, Latteri F, et al. Three-week versus four-week schedule of cisplatin and gemcitabine: results of a randomized phase II study. Ann Oncol 2002;13:1080–6.

22. Hiramatsu A, Iwasaki Y, Koyama Y, et al. Phase II trial of weekly gemcitabine and split-dose cisplatin for advanced non-small-cell lung cancer. Jpn J Clin Oncol 2009;39:779–83.

23. Hussain SA, Stocken DD, Riley P, et al. A phase I/II study of gemcitabine and fractionated cisplatin in an outpatient setting using a 21-day schedule in patients with advanced and metastatic bladder cancer. Br J Cancer 2004;91:844–9.

24. Kim JH, Lee DH, Shin HC, et al. A phase II study with gemcitabine and split-dose cisplatin in patients with advanced non-small cell lung cancer. Lung Cancer 2006;54:57–62.

25. Carles J, Esteban E, Climent M, et al. Gemcitabine and oxaliplatin combination: a multicenter phase II trial in unfit patients with locally advanced or metastatic urothelial cancer. Ann Oncol 2007;18:1359–62.

26. Theodore C, Bidault F, Bouvet-Forteau N, et al. A phase II monocentric study of oxaliplatin in combination with gemcitabine (GEMOX) in patients with advanced/metastatic transitional cell carcinoma (TCC) of the urothelial tract. Ann Oncol 2006;17:990–4.

27. Bellmunt J, Ribas A, Eres N, et al. Carboplatin-based versus cisplatin-based chemotherapy in the treatment of surgically incurable advanced bladder carcinoma. Cancer 1997;80:1966–72.

28. Dreicer R, Manola J, Roth BJ, et al. Phase III trial of methotrexate, vinblastine, doxorubicin, and cisplatin versus carboplatin and paclitaxel in patients with advanced carcinoma of the urothelium. Cancer 2004;100:1639–45.

29. Dogliotti L, Carteni G, Siena S, et al. Gemcitabine plus cisplatin versus gemcitabine plus carboplatin as first-line chemotherapy in advanced transitional cell carcinoma of the urothelium: results of a randomized phase 2 trial. Eur Urol 2007;52:134–41.

30. Galsky MD, Hahn NM, Rosenberg J, et al. A consensus definition of patients with metastatic urothelial carcinoma who are unfit for cisplatin-based chemotherapy. Lancet Oncol 2011;12:211–4.

31. De Santis M, Bellmunt J, Mead G, et al. Randomized phase II/III trial assessing gemcitabine/carboplatin and methotrexate/carboplatin/vinblastine in patients with advanced urothelial cancer who are unfit for cisplatin-based chemotherapy: EORTC study 30986. J Clin Oncol 2012;30:191–9.

32. Hussain M, Vaishampayan U, Du W, et al. Combination paclitaxel, carboplatin, and gemcitabine is an active treatment for advanced urothelial cancer. J Clin Oncol 2001;19:2527–33.

33. Ghosh M, Brancato SJ, Agarwal PK, et al. Targeted therapies in urothelial carcinoma. Curr Opin Oncol 2014;26:305–20.

34. Hahn NM, Stadler WM, Zon RT, et al. Phase II trial of cisplatin, gemcitabine, and bevacizumab as first-line therapy for metastatic urothelial carcinoma: Hoosier Oncology Group GU 04-75. J Clin Oncol 2011;29:1525–30.

35. Balar AV, Apolo AB, Ostrovnaya I, et al. Phase II study of gemcitabine, carboplatin, and bevacizumab in patients with advanced unresectable or metastatic urothelial cancer. J Clin Oncol 2013;31:724–30.

36. Page DB, Postow MA, Callahan MK, et al. Immune modulation in cancer with antibodies. Annu Rev Med 2014;65:185–202.

37. Chalasani V, Chin JL, Izawa JI. Histologic variants of urothelial bladder cancer and nonurothelial histology in bladder cancer. Can Urol Assoc J 2009;3:S193–8.

38. Pons F, Orsola A, Morote J, et al. Variant forms of bladder cancer: basic considerations on treatment approaches. Curr Oncol Rep 2011;13:216–21.

39. Hong JY, Choi MK, Uhm JE, et al. Palliative chemotherapy for non-transitional cell carcinomas of the urothelial tract. Med Oncol 2009;26:186–92.

40. Siefker-Radtke AO, Gee J, Shen Y, et al. Multimodality management of urachal carcinoma: the M. D. Anderson Cancer Center experience. J Urol 2003;169:1295–8.

41. Galsky MD, Iasonos A, Mironov S, et al. Prospective trial of ifosfamide, paclitaxel, and cisplatin in patients with advanced non-transitional cell carcinoma of the urothelial tract. Urology 2007;69:255–9.

42. Bex A, Nieuwenhuijzen JA, Kerst M, et al. Small cell carcinoma of bladder: a single-center prospective study of 25 cases treated in analogy to small cell lung cancer. Urology 2005;65:295–9.

43. Mukesh M, Cook N, Hollingdale AE, et al. Small cell carcinoma of the urinary bladder: a 15-year retrospective review of treatment and survival in the Anglian Cancer Network. BJU Int 2009;103:747–52.
44. Bajorin DF, Dodd PM, Mazumdar M, et al. Long-term survival in metastatic transitional-cell carcinoma and prognostic factors predicting outcome of therapy. J Clin Oncol 1999;17:3173–81.
45. Bellmunt J, Albanell J, Paz-Ares L, et al. Pretreatment prognostic factors for survival in patients with advanced urothelial tumors treated in a phase I/II trial with paclitaxel, cisplatin, and gemcitabine. Cancer 2002;95:751–7.
46. Lin CC, Hsu CH, Huang CY, et al. Prognostic factors for metastatic urothelial carcinoma treated with cisplatin and 5-fluorouracil-based regimens. Urology 2007; 69:479–84.
47. Galsky MD, Moshier E, Krege S, et al. Posttreatment prognostic nomogram for patients with metastatic urothelial cancer completing first-line cisplatin-based chemotherapy. Urol Oncol 2014;32:48.e1–8.
48. Bellmunt J, Paz-Ares L, Cuello M, et al. Gene expression of ERCC1 as a novel prognostic marker in advanced bladder cancer patients receiving cisplatin-based chemotherapy. Ann Oncol 2007;18:522–8.
49. Li S, Wu J, Chen Y, et al. ERCC1 expression levels predict the outcome of platinum-based chemotherapies in advanced bladder cancer: a meta-analysis. Anticancer Drugs 2014;25:106–14.
50. Kim KH, Do IG, Kim HS, et al. Excision repair cross-complementation group 1 (ERCC1) expression in advanced urothelial carcinoma patients receiving cisplatin-based chemotherapy. APMIS 2010;118:941–8.
51. Matsumura N, Nakamura Y, Kohjimoto Y, et al. The prognostic significance of human equilibrative nucleoside transporter 1 expression in patients with metastatic bladder cancer treated with gemcitabine-cisplatin-based combination chemotherapy. BJU Int 2011;108:E110–6.
52. Friboulet L, Olaussen KA, Pignon JP, et al. ERCC1 isoform expression and DNA repair in non-small-cell lung cancer. N Engl J Med 2013;368:1101–10.
53. Van Allen EM, Mouw KW, Kim P, et al. Somatic ERCC2 Mutations Correlate with Cisplatin Sensitivity in Muscle-Invasive Urothelial Carcinoma. Cancer Discov 2014;4:1140–53.
54. Choi W, Porten S, Kim S, et al. Identification of distinct basal and luminal subtypes of muscle-invasive bladder cancer with different sensitivities to frontline chemotherapy. Cancer Cell 2014;25:152–65.
55. Lee JK, Havaleshko DM, Cho H, et al. A strategy for predicting the chemosensitivity of human cancers and its application to drug discovery. Proc Natl Acad Sci U S A 2007;104:13086–91.
56. Takata R, Katagiri T, Kanehira M, et al. Validation study of the prediction system for clinical response of M-VAC neoadjuvant chemotherapy. Cancer Sci 2007;98: 113–7.
57. Takata R, Katagiri T, Kanehira M, et al. Predicting response to methotrexate, vinblastine, doxorubicin, and cisplatin neoadjuvant chemotherapy for bladder cancers through genome-wide gene expression profiling. Clin Cancer Res 2005;11:2625–36.
58. Williams PD, Cheon S, Havaleshko DM, et al. Concordant gene expression signatures predict clinical outcomes of cancer patients undergoing systemic therapy. Cancer Res 2009;69:8302–9.
59. Cancer Genome Atlas Research Network. Comprehensive molecular characterization of urothelial bladder carcinoma. Nature 2014;507:315–22.

60. Iyer G, Al-Ahmadie H, Schultz N, et al. Prevalence and co-occurrence of actionable genomic alterations in high-grade bladder cancer. J Clin Oncol 2013;31: 3133–40.
61. Scosyrev E, Yao J, Messing E. Urothelial carcinoma versus squamous cell carcinoma of bladder: is survival different with stage adjustment? Urology 2009;73: 822–7.
62. Logothetis CJ, Dexeus FH, Chong C, et al. Cisplatin, cyclophosphamide and doxorubicin chemotherapy for unresectable urothelial tumors: the M.D. Anderson experience. J Urol 1989;141:33–7.

First-line Treatment of Metastatic Disease
Cisplatin-ineligible Patients

Richard Cathomas, MD[a], Maria De Santis, MD[b],
Matthew D. Galsky, MD[c],*

KEYWORDS

- Urothelial carcinoma • Unfit for cisplatin • Prognostic factors • Carboplatin
- Gemcitabine

KEY POINTS

- Patients not eligible for cisplatin are defined by one of the following: Eastern Cooperative Oncology Group performance status (PS) greater than or equal to 2, creatinine clearance (glomerular filtration rate [GFR]) less than 60 mL/min, hearing loss greater than or equal to grade 2, peripheral neuropathy greater than or equal to grade 2, heart failure greater than or equal to New York Heart Association class III.
- Patients unfit for cisplatin generally have a poor prognosis. Within this group PS 2, presence of visceral metastases, liver metastases, and low baseline hemoglobin are prognostic factors of poor outcome.
- Treatment decisions in patients who are unfit for cisplatin are mainly based on 2 factors: PS and renal function. In case of PS greater than or equal to 2 and GFR less than 60 mL/min, treatment consists of best supportive care or single-agent chemotherapy. In case of 0 or 1 risk factor, carboplatin-based combination chemotherapy is the preferred option with the highest level of evidence. Patient inclusion in clinical trials is highly recommended.

INTRODUCTION

Cisplatin-based combination chemotherapy is effective and can considerably improve outcomes in patients with advanced urothelial carcinoma (UC), with response rates of

Conflicts of interest: Advisory role for Pierre Fabre (R. Cathomas). Bristol-Myers Squibb, advisory role and research funding; Novartis, research funding; BioMotiv, research funding (M.D. Galsky).
[a] Division of Oncology/Hematology, Kantonsspital Graubünden, Chur CH-7000, Switzerland; [b] Ludwig Boltzmann Institute for Applied Cancer Research (LBI-ACR VIEnna) - LBCTO, 3rd Medical Department, Centre for Oncology and Haematology, Kaiser Franz Josef Hospital, Vienna, Austria; [c] The Tisch Cancer Institute, Icahn School of Medicine at Mount Sinai, 1470 Madison Avenue, New York, NY 10029, USA
* Corresponding author.
E-mail address: matthew.galsky@mssm.edu

hemonc.theclinics.com

more than 50% and 5-year survival rates of 33% in patients with good performance status (PS; ie, Karnofsky score >80%) and no evidence of visceral metastases.[1,2] Patients fit for cisplatin, but with 1 or both of these poor prognostic factors, experience considerably worse outcomes.[1] Poor outcomes have also been shown when carboplatin is substituted for cisplatin. Although no adequately powered randomized trials have been completed comparing cisplatin-based with carboplatin-based chemotherapy combinations, a meta-analysis showed a significantly increased likelihood of achieving an objective response with cisplatin-based chemotherapy.[3] All practice guidelines therefore support the use of cisplatin-based regimens in advanced UC.[4,5] In clinical practice, greater than 50% of all patients with advanced UC have contraindications for treatment with cisplatin and alternative treatment options are necessary.[6] There is no consensus on the standard chemotherapy treatment of patients who are unfit for cisplatin.[4] This article reviews the definition of patients not eligible for cisplatin; clinical, pathologic, and molecular prognostic factors for this patient group; as well as different treatment options based on baseline patient characteristics.

DEFINING PATIENTS NOT ELIGIBLE FOR CISPLATIN

Although the human condition and the heterogeneity of disease necessitates a degree of vagueness and instinct in the practice of medicine, uniformly defining disease states, conditions, and end points is critical to drug development and integral to regulatory science. Several prior clinical trials, discussed in this article, have explored the development of therapeutic regimens in patients with metastatic UC who were considered ineligible for cisplatin.[7] However, these trials generally used variable eligibility criteria, complicating interpretation of the results. In 2011, an expert panel was convened to establish a uniform definition of cisplatin ineligibility to facilitate clinical trials in this patient population for the future.[8] Through consensus, this panel established the definition presented in **Box 1**. Although clinical judgment is essential when applying rigid guidelines such as these, to routine patient management, consistency in how patient populations are defined is critical for clinical trial purposes. The definition shown in **Box 1** has been adopted in the design of several ongoing clinical trials.

PROGNOSTIC FACTORS IN PATIENTS NOT ELIGIBLE FOR CISPLATIN

Similar to cisplatin-eligible patients with metastatic UC, cisplatin-ineligible patients also represent a heterogeneous group with variable outcomes to treatment. Several

---

Box 1
Consensus definition of cisplatin ineligibility for clinical trial design

At least 1 of the following:

- ECOG PS of 2 (KPS of 60%–70%)
- Creatinine clearance less than 60 mL/min
- CTCAE v4 grade greater than or equal to 2 audiometric hearing loss
- CTCAE v4 grade greater than or equal to 2 peripheral neuropathy
- NYHA class III heart failure

Abbreviations: CTCAE v4, common terminology criteria for adverse events, version 4; ECOG, Eastern Cooperative Oncology Group; KPS, Karnofsky performance status; NYHA, New York Heart Association.

analyses have defined baseline prognostic factors in patients with metastatic UC treatment with cisplatin-based chemotherapy. However, baseline prognostic factors have been explored less commonly in the cisplatin-ineligible patient population. Collette and colleagues[9] analyzed the cohort of patients enrolled in EORTC (European Organisation for Research and Treatment of Cancer) 30986, a phase II/III trial of gemcitabine plus carboplatin (GCa) versus methotrexate, carboplatin, plus vinblastine, to identify baseline factors associated with patient survival. On multivariate analysis, the risk of death was significantly increased in patients with a PS of 2, visceral metastases, liver metastases, and a lowered hemoglobin level ($\leq$12 g/dL for women and $\leq$13.6 g/dL for men). The median survival was 17.4 months in patients with no poor prognostic factors versus 5.5 months in patients with 3 or more poor prognostic factors. Whether impaired renal function is an independent poor prognostic factor in patients with metastatic UC is unclear, given the limitations of the datasets available to address this question.

FIRST-LINE TREATMENT OPTIONS IN PATIENTS NOT ELIGIBLE FOR CISPLATIN

Although a considerable number of patients with metastatic UC are unfit for cisplatin, few trials in general, and only 1 randomized phase III trial in particular, have been performed. Interpretation of the published trials is difficult in view of the lack of a consensus definition for this patient group until 2011. In addition, assessment of PS is complicated because it can be related to the underlying malignancy or related to comorbidities and age. It is unclear whether these different underlying causes of functional impairment confer similar prognostic and treatment implications. A response to chemotherapy could theoretically result in an improvement in the former but not necessarily the latter. In general, constitutional symptoms such as fatigue, weight loss, anorexia, and failure to thrive are typical signs of advanced or metastatic disease and denote a poor prognosis. In rare cases, patients may have constitutional symptoms caused by potentially reversible complications of cancer or other comorbidities, such as renal failure caused by bilateral ureteral obstruction. In such situations, identifying the cause of the deterioration may help to improve symptoms and functional status, and increase the likelihood of delivery of standard anticancer therapy with subsequent improved prognosis. Therefore, exploring the cause of a patient's symptoms, rather than assuming that all symptoms in patients with advanced cancer are direct systemic manifestations of the cancer itself, is important for optimizing care.

Clinical trials in cisplatin-ineligible patients have explored both single-agent and combination regimens, which are discussed in further detail later.

Single-agent Chemotherapy

Several chemotherapeutic agents have shown activity in UC when used as single agents. Few trials have included predominantly patients with impaired renal function, reduced PS, or both. All these trials are small and the publications date back 20 years. The patient populations included were heterogeneous and some factors, such as renal function, are not uniformly reported across trials. Several patients included in these trials may be considered cisplatin eligible based on contemporary standards. No randomized trials comparing single-agent therapy with best supportive care or trials comparing one agent with another have been published. The results of these trials must be interpreted with caution and cross-trial comparisons are problematic.

Although some of the monotherapy trials included a large number of patients with PS 2, few patients with PS 3 were included. In these latter patients, the risks of cytotoxic chemotherapy likely outweigh any potential benefits and these patients may be best managed with supportive care alone.

The trials discussed are summarized in **Table 1**.

Single-agent chemotherapy with gemcitabine

Several trials explored the efficacy and safety of gemcitabine monotherapy[10–12]: response rates of up to 46% have been reported, usually short lived and few were complete. The most recent and stringent data derive from the trial of Culine and colleagues.[12] This randomized phase II trial tested monotherapy for gemcitabine against the combination of gemcitabine and oxaliplatin. The population was restricted to patients unfit for cisplatin, and almost half of the patients included had PS 2. The results show the limited efficacy of single-agent gemcitabine, with an overall survival (OS) of only 5.4 months despite a response rate of 43%. In addition, patients in this trial experienced substantial toxicity.

Single-agent chemotherapy with taxanes

Both docetaxel and paclitaxel have been tested as monotherapy in cisplatin-ineligible patients with results similar to those of gemcitabine.[13–15] High response rates were reported in these studies; however, OS remained short. Roth and colleagues[14] reported complete remissions in 27% of patients treated with paclitaxel lasting up to 16 months. The number of patients with impaired renal function was not reported in this trial. Monotherapy with taxanes causes toxicity with febrile neutropenia in up to 23% of patients. In the reported trials growth factors were not used prophylactically.

Summary of single-agent chemotherapy

Monotherapy with either gemcitabine or taxanes can achieve objective responses in a large proportion of chemonaive patients with advanced UC; however, OS remains poor. In cisplatin-ineligible patients with advanced UC who are also considered poor candidates for carboplatin-based combination chemotherapy, decisions regarding single-agent chemotherapy versus best supportive care require careful consideration of the risks and benefits of each approach.

Combination Chemotherapy

For patients eligible for cisplatin, combination chemotherapy regimens such as methotrexate, doxorubicin, vinblastine, and cisplatin or gemcitabine plus cisplatin have become the standard of care. In view of the modest benefits with single-agent chemotherapy, the use of combination regimens has also been explored in patients unfit for cisplatin. A logical choice was to replace cisplatin with the less nephrotoxic, and generally better tolerated, platinum agent, carboplatin. Another strategy has been to use split doses or lower doses of cisplatin in patients with only mildly impaired renal function.[16,17] Non–platinum-containing combination regimens have also been explored.

Carboplatin-containing combination chemotherapy

Combination chemotherapy in cisplatin-ineligible patients may be associated with an increase in toxicity compared with combination regimens in fitter patient groups. This association was shown by the dose finding study for the trial EORTC 30986.[18] Based on phase II data obtained in patients with non–small cell lung cancer,[19] an initial dose level of gemcitabine 1000 mg/m^2 on days 1 and 8 and carboplatin area under the curve (AUC) 5 on day 1 every 21 days was selected. This regimen proved poorly tolerated in a frail patient population with metastatic UC: dose-limiting myelotoxicity was observed in 6 of 8 patients, requiring dose reduction or delay in 5 patients. After reducing the carboplatin dose to AUC 4.5, while maintaining the gemcitabine dose

Table 1
Overview of phase II trials using first-line single-agent chemotherapy in cisplatin-unfit patients with urothelial cancer

Combination (Doses mg/m²)	N	Design	Cisplatin Unfit	ORR (%)	Median PFS (mo)	Median OS (mo)	Reference
Gem (1000) day 1, day 8, day 15, q4w	40	Phase II Single arm	25% Karnofsky ≤80% S-Creat ≤2 mg/dL for inclusion	28	4.6	12.4	10
Gem (1200) day 1, day 8, q3w	25	Phase II Single arm	52% PS 2 Median age 76 y	46	5	8	11
Gem (1200) day 1, day 8, day 15, q4w vs	22	Phase II randomized	41% PS 2 84% GFR<60	43	3.8	5.4	12
Gem (1000) day 1, day 15 Oxali (100) day 2, day 16, q4w	22		25% both factors	28	3.4	8.1	
Docetaxel (100) d1, q3w (+G-CSF)	11	Phase II Single arm	26% PS ≥2 100% Creat >1.6 mg/dL	36	NR	11	13
Paclitaxel (225) d1, 24-h infusion q3w	26	Phase II Single arm	14% PS 2 S-Creat up to ≤2 mg/dL for inclusion	42	NR	8.4	14
Paclitaxel (175) d1, q3w	13	Phase II Single arm	69% PS ≥2 54% S-Creat >1.5 mg/dL	31	NR	9	15

Abbreviations: Gem, gemcitabine; GFR, glomerular filtration rate in mL/min; NR, not reported; ORR, overall response rate; OS, overall survival; Oxali, oxaliplatin; PFS, progression-free survival; q3w, every 3 weeks; q4w, every 4 weeks; S-Creat, serum creatinine.

at 1000 mg/m^2, hematological toxicity was less pronounced and this dose and schedule were chosen for the randomized study. Another trial using carboplatin and gemcitabine in a frail and elderly patient population used an even lower dose of carboplatin (AUC 4). Despite these lower doses, patients experienced considerable toxicity.[20] The EORTC performed the first randomized phase III trial in cisplatin-ineligible patients with metastatic UC. Patients were eligible for this trial based on a World Health Organization PS of 2, and/or impaired renal function with GFR less than 60 mL/min, or both. This pivotal trial was performed in 2 steps as a phase II/phase III trial allowing for premature termination in case of inadequate response rate or excessive toxicity.[21] Patients were randomized to receive methotrexate, carboplatin, vinblastine (M-CAVI) or GCa. The main results are shown in **Table 2**. Both regimens showed objective responses in a large proportion of patients, with a numerical advantage for GCa. A statistically significant difference was seen only for the confirmed response rate in favor of GCa. OS and progression-free survival (PFS) were disappointingly low in both treatment arms (9.3 and 8.1 months for GCa and M-CAVI, respectively) in the context of contemporary studies using cisplatin-based chemotherapy. No statistically significant difference between GCa and M-CAVI was seen in either PFS or OS.[22] Severe acute toxicity was higher in the M-CAVI arm. Therefore the use of carboplatin in combination with gemcitabine is a reasonable choice in patients unfit for cisplatin with either PS 2 or impaired renal function with GFR less than 60 mL/min. For patients with both of these factors the response rate was low and OS short. Moreover, severe acute toxicity was high (25%) and the likelihood of receiving only 1 cycle of therapy was 20%.[22]

Combining chemotherapy with antiangiogenic treatment has also been studied in cisplatin-ineligible patients with metastatic UC. Balar and colleagues[23] explored the combination of gemcitabine, carboplatin, and bevacizumab (beva) followed by beva maintenance in patients defined as being unfit for cisplatin based on at least 1 of the following: impaired renal function, solitary kidney, Karnofsky score 60% to 70%, or visceral metastases. In this trial, the response rate was 49% and OS 13.9 months. Similar results were seen in a randomized phase II screening trial comparing vinflunine (VFL) and carboplatin with VFL and gemcitabine.[24] All patients had impaired renal function but a PS of 0 to 1. The OS rates were 12.8 versus 13.9 months for VFL-carboplatin and VFL-gemcitabine, respectively. Whether or not these combination regimens represent an improvement compared with GCa, or whether the outcomes in these trials are a result of more favorable baseline prognostic factors, is unknown and requires assessment in definitive randomized trials.

Further results of carboplatin combination chemotherapy are summarized in **Table 2**.

Nonplatinum combination chemotherapy

Gemcitabine has formed the basis of most nonplatinum combinations and is a reasonable choice in view of the single-agent activity and mechanism of action.[12,28–32] Combinations of gemcitabine with paclitaxel, pemetrexed, oxaliplatin, epirubicin, doxorubicin, and vinblastine have been tested and results are summarized in **Table 3**. All of these trials were small and, with the exception of a single trial, non-randomized, limiting the interpretation of the results. Although all combinations achieved high response rates, responses have generally been short lived. None of the combinations stands out in terms of efficacy or safety. A small, randomized, phase II trial of gemcitabine versus gemcitabine plus oxaliplatin showed similar anticancer activity with the 2 regimens but higher rates of adverse events with the combination.[12] This trial included mainly patients with a PS of 2% and 25% had both PS 2 and

Table 2
Overview of trials with first-line carboplatin-based combination chemotherapy in cisplatin–unfit patients with urothelial cancer

Combination (Doses mg/m²)	N	Design	Reason for Being Cisplatin Unfit	ORR (%)	Median PFS (mo)	Median OS (mo)	Reference
Gem (1000) day 1, day 8 Carbo AUC 4.5 (5) day 1, q3w	16	Feasibility Single arm	PS 2 and/or GFR<60	44	NR	NR	18
Gem (1000) day 1, day 8 Carbo AUC 4 day 1, q3w	56	Phase II Single arm	PS 2 and/or GFR<50 and/or age >75 y	36	4.8	7.2	20
Gem (1000) day 1, day 8 Carbo AUC 4.5 day 1, q3w vs MTX (30) day 1, day 15, day 22 Vinblast (3) day 1, day 15, day 22 Carbo AUC 4.5 day 1, q4w	119 119	Phase II/III randomized	PS 2 and/or GFR<60 mL/min	41 30	5.8 4.2	9.3 8.1	21,22
Gem (1000) day 1, day 8 Carbo AUC 5 day 1, q3w	17	Phase II Single arm	Renal impairment and/or KPS ≥80%	56	NR	10.0	25
Gem (1000) day 1, day 8 Carbo AUC 5 day 1, q3w	34	Phase II Single arm	PS 2–3 and/or GFR<50	24	4.4	9.8	26
Pacli (225) day Carbo AUC 6 day 1, q3w	37	Phase II Single arm	S-Creat 1.6–4 mg/dL	24	3.0	7.1	27
Gem (2000) q2w + Doxo (50) q2w ×5 Then: Pacli (65) + Carbo AUC 1.7 weekly ×12	25	Phase II Single arm	GFR<60 mL/min and/or prior nephrectomy	56	NR	15	28
Gem (1000) day 1, day 8 Carbo AUC 5 day 1, q3w Beva 15 mg/kg day 1, q3w (including maintenance)	51	Phase II Single arm	GFR<60 and/or solitary kidney and/or PS 2 and/or visceral metastases	49	6.5	13.9	23
VFL (250/280) day 1 Carbo AUC 4.5 day 1, q3w vs VFL (250/280) day 1 Gem (750/1000) day 1, day 8, q3w	35 34	Phase II randomized	GFR<60 mL/min (100%) and/or cardiac impairment PS 0–1	42.9 52.9	6.1 5.9	12.8 13.9	24

Abbreviations: AUC, area under the curve; Carbo, carboplatin; Doxo, doxorubicin; MTX, methotrexate; Pacli, Paclitaxel; q2w, every 2 weeks; VFL, vinflunine; Vinblast, vinblastine.

Table 3
Overview of trials with first-line non–platinum-containing combination chemotherapy in cisplatin-unfit patients with urothelial cancer

Combination (Doses mg/m²)	N	Design	Cisplatin Unfit	ORR (%)	Median PFS (mo)	Median OS (mo)	Reference
Gem (2500) q2w Pacli (150) q2w	54	Phase II single arm	13% PS 2 GFR>40 (no numbers, median GFR 62)	37	5.8	13.2 4.1 (PS 2)	29
Gem (1200) day 1, day 8, day 15, q4w vs Gem (1000) day 1, day 15 Oxali (100) day 2, day 16, q4w	22 22	Phase II randomized	41% PS 2 84% GFR<60 25% both factors	43 28	3.8 3.4	5.4 8.1	12
Gem (1000) day 1, day 8 Pemetrexed (500) day 1, q3w	46	Phase II single arm	7% PS 2 GFR>45 (no numbers provided)	32	5.8	13.4	30
Gem (1000) day 1, day 8 Epirubicin 70 day 1, day 8, q3w	38	Phase II single arm	24% PS 2 79% GFR<60 Median age 72 y	40	4.8	8.0	31
Gem (2000) 2qw + Doxo (50) 2qw ×5 Then: Pacli (65) + Carbo AUC 1.7 weekly × 12	25	Phase II single arm	100% GFR<60 or S-Creat>1.5 mg/dL	56	NR	15	28
Gem (1000) day 1, day 8 Vinorelbine (30) day 1, day 8, q3w	21	Phase II single arm	100% GFR<50	48	5	15	32

impaired renal function. The results are similar to those of EORTC 30986, reinforcing that combination chemotherapy in this latter group of patients may be associated with an unfavorable risk/benefit profile.

NOVEL THERAPIES IN PATIENTS NOT ELIGIBLE FOR CISPLATIN

Given the modest response durations with traditional cytotoxic chemotherapy in cisplatin-ineligible patients with metastatic UC, there has been an interest in exploring novel targeted therapies in this patient population. Bellmunt and colleagues[33] performed a phase II trial of the multitargeted tyrosine kinase inhibitor sunitinib as first-line treatment in cisplatin-ineligible patients with metastatic UC. Although objective responses were uncommon (3 of 38 patients), the median PFS and OS in this cohort compared favorably with trials exploring cytotoxic chemotherapy (notwithstanding the limitations of cross-trial comparisons). Approximately 10% to 20% of invasive bladder cancers harbor activating mutations, or gene fusions, involving fibroblast growth factor receptor (FGFR) 3.[34] Although clinical trials with first-generation small molecule inhibitors of FGFR3 yielded disappointing results,[35,36] more potent and selective second-generation drugs seem promising. Preliminary results with the orally administered small molecule FGFR inhibitor BGJ398 revealed single-agent objective responses in patients with metastatic UC harboring FGFR3 alterations. Although not explored specifically in cisplatin-ineligible patients, a patient showing some of the best responses in a small metastatic UC population from the phase I trial was 86 years old.[37] The anti–Programmed death-ligand 1 (PD-L1) antibody MPDL3280A has also recently shown single-agent activity in metastatic UC, including durable responses, and is being explored further as first-line treatment in cisplatin-ineligible patients.[38]

Note that categorizing patients as cisplatin eligible or cisplatin ineligible is a function of the current standard therapies used to treat this disease. However, response durations are also inadequate for most patients even with cisplatin-based therapy. As newer therapies emerge that are both more effective and less toxic, this artificial categorization of patients may become irrelevant, replaced by categories that are more relevant to tumor biology (eg, FGFR3 altered UC or PD-L1 overexpressing UC).

SUMMARY

GCa is a reasonable treatment standard for cisplatin-ineligible patients with metastatic UC, based on the only completed phase III trial in this patient population, EORTC 30986. However, for patients with both a borderline PS (PS 2) and impaired renal function (GFR<60 mL/min), combination chemotherapy is associated with substantial toxicity and single-agent chemotherapy, or best supportive care alone, should be considered.

In view of the limited success of single-agent or combination chemotherapy, more effective and better tolerated treatments are needed and patients should be included in clinical trials as first treatment choice whenever possible.

REFERENCES

1. Bajorin DF, Dodd PM, Mazumdar M, et al. Long-term survival in metastatic transitional-cell carcinoma and prognostic factors predicting outcome of therapy. J Clin Oncol 1999;17:3173–81.
2. von der Maase H, Hansen SW, Roberts JT, et al. Gemcitabine and cisplatin versus methotrexate, vinblastine, doxorubicin and cisplatin in advanced or

metastatic bladder cancer: results of a large, randomized, multinational, multi-center, phase III study. J Clin Oncol 2000;18:3068–77.

3. Galsky MD, Chen GJ, Oh WK, et al. Comparative effectiveness of cisplatin-based and carboplatin-based chemotherapy for treatment of advanced urothelial carcinoma. Ann Oncol 2012;23:406–10.

4. Witjes JA, Comperat E, Cowan NC, et al. Guidelines on muscle-invasive and metastatic bladder cancer. EAU European Association of Urology. 2014. Available at: www.uroweb.org. Accessed July 30, 2014.

5. NCCN clinical practice guidelines in Oncology. Bladder cancer version 2. 2014. Available at: www.nccn.org. Accessed July 30, 2014.

6. Dash A, Galsky MD, Vickers AJ, et al. Impact of renal impairment on eligibility for adjuvant cisplatin-based chemotherapy in patients with urothelial carcinoma of the bladder. Cancer 2006;107:506–13.

7. Galsky MD, Hahn NM, Rosenberg J, et al. Treatment of patients with metastatic urothelial cancer "unfit" for cisplatin-based chemotherapy. J Clin Oncol 2011; 29(17):2432–8.

8. Galsky MD, Hahn NM, Rosenberg J, et al. A consensus definition of patients with metastatic urothelial carcinoma who are unfit for cisplatin-based chemotherapy. Lancet Oncol 2011;12(3):211–4.

9. Collette S, Sylvester R, Bellmunt J, et al. Prognostics factors in previously untreated urothelial cancer patients ineligible for cisplatin-based chemotherapy: An external validation of the Bajorin risk groups. J Clin Oncol 2013;31(Suppl) [abstract: 4529].

10. Stadler WM, Kruzel T, Roth B, et al. Phase II study of single-agent gemcitabine in previously untreated patients with metastatic urothelial cancer. J Clin Oncol 1997; 15:3394–8.

11. Castagneto B, Zai S, Marenco D, et al. Single-agent gemcitabine in previously untreated elderly patients with advanced bladder carcinoma: response to treatment and correlation with the comprehensive geriatric assessment. Oncology 2004;67:27–32.

12. Culine S, Flechon A, Guillot A, et al. Gemcitabine or gemcitabine plus oxaliplatin in the first-line treatment of patients with advanced transitional cell carcinoma of the urothelium unfit for cisplatin-based chemotherapy: a randomized phase II study of the French Genitourinary Tumor Group (GETUG V01). Eur Urol 2011; 60:1251–7.

13. Dimopoulos MA, Deliveliotis C, Moulopoulos LA, et al. Treatment of patients with urothelial carcinoma and impaired renal function with single-agent docetaxel. Urology 1998;52:56–60.

14. Roth B, Dreicer R, Einhorn LH, et al. Significant activity of paclitaxel in advanced transitional cell carcinoma of the urothelium: a phase II trial of the Eastern Cooperative Oncology Group. J Clin Oncol 1994;12:2264–70.

15. Yang MH, Yen CC, Chang YH, et al. Single-agent paclitaxel as a first-line therapy in advanced urothelial carcinoma: its efficacy and safety in patients even with pretreatment renal insufficiency. Jpn J Clin Oncol 2000;310:547–52.

16. Maughan BL, Agarwal N, Husssain SA, et al. Pooled analysis of phase II trials evaluating weekly or conventional cisplatin as first-line therapy for advanced urothelial carcinoma. Clin Genitourin Cancer 2013;11:316–20.

17. Morales-Barrera R, Bellmunt J, Suarez C, et al. Cisplatin and gemcitabine administered every two weeks in patients with locally advanced or metastatic urothelial carcinoma and impaired renal function. Eur J Cancer 2012;48: 1816–21.

18. Bellmunt J, de Wit R, Albanell J, et al. A feasibility study of carboplatin with fixed dose of gemcitabine in "unfit" patients with advanced bladder cancer. Eur J Cancer 2001;37:2212–5.

19. Iaffaioli RV, Tortoriello A, Facchini G, et al. Phase I-II study of gemcitabine and carboplatin in stage IIIB-IV non-small-cell lung cancer. J Clin Oncol 1999;17:921–6.

20. Linardou H, Aravantinos G, Efstathiou E, et al. Gemcitabine and carboplatin combination as first-line treatment in elderly patients and those unfit for cisplatin-based chemotherapy with advanced bladder carcinoma: a phase II study of the Hellenic CO-operative Oncology group. Urology 2004;64:479–84.

21. De Santis M, Bellmunt J, Mead G, et al. Randomized phase II/III trial assessing gemcitabine/carboplatin and methotrexate/carboplatin/vinblastine in patients with advanced urothelial cancer "unfit" for cisplatin-based chemotherapy: phase II-results of EORTC Study 30986. J Clin Oncol 2009;27:5634–9.

22. De Santis M, Bellmunt J, Mead G, et al. Randomized phase II/III trial assessing gemcitabine/carboplatin and methotrexate/carboplatin/vinblastine in patients with advanced urothelial cancer who are unfit for cisplatin-based chemotherapy: EORTC study 30986. J Clin Oncol 2012;30:191–9.

23. Balar AV, Apolo AB, Ostrovnaya I, et al. Phase II study of gemcitabine, carboplatin, and bevacizumab in patients with advanced unresectable or metastatic urothelial cancer. J Clin Oncol 2013;31:724–30.

24. De Santis M, Wiechno PJ, Lucas C, et al. Feasibility and activity of two vinflunine (VFL)-based combinations as first-line chemotherapy in CDDP-unfit patients with advanced urothelial carcinoma: VFL-gemcitabine (GEM) or VFL-CBDCA in a randomized international phase II trial (JASINT). J Clin Oncol 2014;32(5s (Suppl)) [abstract: 4534].

25. Carles J, Nogué M, Doménech M, et al. Carboplatin-gemcitabine treatment of patients with transitional cell carcinoma of the bladder and impaired renal function. Oncology 2000;59:24–7.

26. Bamias A, Moulopoulos LA, Koutras A, et al. The combination of gemcitabine and carboplatin as first-line treatment in patients with advanced urothelial carcinoma. A Phase II study of the Hellenic Cooperative Oncology Group. Cancer 2006;106: 297–303.

27. Vaughn DJ, Manola J, Dreicer R, et al. Phase II study of paclitaxel plus carboplatin in patients with advanced carcinoma of the urothelium and renal dysfunction (E2896): a trial of the Eastern Cooperative Oncology Group. Cancer 2002;95:1022–7.

28. Galsky MD, Iasonos A, Mironov S, et al. Phase II trial of dose-dense doxorubicin plus gemcitabine followed by paclitaxel plus carboplatin in patients with advanced urothelial carcinoma and impaired renal function. Cancer 2007;109: 549–55.

29. Calabaro F, Lorusso V, Rosati G, et al. Gemcitabine and paclitaxel every 2 weeks in patients with previously untreated urothelial carcinoma. Cancer 2009;115: 2652–9.

30. Dreicer R, Li H, Cooney MM, et al. Phase 2 trial of pemetrexed disodium and gemcitabine in advanced urothelial cancer (E4802): a trial of the Eastern Cooperative Oncology Group. Cancer 2008;112:2671–5.

31. Ricci S, Galli L, Chioni A, et al. Gemcitabine plus epirubicin in patients with advanced urothelial carcinoma who are not eligible for platinum-based agents. Cancer 2002;95:1444–50.

32. Turkolmez K, Bduk Y, Baltaci S, et al. Gemcitabine plus vinorelbine chemotherapy in patients with advanced bladder carcinoma who are medically unsuitable for or who have failed cisplatin-based chemotherapy. Eur Urol 2003;44:682–6.

33. Bellmunt J, Gonzalez-Larriba JL, Prior C, et al. Phase II study of sunitinib as first-line treatment of urothelial cancer patients ineligible to receive cisplatin-based chemotherapy: baseline interleukin-8 and tumor contrast enhancement as potential predictive factors of activity. Ann Oncol 2011;22:2646–53.

34. Cancer Genome Atlas Research Network. Comprehensive molecular characterization of urothelial bladder carcinoma. Nature 2014;507:315–22.

35. Milowsky MI, Dittrich C, Duran Martinez I, et al. Final results of a multicenter, open-label phase II trial of dovitinib (TKI258) in patients with advanced urothelial carcinoma with either mutated or nonmutated FGFR3. J Clin Oncol 2013; 31(Suppl 6) [abstract: 255].

36. Galsky MD, Posner M, Holcombe RF, et al. Phase Ib study of dovitinib in combination with gemcitabine plus cisplatin or gemcitabine plus carboplatin in patients with advanced solid tumors. Cancer Chemother Pharmacol 2014. http://dx.doi.org/10.1007/s00280-014-2518-5.

37. Sequist LV, Cassier P, Varga A, et al. Phase I study of BGJ398, a selective pan-FGFR inhibitor in genetically preselected advanced solid tumors. In: American Association for Cancer Research 2014 Annual Meeting. 2014:CT326. San Diego, CA – April 08, 2014.

38. Powles T, Vogelzang NJ, Fine GD, et al. Inhibition of PD-L1 by MPDL3280A and clinical activity in pts with metastatic urothelial bladder cancer (UBC). J Clin Oncol 2014;32(5s (Suppl)) [abstract: 5011].

Second-Line Therapies in Metastatic Urothelial Carcinoma

Sujata Narayanan, MD[a], Lauren C. Harshman, MD[b],
Sandy Srinivas, MD[a],*

KEYWORDS

- Refractory • Therapies in urothelial cancer • Chemotherapy • Targeted
- Immunotherapy

KEY POINTS

- There is no standard of care treatment that improves patient survival.
- Taxanes in the US and Vinflunine in Europe are the most commonly used agents.
- Participation in clinical trials is critical.

INTRODUCTION

Platinum-based chemotherapy regimens have shown significant clinical activity against urothelial carcinomas (UC) and are generally used in the first-line setting. These regimens include combinations such as gemcitabine and cisplatin (GC) and methotrexate, vinblastine adriamycin, cisplatin (MVAC). Although these regimens have initial high response rates (RRs), ranging from 40% to 70%, they are generally not curative, with median progression-free survival (PFS) of approximately 8 months and a 5-year overall survival (OS) of 15%.[1,2] Most of these patients relapse and require additional therapy, but often, in the setting of decreased performance status and impaired renal function, precluding further administration of cisplatin.

Once patients progress or relapse after initial platinum-based chemotherapy, there is no standard of care treatment in the United States, despite scores of trials attempting to identify agents that improve patient survival. Further complicating matters, these patients tend to be older (median age, 70s), with multiple comorbidities. Selection of second-line or salvage treatment requires careful consideration of their prognosis, performance status, and organ function.

[a] Department of Medicine, Stanford University School of Medicine, Blake Wilbur Drive, Stanford, CA 94305, USA; [b] Lank Center for Genitourinary Oncology, Dana-Farber Cancer Institute, Harvard Medical School, 450 Brookline Ave, DANA 1230, Boston, MA 02215, USA
* Corresponding author.
E-mail address: sandysri@stanford.edu

Hematol Oncol Clin N Am 29 (2015) 341–359
http://dx.doi.org/10.1016/j.hoc.2014.10.007
0889-8588/15/$ – see front matter © 2015 Elsevier Inc. All rights reserved.

CLINICAL PROGNOSTIC FACTORS

Various clinical prognostic factors have been identified in patients with advanced UC. In a retrospective analysis of patients treated with first-line MVAC,[3] Karnofsky Performance Score less than 80% and presence of visceral (lung, liver, or bone) were found to be 2 independent risk factors in predicting survival. When classified by the number of risk factors, 3 groups clearly emerged, with differential survival estimates. Patients with zero, 1, or 2 risk factors were found to have a median OS of 33, 13.4, and 9.3 months, respectively.

In the platinum-refractory second-line setting, performance status and liver metastasis continue to portend worse survival. In addition to these factors, Bellmunt and colleagues[4] identified anemia, defined as a hemoglobin level less than 10 g/dL, as an additional prognostic factor in patients with platinum-refractory UC who were treated with vinflunine. Based on the presence of zero, 1, 2, or 3 prognostic factors; the median OS was 14.2, 7.3, 3.8, and 1.7 months ($P<.001$), respectively. In a retrospective review of 7 prospective second-line phase 2 trials, shorter time from previous cisplatin therapy to start of subsequent therapy also portended worse survival.[5] In the randomized phase 3 trial comparing vinflunine in combination with best supportive care (BSC) with BSC in patients relapsing after first-line platinum-based chemotherapy, patients who had received previous cisplatin had overall more favorable prognostic criteria (better performance status and absence of visceral metastasis or anemia) and improved OS.[6,7]

BIOLOGY OF ADVANCED UROTHELIAL CARCINOMA

Until recently, the biology of progression in UC after response to previous therapy was poorly understood. Accumulating molecular data have now provided an improved understanding of the underlying tumor biology, and multiple candidate genes have been implicated in the pathogenesis and resistance mechanisms of UC. In advanced UC, alterations in various signaling pathways have been observed, involving angiogenesis (VEGFR [vascular endothelial growth factor receptor], FGFR [fibroblast growth factor receptor], angiopoietin receptor 1 and 2), survival (PI3K/AKT/mTOR [phosphatidylinositol 3-kinase/protein kinase B/mammalian target of rapamycin] pathway, phosphatase and tensin homolog [PTEN], tumor protein p53), and proliferation (MAPK/ERK [mitogen activated protein kinase/extracellular signal-regulated kinases], EGFR [epithelial growth factor receptor], HER2 [human epidermal growth factor receptor 2], JAK-STAT [Janus kinase and signal transducer and activator of transcription]), have been observed, and are frequently associated with poor outcomes.[8–11]

Recently, a comprehensive profiling of muscle-invasive UCs by The Cancer Genome Atlas (TCGA) project showed 29 recurrently mutated genes, and several potential therapeutic targets in UC, including alterations in PIK3CA, HER2, FGFR3, TSC1 and HER3, as well as mutations in chromatin-regulating genes MLL, MLL2, MLL3, CREBBP, CHD7, SRCAP, ARID1A, KDM6A (UTX), and EP300.[12] Several of the genomic alterations identified in this study, particularly those involving the PI(3) K/AKT/mTOR, , MAPK, HER2, HER3, FGFR3 and CCND1 (cyclin D1) are amenable in principle to therapeutic targeting.

Encouraging preclinical and clinical data have recently emerged in tumor immunology with therapies focused on enhancing T-cell responses against cancer.[13–15] PD-L1 (programmed death ligand 1) is an extracellular protein that downregulates immune responses primarily in peripheral tissues by binding to its receptor, PD-1 (pro- grammed death 1). The interaction of PD-L1 with PD-1 inhibits T-cell proliferation, cytokine production, and cytolytic activity, leading to the functional inactivation or exhaustion of T cells.[16]

Overexpression of PD-L1 on tumor cells is believed to impede antitumor immunity by inactivating the host cytotoxic T lymphocytes, resulting in immune evasion.[17] PD-L1 expression is prevalent in many human tumors, and increased PD-L1 expression on tumor cells is associated with a poor prognosis in patients with UC.[18] Therefore, interruption of the PD-L1/PD-1 pathway represents an attractive strategy to reinvigorate tumor-specific T-cell immunity.

Identification of these molecular drivers and escape mechanisms has paved the way for rational investigation and potential development of novel targeted therapeutics in bladder cancer. However, genomic testing of tumors still remains in its nascent stages and requires standardization, replication, and implementation in clinical trials to become standard of care for management of advanced UC.

APPROACH TO PATIENTS

In the absence of definitive guidelines, treatment of patients requiring second-line or salvage chemotherapy has distinct challenges, and multiple host-related, disease-related, and therapy-related factors must be considered in formulating a treatment plan. Consideration of a patient's prognosis forms the backbone of decision making in the salvage setting, in which options include available chemotherapies, enrollment in clinical trials, and BSC. Multiple clinical trials[3,4] have implicated the patient's performance status as a strong determinant of their OS. Age and end-organ function also influence the choice of second-line chemotherapy, along with patient eligibility for clinical trials.

Adequate cardiac and renal function, neurologic status, and hearing ability are important components when determining suitability for platinum-based regimens.[19,20] Carboplatin-based combinations are feasible in patients unsuitable for cisplatin, but small randomized trials[19] have suggested that they are suboptimal compared with cisplatin-based regimens. Previous cisplatin or taxane use can induce significant neuropathy, which may limit the use of these agents in the second-line setting. Retreatment with a previous regimen is a viable option, especially if it is offered after long duration of disease remission. Because platinum-based regimens are often applied in the first-line setting, it is important to define whether the patients are platinum sensitive or refractory. Although not uniformly defined for UC, a relapse-free interval greater or equal to 6 months after the last dose of platinum treatment, a rule generally applied in ovarian cancer, could be used to define platinum sensitivity in UC.[21,22]

Given the absence of a second-line agent with meaningful improvement in survival, clinical trials should be considered in every patient who is amenable. With the advent of molecular testing and targeted therapies, clinical trials offer a unique opportunity for patient care and also enrich our knowledge of UC pathogenesis.

RESULTS OF SECOND-LINE CHEMOTHERAPY IN ADVANCED UROTHELIAL CANCER

There is no standard second-line chemotherapy in the United States that is recommended for advanced UC. The evidence for the use of chemotherapy in the second-line setting comes from mostly small phase 2 trials evaluating single agents and combination regimens and 2 phase 3 trials.

SINGLE AGENTS

Several chemotherapeutics have been evaluated in the second-line setting, with modest responses between 8% and 30% (**Table 1**).[23–38]

Gemcitabine as a single agent, in varying doses, has shown good RRs, with a low toxicity profile in the second-line setting. In a phase 2 study of 30 patients who had

Table 1
Phase 2/3 trials of single agents used for second-line treatment of UC

Drug	Type of Study	Number of Patients	RR (%)	Time to Progression (mo)	Overall Survival (mo)
Paclitaxel[23]	Phase 2	31	10	2.2	7.2
Nanoparticle albumin-bound paclitaxel[24]	Phase 2	47	27.7	6	10.8
Pemetrexed[25]	Phase 2	13	8	—	—
Pemetrexed[26]	Phase 2	47	27.7	2.9	9.6
Docetaxel[27]	Phase 2	30	13.3	—	9
Gemcitabine[28]	Phase 2	28	11	4.9	8.7
Gemcitabine[29]	Phase 2	35	22.5	—	5
Vinflunine[30]	Phase 2	51	18	3	6.6
Vinflunine[31]	Phase 2	151	15	2.8	8.2
Vinflunine[6]	Phase 3	370	8.6	3	—
Oxaliplatin[32]	Phase 2	18	6	1.5	7
Irinotecan[33]	Phase 2	40	5	2.1	5.4
Ixabepilone[34]	Phase 2	42	11.9	2.7	8
Bortezomib[35]	Phase 2	25	0	1.4	5.7
Ifosfamide[36]	Phase 2	56	20	2.4	5.5
Lapatinib[37]	Phase 2	34	3	2	4.5
Topotecan[38]	Phase 2	44	9.1	1.5	6.3

received previous cisplatin-based chemotherapy,[28] gemcitabine 1250 mg/m^2 administered on days 1 and 8 of a 21-day schedule for a maximum of 6 cycles was able to achieve an objective RR of 11%, a mean time to progression (TTP) of 4.9 months, and disease-specific survival of 8.7 months. Previous nonresponders to cisplatin had a significantly lower frequency of response to gemcitabine. Another phase 2 trial[29] with a similar cohort of patients who received gemcitabine 1200 mg/m^2 on day 1, 8, and 15 of a 28-day cycle showed a promising overall response of 22.5%, with a median survival of 5 months.

Taxanes are also frequently implemented after previous use of cisplatin-based chemotherapy. In this setting, docetaxel can elicit an RR of 13.3% and a median survival of 9 months.[27] Paclitaxel monotherapy has been evaluated in several phase 2 trials, with paltry RRs of 5% to 10%.[23,39,40] In a phase 2 study evaluating weekly paclitaxel dosing,[23] an RR of 10% with a PFS of 2.2 months and median survival of 7.2 months were noted. The nanoparticle albumin-bound paclitaxel was studied in a phase 2 trial involving 48 patients who had received previous cisplatin-based therapy.[24] The agent elicited an encouraging overall RR of 27·7%, median PFS of 6 months, and a median OS of 10.8 months.

Vinflunine is a microtubule inhibitor that has been evaluated in phase 2 and 3 studies in patients with platinum-refractory advanced UC. In phase 2 studies,[30,31] vinflunine produced an objective RR of 15% to 18%, a median PFS around 3 months, and a median OS of 6 to 9 months. The promising survival results prompted a phase 3 trial comparing vinflunine plus BSC with BSC alone in 370 patients progressing after first-line platinum-based chemotherapy.[6] Although the median 2-month survival advantage (6.9 months for vinflunine + BSC vs 4.6 months for BSC) was not significant in the intent to treat population (hazard ratio [HR] = 0.88; 95% confidence interval [CI], 0.69–1.12) (P = .287), in the eligible population (n = 357), the median OS was statistically significantly longer for vinflunine + BSC than BSC (6.9 vs 4.3 months, respectively, $P = .04$). The overall RR, disease control, and PFS all statistically favored the vinflunine plus BSC group (overall RR [ORR]: 8.6% vs 0%, respectively; $P = .006$; disease control rate: 41.1% vs 24.8%, respectively; $P = .002$; median PFS: 3.0 vs 1.5 months, respectively; $P = .001$; HR = 0.68; 95% CI, 0.54–0.86). Based on this study, vinflunine is approved in Europe as a second-line treatment option for patients with advanced UC who have failed a previous platinum-containing regimen.

Pemetrexed has also shown promise as a well-tolerated, single agent with an RR of 27.7%, PFS of 2.9 months, and a median survival of 9.6 months.[26] Ifosfamide can induce considerable RRs, but at the expense of significant toxicity (RR, 20%; PFS, 2.4 months; OS, 5.5 months).[36] Other agents with modest activity in the second-line setting include ixabepilone[34] and oxaliplatin (see **Table 1**).[32]

COMBINATION REGIMENS

Multiple second-line combination regimens have been evaluated in bladder cancer and frequently include platinums, taxanes, and gemcitabine as backbone agents (**Table 2**).[20,41–57] Although combination regimens have generally shown better RRs, they have not shown improved survival and are frequently associated with higher toxicity.

The combination of gemcitabine and paclitaxel has been the most extensively evaluated regimen in the second-line setting in advanced UC.[41–46] Although the phase 2 studies have all used different dosing and treatment schedules, this combination can elicit objective responses ranging from 30% to 60% and a median OS of 11 to 14 months (see **Table 2**). A German phase 3 trial[47] randomized patients to receive 6 cycles of gemcitabine and paclitaxel (group A) versus an additional maintenance therapy for gemcitabine and paclitaxel every 3 weeks until progression (group B). No significant difference in OS (group A, 7.5 months; group B, 6.8 months, $P = .8$) or overall RRs (group A, 34.5%; group B, 50.0%) was observed with the added maintenance dosing. It was also noted in the study that patients who had a previous major response to first-line chemotherapy had a trend toward a higher chance of response to second-line treatment ($P = .06$), and patients with a median duration of response greater than 7.1 months to first-line therapy also had a significantly better response to second-line treatment.

In contrast, the combination of carboplatin and paclitaxel has modest efficacy, with RRs of only 16%, median PFS of 4 months, and median OS of 6 months.[20] The triplet combination of carboplatin, docetaxel, and gemcitabine produced a high RR of 45% but was limited by significant dose-limiting neutropenia.[55]

Studies have also evaluated the use of GC or methotrexate, vinblastine, adriamycin, and cisplatin (MVAC) as second-line regimens. In a study that enrolled 30 patients, who had progressed or relapsed after treatment with GC,[58] the use of second-line MVAC produced an RR of 30% with a median PFS of 5.3 months and OS of 10.9 months, with grade 3 to 4 neutropenia, thrombocytopenia, and anemia occurring in 63.3%, 30%, and 16.7% of the patients, respectively. Similarly, GC after first-line MVAC produced an objective RR of 39.4% in 33 patients with a median survival of 10.5 months with similar rates of neutropenia (66.7%) and thrombocytopenia (30.3%).[59]

EVALUATION OF TARGETED THERAPIES IN UROTHELIAL CANCER

In recent years, genomic studies have shown the heterogeneous nature of UC.[60] Many somatic mutations are expressed that may provide rational targets for novel targeted therapies.[61] Multiple candidate genes with potential diagnostic and prognostic relevance from oncogenic signaling, cell cycle, tumor suppressor, and stromal angiogenesis pathways have been identified for both non–muscle-invasive and muscle-invasive bladder cancers.[12,62–64]

Table 2
Phase 1/2 studies evaluating combination second-line chemotherapy in advanced UC

Agents	Chemotherapy and Dosing	Study Type	N	RR (%)	OS (mo)
Gemcitabine/Paclitaxel					
Meluch et al,[41] 2001	Gemcitabine 1000 mg/m^2 (D 1, 8, 15) Paclitaxel 200 mg/m^2 (D 1) Every 3 wk	Phase 2	54	54	14.4
Sternberg et al,[42] 2001	Gemcitabine 2500–3000 mg/m^2 Paclitaxel 150 mg/m^2 Every 2 wk	Phase 2	41	60	14.4
Fechner et al,[43] 2006	Gemcitabine 1000 mg/m^2 (D 1, 8) Paclitaxel 175 mg/m^2 (D 1) Every 3 wk or Gemcitabine 1250 mg/m^2 (D 1) Paclitaxel 120 mg/m^2 (D 2) Every 2 wk	Randomized Phase 2	30	44	—
Takahashi et al,[44] 2006	Gemcitabine 2500 mg/m^2 Paclitaxel 150 mg/m^2 Every 2 wk	Phase 2	23	30	12.1
Kanai et al,[45] 2008	Gemcitabine 2500 mg/m^2 Paclitaxel 150 mg/m^2 Every 2 wk	Phase 2	20	30	11.5
Suyama et al,[46] 2009	Gemcitabine 1000 mg/m^2 (D 1, 8, 15) Paclitaxel 180 mg/m^2 Every 4 wk	Phase 2	30	33.3	11.3
5-Fluorouracil/α-Interferon/Cisplatin		—	—	—	—
Logothetis et al,[48] 1992	—	Phase 2	28	61	—
De Mulder et al,[49] 2000	—	Phase 2	40	12.5	—
Paclitaxel/methotrexate/cisplatin[50]	Paclitaxel 200 mg/m^2, methotrexate 30 mg/m^2, cisplatin 70 mg/m^2 Every 3 wk	Phase 2	25	40	—

	Dosing	Phase			
Paclitaxel/ifosfamide[51]	Ifosfamide 1.0 gm/m² D 1–4, Paclitaxel 135 mg/m² (24-h infusion, D 4), Every 3 wk	Phase 2	26	15	8
Docetaxel/ifosfamide[52]	Docetaxel 60 mg/m², Ifosfamide 2.5 g/m² (24-h infusion), Every 3 wk	Phase 2	20	25	4
Methotrexate/paclitaxel[53]	Methotrexate 30 mg/m² and paclitaxel 175 mg/m², Every 3 wk	Phase 2	19	32	5
Cisplatin/gemcitabine/ifosfamide[54]	Cisplatin 30 mg/m², gemcitabine 800 mg/m², ifosfamide 1 g/m² (D 1, 8, 15), Every 4 wk	Phase 2	49	41	9.5
Docetaxel/gemcitabine/carboplatin[55]	Docetaxel 50 mg/m² (D 1), Carboplatin AUC = 5 (D 1), Gemcitabine 800 mg/m² (D 1, 8), Every 21 d or Docetaxel 50 mg/m² (D 1), Carboplatin AUC = 5 (D 1), Gemcitabine 800 mg/m² (D 2, 8, or 15), Every 21 d	Phase 1/2	20	45	—
Carboplatin/paclitaxel[20]	Carboplatin AUC 5, Paclitaxel 200 mg/m², Every 3 wk	Phase 2	44	16	6
Gemcitabine/Ifosfamide	—	—	—	—	—
Pectasides et al,[57] 2001	Gemcitabine 800 mg/m², Ifosfamide 2 g/m² (D 1, 8), Every 3 wk	Phase 2	34	21	9
Lin et al,[56] 2007	Gemcitabine 800 mg/m² (D 1, 8, 15), Ifosfamide 1500 mg/m² (24-h infusion D 8–10), Every 4 wk	Phase 2	23	22	4.8

Abbreviations: AUC, area under the curve; D, day; N, sample size.

For example, profiling of muscle-invasive UCs by TCGA identified the FGFR3, PI3-kinase/mTOR/AKT/TSC1, and ERBB2 (or HER2) pathways as potential targets for novel therapeutics based on the frequency of these alterations (**Fig. 1**).[12]

UCs that progress after cisplatin-based chemotherapy regimens are frequently resistant to other available chemotherapies, and, therefore, addition of targeted agents alone or in combination is a rational treatment strategy. Clinical trials have evaluated several novel agents, including those targeting angiogenesis (VEGF), growth factor receptors (EGFR, HER2, FGFR), and immunomodulatory agents in UC with variable levels of success.[65,66] **Table 3** lists the recently concluded trials evaluating targeted therapies in UC.[35,37,67–80]

Vandetanib is a selective tyrosine kinase inhibitor of vascular endothelial growth factor receptor (VEGFR)-2 and EGFR that has shown significant antitumor activity in preclinical and early clinical trials.[74] However, Choueiri and colleagues[74] in a randomized phase 2 study compared the combination of docetaxel with vandetanib with docetaxel and placebo and failed to show any significant improvement in PFS, RR, or OS. In this trial, patients receiving docetaxel plus placebo had the option to cross over to single-agent vandetanib at progression, allowing the analysis of a sequence of therapies. Of the 37 patients who crossed over to vandetanib therapy, the RR was 3% and OS was 5.2 months.

Sunitinib is an oral tyrosine kinase inhibitor targeting the VEGF receptor with antitumor activity in UC.[81] In a phase 2 study,[70] sunitinib was administered as a

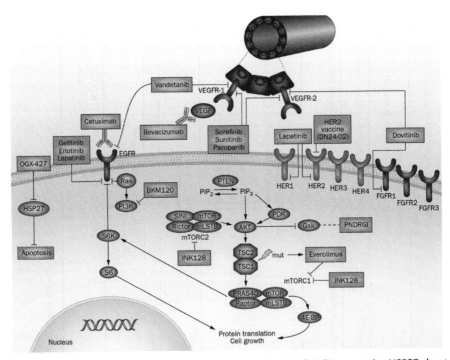

Fig. 1. Therapeutic targets in urothelial tumors. 4E-BP, IF4E-binding protein; HSP27, heat shock 27 kDa protein; mTORC1/2, mammalian target of rapamycin complex 1/2; PDK, phosphoinositide-dependent kinase; PI3K, phosphatidylinositol-3-kinase; PRAS40, proline-rich AKT1 substrate 1 40 kDa; S6K, S6 kinase; SIN1, stress-activated protein kinase interaction protein 1; TSC1/2, tuberous sclerosis protein 1/2. (*From* Bellmunt J, Teh BT, Tortora G, et al. Molecular targets on the horizon for kidney and urothelial cancer. Nat Rev Clin Oncol 2013;10(10):561; with permission.)

Table 3
Completed trials using targeted agents in the second-line setting for advanced UC

Target	Agent	Type of Study	Chemotherapy	Number of Patients	RR (%)	OS (mo)
EGFR	Cetuximab[67]	Randomized phase 2	Paclitaxel and cetuximab vs	39	25	10.5
			Cetuximab alone		0	1.3
	Lapatinib[37]	Phase 2	None	59	3	4.5
	Gefitinib[68]	Phase 2	None	31	3	3
VEGF	Sorafenib[69]	Phase 2	None	27	0	6.8
	Sunitinib[70]	Phase 2	None	45	7	6.9
	Aflibercept[71]	Phase 2	None	22	4.5	NR
	Pazopanib[72]	Phase 2	None	19	0	NR
	Pazopanib[73]	Phase 2	None	41	17	4.7
VEGFR, EGFR	Vandetanib[74]	Randomized phase 2	Docetaxel and vandetanib vs	142	7	5.56
			Docetaxel and placebo		11	7.39
FGFR3	Dovitinib[75]	Phase 2	None	44	0	NR
PI3k/Akt/mTOR	Everolimus[76]	Phase 2	None	45	5	10.5
SAHA: histone deacetylase	Vorinostat[77]	Phase 2	None	14	0	4.3
Pololike kinase 1	Volasertib[78]	Phase 2	None	31	19	NR
Farnesyl transferase	Lonafarnib[79]	Phase 2	Gemcitabine	31	32	NR
Proteasome inhibitor	Bortezomib[80]	Phase 2	None	20	0	NR
	Bortezomib[35]	Phase 2	None	25	0	5.7

Abbreviations: NR, not reported; V, vascular endothelial growth factor receptor.

second-line agent to 77 patients with advanced UC and showed clinical regression or stable disease in 43% of the patients. In a recently published phase 2 trial,[82] 26 patients with relapsed UC were treated with the combination of pazopanib, an oral multityrosine kinase inhibitor, and paclitaxel. This study reported a high objective RR of 60%, with complete response in 2 (8%) patients and partial response in 12 (52%) patients.

Strong expression of EGFR is found in 50% of bladder cancers, with higher expression in invasive tumors (pT2-4) and high-grade tumors. Higher EGFR expression has also been associated with tumor progression and shorter disease-free survival.[83-87] Cetuximab is a monoclonal antibody directed against EGFR. A randomized phase 2 study[67] compared cetuximab monotherapy with the combination therapy with paclitaxel and noted disappointing results of no objective responses for cetuximab alone and 25% for the combination in this unselected patient population.

Receptor tyrosine-protein kinase erbB-2 (*ERBB2*), also frequently called *HER2* (from human EGFR2) or *HER2/neu*, is the most studied of the 4 receptors in the EGFR family that regulates multiple processes, including cell proliferation. In advanced UC, up to 50% of the tumors have been shown to overexpress the HER2 protein,[88] and their expression correlates with increased number of metastatic sites.[88] A phase 2 trial[88] evaluated the combination of trastuzumab (HER2/neu receptor-targeted monoclonal antibody) with paclitaxel, carboplatin, and gemcitabine in HER2-positive patients with urothelial carcinoma in the first-line setting. This study reported a promising RR of 70%, median response duration of 7 months, median TTP of 9.3 months, and a median survival of 14 months. This study highlights the importance of identifying predictive biomarkers that may enhance outcomes for patients.

Gefitinib and lapatinib (dual TKI-targeting HER2/neu and EGFR) have been tested as single agents in the second-line treatment of metastatic urothelial carcinoma, with disappointingly low RRs of less than 5%.[37,68]

Several trials have recently evaluated targeted agents in UC,[89-101] and a summary of ongoing trials is provided in **Table 4**.

IMMUNOTHERAPY

The concept of immune surveillance in controlling outgrowth of neoplastic transformations has been debated for decades. The physiologic function of PD-1, expressed on the cell surface of activated T cells under healthy conditions, is to downmodulate unwanted or excessive immune responses, such as during viral infection or to prevent autoimmune reactions.[102] PD-1 is an inhibitory receptor expressed on T cells after T-cell activation. Tumors can express the PD-L1 ligand, which, when it binds to PD-1 on the T cells, can result in functional deactivation.[16] UC has been shown to express the PD-L1 ligands in 12% to 25% of UCs.[18,103,104] Blocking the interaction between PD-1 and PD-L1 can enhance the functional activity of these effector lymphocytes, facilitating tumor regression and immune rejection. Several antibodies are being evaluated in clinical trials, such as the anti-PD-1 antibodies nivolumab and pembrolizumab and anti-PD-L1 antibodies, such as MPDL3280A.

A recently conducted phase 1 study[105] investigating the anti-PD-L1 monoclonal antibody MPDL3280A achieved promising overall RRs in patients with previously treated metastatic urothelial bladder cancer whose tumors expressed the PD-L1 ligand. This study recruited 31 patients with UC, most of whom (71%) had received more than 2 previous lines of therapy (>97% platinum based). Twenty patients were available for evaluation at a median follow-up of 2.8 months and showed a promising ORR of 50%. In this study, a higher degree of PD-L1 expression in the tumor cells as

Table 4
Recent trials evaluating targeted therapies in advanced UC

Target	Drug	Trial	Clinicaltrials.gov Identifier	Status
VEGF	Ramucirumab[89]	Randomized phase 2; ramucirumab or IMC-18F1 with docetaxel or docetaxel alone	NCT01282463	Active
	Pazopanib[90]	Phase 2; pazopanib and vinflunine	NCT01265940	Completed, results unavailable
	Pazopanib[91]	Phase 2; pazopanib with paclitaxel	NCT01108055	Active
VEGF/c-Met	Cabozantinib[92]	Phase 2	NCT01688999	Active
EGFR	Lapatinib[93]	Phase 2; docetaxel and lapatinib	NCT01382706	Terminated
	Lapatinib[94]	Randomized phase 2/3; lapatinib vs placebo	NCT00949455	Active
	Trastuzumab[95]	Phase 2	NCT02013765	Completed, results unavailable
Hsp27	OGX-427[96]	Randomized phase 2; docetaxel with OGX-427 vs docetaxel alone	NCT01780545	Active
LHRH (linked to doxorubicin)	AEZS-108[97]	Phase 1/2	NCT01234519	Terminated
CD105	TRC105[98]	Phase 2	NCT01328574	Active
PI3K	BKM120[99]	Phase 2	NCT01551030	Active
TGFbR/ALK1	PF-03446962[100]	Phase 2	NCT01620970	Unknown
SLITRK6	ASG-15ME[101]	Phase 1	NCT01963052	Active

Abbreviation: IMC, Icrucumab.

assessed by immunohistochemistry was associated with increased objective response to MPDL3280A. This drug has been granted a breakthrough therapy designation by the US Food and Drug Administration, and further follow-up results from the study are awaited.

Preclinical studies have also implicated CD47 as a potential target for solid tumors. CD47 is a widely expressed transmembrane protein that functions as a ligand for signal regulatory protein α (SIRPα), a protein expressed on macrophages and dendritic cells.[106] On binding CD47, SIRPα initiates a signaling cascade, which results in the inhibition of phagocytosis. CD47 is a commonly expressed molecule on all cancers, and its blockade leads to tumor cell phagocytosis and elimination. In vitro and in vivo studies using monoclonal antibodies against CD47 have shown promising results in solid tumors, including UC.[107]

BEST SUPPORTIVE CARE AND PALLIATION

Patients with recurrent urothelial carcinoma often have multiple comorbidities and complications secondary to metastatic disease, such as pain, bleeding, and end-organ dysfunction. Careful attention to the patient's quality of life should be the foremost consideration before choosing any systemic therapy, and the choice of BSC with transition to hospice instead of further anticancer therapy is reasonable.

Radiation is often used as a palliative measure in advanced UC. Patients with urothelial carcinoma can frequently experience pain, bleeding, obstruction secondary to enlarged lymph nodes, and symptomatic metastasis to the brain and bone. Radiation can be useful to control bleeding arising from the urinary tract, local obstruction produced by metastatic disease, symptomatic brain metastases, or pain secondary to osseous metastases.

In a phase 3 trial,[108] patients with muscle-invasive bladder cancer causing local symptoms and deemed unsuitable for curative treatment either because of advanced disease or comorbidities were randomized to receive radiation treatments either as 35 Gy in 10 fractions or 21 Gy in 3 fractions. On follow-up after 3 months, 272 patients were evaluated, and 68% achieved symptomatic improvement (71% for 35 Gy, 64% for 21 Gy), with no evidence of a difference in efficacy or toxicity between the 2 arms. Hematuria improved in 88% of patients, urinary frequency in 82%, dysuria in 72%, and nocturia in 64%. Median survival for this cohort was 7.5 months, and approximately 25% had died by the 3-month time point. These data show that a short course of radiation treatment is effective in palliating local symptoms in most patients with advanced UC.

When treating recurrent pelvic disease with palliative radiation, combining radiation with radiosensitizing chemotherapy can be considered, although it represents an unproven extrapolation from trials testing such combined modality therapy in the treatment of primary bladder tumors. Agents such as cisplatin, taxanes, 5-fluorouracil, 5-fluorouracil with mitomycin, capecitabine, and low-dose gemcitabine have been given concurrently with conventionally fractionated radiation for palliation of metastases or for pelvic recurrence after cystectomy.

Central nervous system metastases can be treated with a multimodality approach, with either a combination of metastatectomy and radiation or radiation alone. Whole brain or stereotactic radiation may be used for the treatment of brain metastases.

The role of radical cystectomy or metastectomy in the palliative setting is rare. Although it may be considered as a palliative approach for relief of symptoms or complications, there are limited data to support the role of metastatectomy for long-term disease control. Examination of a prospective cohort consisting of 31 patients undergoing metastatectomy after chemotherapy with a curative intent showed a 5-year survival rate of 33%.[109]

Although complete responses can be achieved in a subset of metastatic patients after primary chemotherapy, patients undergoing second-line chemotherapy need to be carefully selected as candidates for surgical consolidation.

Managing the myriad of debilitating symptoms of advanced disease, such as pain, cachexia, fatigue, and nausea, often requires a multimodality approach. We recommend the introduction of palliative care specialists early in the advanced disease course to enhance quality of life and aid in the handling of psychosocial issues.

SUMMARY

Patients with UC relapsing after first-line platinum-based regimens have a poor prognosis. There is a dearth of treatment options that improve survival, and the additional toxicities related to chemotherapy may contribute to the decline of the patient's quality of life. However, with recent advances that have further elucidated the genomic background of UC, along with the introduction of investigational targeted therapies and immunotherapies, the treatment paradigm for UC continues to evolve. By carefully selecting patients for salvage therapies and by encouraging participation in clinical trials, physicians have the opportunity to significantly improve the overall outlook for patients with advanced UC.

REFERENCES

1. von der Maase H, Hansen SW, Roberts JT, et al. Gemcitabine and cisplatin versus methotrexate, vinblastine, doxorubicin, and cisplatin in advanced or metastatic bladder cancer: results of a large, randomized, multinational, multicenter, phase III study. J Clin Oncol 2000;18:3068–77.
2. von der Maase H, Sengelov L, Roberts JT, et al. Long-term survival results of a randomized trial comparing gemcitabine plus cisplatin, with methotrexate, vinblastine, doxorubicin, plus cisplatin in patients with bladder cancer. J Clin Oncol 2005;23:4602–8.
3. Bajorin DF, Dodd PM, Mazumdar M, et al. Long-term survival in metastatic transitional-cell carcinoma and prognostic factors predicting outcome of therapy. J Clin Oncol 1999;17:3173–81.
4. Bellmunt J, Choueiri TK, Fougeray R, et al. Prognostic factors in patients with advanced transitional cell carcinoma of the urothelial tract experiencing treatment failure with platinum-containing regimens. J Clin Oncol 2010;28:1850–5.
5. Sonpavde G, Pond GR, Fougeray R, et al. Time from prior chemotherapy enhances prognostic risk grouping in the second-line setting of advanced urothelial carcinoma: a retrospective analysis of pooled, prospective phase 2 trials. Eur Urol 2013;63:717–23.
6. Bellmunt J, Theodore C, Demkov T, et al. Phase III trial of vinflunine plus best supportive care compared with best supportive care alone after a platinum-containing regimen in patients with advanced transitional cell carcinoma of the urothelial tract. J Clin Oncol 2009;27:4454–61.
7. Harshman LC, Fougeray R, Choueiri TK, et al. The impact of prior platinum therapy on survival in patients with metastatic urothelial cancer receiving vinflunine. Br J Cancer 2013;109:2548–53.
8. Campbell SC, Volpert OV, Ivanovich M, et al. Molecular mediators of angiogenesis in bladder cancer. Cancer Res 1998;58:1298–304.

9. Wu X, Obata T, Khan Q, et al. The phosphatidylinositol-3 kinase pathway regulates bladder cancer cell invasion. BJU Int 2004;93:143–50.

10. Oka N, Yamamoto Y, Takahashi M, et al. Expression of angiopoietin-1 and -2, and its clinical significance in human bladder cancer. BJU Int 2005;95:660–3.

11. Tomlinson DC, Lamont FR, Shnyder SD, et al. Fibroblast growth factor receptor 1 promotes proliferation and survival via activation of the mitogen-activated protein kinase pathway in bladder cancer. Cancer Res 2009;69:4613–20.

12. Cancer Genome Atlas Research Network. Comprehensive molecular characterization of urothelial bladder carcinoma. Nature 2014;507:315–22.

13. Chen DS, Irving BA, Hodi FS. Molecular pathways: next-generation immunotherapy–inhibiting programmed death-ligand 1 and programmed death-1. Clin Cancer Res 2012;18:6580–7.

14. Hodi FS, O'Day SJ, McDermott DF, et al. Improved survival with ipilimumab in patients with metastatic melanoma. N Engl J Med 2010;363:711–23.

15. Kantoff PW, Higano CS, Shore ND, et al. Sipuleucel-T immunotherapy for castration-resistant prostate cancer. N Engl J Med 2010;363:411–22.

16. Blank C, Gajewski TF, Mackensen A. Interaction of PD-L1 on tumor cells with PD-1 on tumor-specific T cells as a mechanism of immune evasion: implications for tumor immunotherapy. Cancer Immunol Immunother 2005;54:307–14.

17. Blank C, Mackensen A. Contribution of the PD-L1/PD-1 pathway to T-cell exhaustion: an update on implications for chronic infections and tumor evasion. Cancer Immunol Immunother 2007;56:739–45.

18. Nakanishi J, Wada Y, Matsumoto K, et al. Overexpression of B7-H1 (PD-L1) significantly associates with tumor grade and postoperative prognosis in human urothelial cancers. Cancer Immunol Immunother 2007;56:1173–82.

19. Dogliotti L, Carteni G, Siena S, et al. Gemcitabine plus cisplatin versus gemcitabine plus carboplatin as first-line chemotherapy in advanced transitional cell carcinoma of the urothelium: results of a randomized phase 2 trial. Eur Urol 2007;52:134–41.

20. Vaishampayan UN, Faulkner JR, Small EJ, et al. Phase II trial of carboplatin and paclitaxel in cisplatin-pretreated advanced transitional cell carcinoma: a Southwest Oncology Group study. Cancer 2005;104:1627–32.

21. Markman M, Rothman R, Hakes T, et al. Second-line platinum therapy in patients with ovarian cancer previously treated with cisplatin. J Clin Oncol 1991;9:389–93.

22. Gore ME, Fryatt I, Wiltshaw E, et al. Treatment of relapsed carcinoma of the ovary with cisplatin or carboplatin following initial treatment with these compounds. Gynecol Oncol 1990;36:207–11.

23. Vaughn DJ, Broome CM, Hussain M, et al. Phase II trial of weekly paclitaxel in patients with previously treated advanced urothelial cancer. J Clin Oncol 2002;20:937–40.

24. Ko YJ, Canil CM, Mukherjee SD, et al. Nanoparticle albumin-bound paclitaxel for second-line treatment of metastatic urothelial carcinoma: a single group, multicentre, phase 2 study. Lancet Oncol 2013;14:769–76.

25. Galsky MD, Mironov S, Iasonos A, et al. Phase II trial of pemetrexed as second-line therapy in patients with metastatic urothelial carcinoma. Invest New Drugs 2007;25:265–70.

26. Sweeney CJ, Roth BJ, Kabbinavar FF, et al. Phase II study of pemetrexed for second-line treatment of transitional cell cancer of the urothelium. J Clin Oncol 2006;24:3451–7.

27. McCaffrey JA, Hilton S, Mazumdar M, et al. Phase II trial of docetaxel in patients with advanced or metastatic transitional-cell carcinoma. J Clin Oncol 1997;15:1853–7.

28. Albers P, Siener R, Hartlein M, et al. Gemcitabine monotherapy as second-line treatment in cisplatin-refractory transitional cell carcinoma–prognostic factors for response and improvement of quality of life. Onkologie 2002;25:47–52.

29. Lorusso V, Pollera CF, Antimi M, et al. A phase II study of gemcitabine in patients with transitional cell carcinoma of the urinary tract previously treated with platinum. Italian Co-operative Group on Bladder Cancer. Eur J Cancer 1998;34: 1208–12.

30. Culine S, Theodore C, De Santis M, et al. A phase II study of vinflunine in bladder cancer patients progressing after first-line platinum-containing regimen. Br J Cancer 2006;94:1395–401.

31. Vaughn DJ, Srinivas S, Stadler WM, et al. Vinflunine in platinum-pretreated patients with locally advanced or metastatic urothelial carcinoma: results of a large phase 2 study. Cancer 2009;115:4110–7.

32. Winquist E, Vokes E, Moore MJ, et al. A phase II study of oxaliplatin in urothelial cancer. Urol Oncol 2005;23:150–4.

33. Beer TM, Goldman B, Nichols CR, et al. Southwest Oncology Group phase II study of irinotecan in patients with advanced transitional cell carcinoma of the urothelium that progressed after platinum-based chemotherapy. Clin Genitourin Cancer 2008;6:36–9.

34. Dreicer R, Li S, Manola J, et al. Phase 2 trial of epothilone B analog BMS-247550 (ixabepilone) in advanced carcinoma of the urothelium (E3800): a trial of the Eastern Cooperative Oncology Group. Cancer 2007;110:759–63.

35. Rosenberg JE, Halabi S, Sanford BL, et al. Phase II study of bortezomib in patients with previously treated advanced urothelial tract transitional cell carcinoma: CALGB 90207. Ann Oncol 2008;19:946–50.

36. Witte RS, Elson P, Bono B, et al. Eastern Cooperative Oncology Group phase II trial of ifosfamide in the treatment of previously treated advanced urothelial carcinoma. J Clin Oncol 1997;15:589–93.

37. Wulfing C, Machiels JP, Richel DJ, et al. A single-arm, multicenter, open-label phase 2 study of lapatinib as the second-line treatment of patients with locally advanced or metastatic transitional cell carcinoma. Cancer 2009;115:2881–90.

38. Witte RS, Manola J, Burch PA, et al. Topotecan in previously treated advanced urothelial carcinoma: an ECOG phase II trial. Invest New Drugs 1998;16:191–5.

39. Papamichael D, Gallagher CJ, Oliver RT, et al. Phase II study of paclitaxel in pretreated patients with locally advanced/metastatic cancer of the bladder and ureter. Br J Cancer 1997;75:606–7.

40. Joly F, Tchen N, Chevreau C, et al. Clinical benefit of second line weekly paclitaxel in advanced urothelial carcinoma (AUC): a GETUG phase II study. ASCO Annual Meeting Proceedings (Post-Meeting Edition). Journal of Clinical Oncology 2004;22:14S (July 15 Supplement), 2004: 4619.

41. Meluch AA, Greco FA, Burris HA 3rd, et al. Paclitaxel and gemcitabine chemotherapy for advanced transitional-cell carcinoma of the urothelial tract: a phase II trial of the Minnie pearl cancer research network. J Clin Oncol 2001;19: 3018–24.

42. Sternberg CN, Calabro F, Pizzocaro G, et al. Chemotherapy with an every-2-week regimen of gemcitabine and paclitaxel in patients with transitional cell carcinoma who have received prior cisplatin-based therapy. Cancer 2001;92: 2993–8.

43. Fechner G, Siener R, Reimann M, et al. Randomised phase II trial of gemcitabine and paclitaxel second-line chemotherapy in patients with transitional cell carcinoma (AUO Trial AB 20/99). Int J Clin Pract 2006;60:27–31.

44. Takahashi T, Higashi S, Nishiyama H, et al. Biweekly paclitaxel and gemcitabine for patients with advanced urothelial cancer ineligible for cisplatin-based regimen. Jpn J Clin Oncol 2006;36:104–8.

45. Kanai K, Kikuchi E, Ohigashi T, et al. Gemcitabine and paclitaxel chemotherapy for advanced urothelial carcinoma in patients who have received prior cisplatin-based chemotherapy. Int J Clin Oncol 2008;13:510–4.

46. Suyama T, Ueda T, Fukasawa S, et al. Combination of gemcitabine and paclitaxel as second-line chemotherapy for advanced urothelial carcinoma. Jpn J Clin Oncol 2009;39:244–50.

47. Albers P, Siener R, Park S, et al. Randomized phase III trial of 2nd line gemcitabine/paclitaxel chemotherapy in patients with advanced bladder cancer: temporary versus maintenance treatment (German Association of Urologic Oncology (AUO) Trial AB 20/99). ASCO Annual Meeting Proceedings (Post-Meeting Edition). Journal of Clinical Oncology 2008;26:15S (May 20 Supplement), 2008: 5030.

48. Logothetis C, Dieringer P, Ellerhorst J, et al. A 61% response rate with 5-fluorouracil, interferon-a 2b and cisplatin in metastatic chemotherapy refractory transitional cell carcinoma. Proc Am Assoc Cancer Res 1992;33:221.

49. De Mulder PH, Theodore C, Sella A, et al. Phase II EORTC trial with 5-fluorouracil, cisplatin and interferon-alpha as second-line treatment of advanced transitional cell cancer of the urothelial tract. Ann Oncol 2000;11:1391–4.

50. Tu SM, Hossan E, Amato R, et al. Paclitaxel, cisplatin and methotrexate combination chemotherapy is active in the treatment of refractory urothelial malignancies. J Urol 1995;154:1719–22.

51. Sweeney CJ, Williams SD, Finch DE, et al. A phase II study of paclitaxel and ifosfamide for patients with advanced refractory carcinoma of the urothelium. Cancer 1999;86:514–8.

52. Krege S, Rembrink V, Borgermann C, et al. Docetaxel and ifosfamide as second line treatment for patients with advanced or metastatic urothelial cancer after failure of platinum chemotherapy: a phase 2 study. J Urol 2001;165:67–71.

53. Bellmunt J, Cos J, Cleries R, et al. Feasibility trial of methotrexate-paclitaxel as a second line therapy in advanced urothelial cancer. Cancer Invest 2002;20:673–85.

54. Pagliaro LC, Millikan RE, Tu SM, et al. Cisplatin, gemcitabine, and ifosfamide as weekly therapy: a feasibility and phase II study of salvage treatment for advanced transitional-cell carcinoma. J Clin Oncol 2002;20:2965–70.

55. Chen AC, Hovey E, Shelton G, et al. Phase I/II study of docetaxel (D), gemcitabine (G), carboplatin (C) in poor prognosis and previously treated patients (pts) with urothelial carcinoma (UTC). ASCO Annual Meeting Proceedings (Post-Meeting Edition). Journal of Clinical Oncology 2004;22:14S (July 15 Supplement), 2004: 4580.

56. Lin CC, Hsu CH, Huang CY, et al. Gemcitabine and ifosfamide as a second-line treatment for cisplatin-refractory metastatic urothelial carcinoma: a phase II study. Anticancer Drugs 2007;18:487–91.

57. Pectasides D, Aravantinos G, Kalofonos H, et al. Combination chemotherapy with gemcitabine and ifosfamide as second-line treatment in metastatic urothelial cancer. A phase II trial conducted by the Hellenic Cooperative Oncology Group. Ann Oncol 2001;12:1417–22.

58. Han KS, Joung JY, Kim TS, et al. Methotrexate, vinblastine, doxorubicin and cisplatin combination regimen as salvage chemotherapy for patients with advanced or metastatic transitional cell carcinoma after failure of gemcitabine and cisplatin chemotherapy. Br J Cancer 2008;98:86–90.

59. Gondo T, Ohori M, Hamada R, et al. The efficacy and safety of gemcitabine plus cisplatin regimen for patients with advanced urothelial carcinoma after failure of M-VAC regimen. Int J Clin Oncol 2011;16:345–51.
60. Morrison CD, Liu P, Woloszynska-Read A, et al. Whole-genome sequencing identifies genomic heterogeneity at a nucleotide and chromosomal level in bladder cancer. Proc Natl Acad Sci U S A 2014;111:E672–81.
61. Ghosh M, Brancato SJ, Agarwal PK, et al. Targeted therapies in urothelial carcinoma. Curr Opin Oncol 2014;26:305–20.
62. Sjodahl G, Lauss M, Lovgren K, et al. A molecular taxonomy for urothelial carcinoma. Clin Cancer Res 2012;18:3377–86.
63. Choi W, Porten S, Kim S, et al. Identification of distinct basal and luminal subtypes of muscle-invasive bladder cancer with different sensitivities to front-line chemotherapy. Cancer Cell 2014;25:152–65.
64. Cheng L, Davison DD, Adams J, et al. Biomarkers in bladder cancer: translational and clinical implications. Crit Rev Oncol Hematol 2014;89:73–111.
65. Abou-Jawde R, Choueiri T, Alemany C, et al. An overview of targeted treatments in cancer. Clin Ther 2003;25:2121–37.
66. Mitra AP, Datar RH, Cote RJ. Molecular pathways in invasive bladder cancer: new insights into mechanisms, progression, and target identification. J Clin Oncol 2006;24:5552–64.
67. Wong YN, Litwin S, Vaughn D, et al. Phase II trial of cetuximab with or without paclitaxel in patients with advanced urothelial tract carcinoma. J Clin Oncol 2012;30:3545–51.
68. Petrylak DP, Tangen CM, Van Veldhuizen PJ Jr, et al. Results of the Southwest Oncology Group phase II evaluation (study S0031) of ZD1839 for advanced transitional cell carcinoma of the urothelium. BJU Int 2010;105: 317–21.
69. Dreicer R, Li H, Stein M, et al. Phase 2 trial of sorafenib in patients with advanced urothelial cancer: a trial of the Eastern Cooperative Oncology Group. Cancer 2009;115:4090–5.
70. Gallagher DJ, Milowsky MI, Gerst SR, et al. Phase II study of sunitinib in patients with metastatic urothelial cancer. J Clin Oncol 2010;28:1373–9.
71. Twardowski P, Stadler WM, Frankel P, et al. Phase II study of aflibercept (VEGF-Trap) in patients with recurrent or metastatic urothelial cancer, a California Cancer Consortium Trial. Urology 2010;76:923–6.
72. Pili R, Qin R, Flynn PJ, et al. A phase II safety and efficacy study of the vascular endothelial growth factor receptor tyrosine kinase inhibitor pazopanib in patients with metastatic urothelial cancer. Clin Genitourin Cancer 2013;11:477–83.
73. Necchi A, Mariani L, Zaffaroni N, et al. Pazopanib in advanced and platinum-resistant urothelial cancer: an open-label, single group, phase 2 trial. Lancet Oncol 2012;13:810–6.
74. Choueiri TK, Ross RW, Jacobus S, et al. Double-blind, randomized trial of docetaxel plus vandetanib versus docetaxel plus placebo in platinum-pretreated metastatic urothelial cancer. J Clin Oncol 2012;30:507–12.
75. Milowsky MI, Dittrich C, Martinez ID, et al. Final results of a multicenter, open-label phase II trial of dovitinib (TKI258) in patients with advanced urothelial carcinoma with either mutated or nonmutated FGFR3. Ann Oncol 2001 Oct;12(10): 1417–22.
76. Milowsky MI, Iyer G, Regazzi AM, et al. Phase II study of everolimus in metastatic urothelial cancer. BJU Int 2013;112:462–70.

77. Barbone D, Cheung P, Battula S, et al. Vorinostat eliminates multicellular resistance of mesothelioma 3D spheroids via restoration of Noxa expression. PLoS One 2012;7:e52753.

78. Stadler WM, Vaughn DJ, Sonpavde G, et al. An open-label, single-arm, phase 2 trial of the Polo-like kinase inhibitor volasertib (BI 6727) in patients with locally advanced or metastatic urothelial cancer. Cancer 2014;120:976–82.

79. Theodore C, Geoffrois L, Vermorken JB, et al. Multicentre EORTC study 16997: feasibility and phase II trial of farnesyl transferase inhibitor & gemcitabine combination in salvage treatment of advanced urothelial tract cancers. Eur J Cancer 2005;41:1150–7.

80. Gomez-Abuin G, Winquist E, Stadler WM, et al. A phase II study of PS-341 (Bortezomib) in advanced or metastatic urothelial cancer. A trial of the Princess Margaret Hospital and University of Chicago phase II consortia. Invest New Drugs 2007;25:181–5.

81. Sonpavde G, Jian W, Liu H, et al. Sunitinib malate is active against human urothelial carcinoma and enhances the activity of cisplatin in a preclinical model. Urol Oncol 2009;27:391–9.

82. Srinivas S, Narayanan S, Harshman LC, et al. Phase II trial of pazopanib and weekly paclitaxel in metastatic urothelial cancer. J Clin Oncol 2014;32(Suppl 4) [abstract: 299].

83. Chow NH, Chan SH, Tzai TS, et al. Expression profiles of ErbB family receptors and prognosis in primary transitional cell carcinoma of the urinary bladder. Clin Cancer Res 2001;7:1957–62.

84. Lipponen P, Eskelinen M. Expression of epidermal growth factor receptor in bladder cancer as related to established prognostic factors, oncoprotein (c-erbB-2, p53) expression and long-term prognosis. Br J Cancer 1994;69:1120–5.

85. Mellon K, Wright C, Kelly P, et al. Long-term outcome related to epidermal growth factor receptor status in bladder cancer. J Urol 1995;153:919–25.

86. Popov Z, Gil-Diez-de-Medina S, Ravery V, et al. Prognostic value of EGF receptor and tumor cell proliferation in bladder cancer: therapeutic implications. Urol Oncol 2004;22:93–101.

87. Sauter G, Haley J, Chew K, et al. Epidermal-growth-factor-receptor expression is associated with rapid tumor proliferation in bladder cancer. Int J Cancer 1994; 57:508–14.

88. Hussain MH, MacVicar GR, Petrylak DP, et al. Trastuzumab, paclitaxel, carboplatin, and gemcitabine in advanced human epidermal growth factor receptor-2/neu-positive urothelial carcinoma: results of a multicenter phase II National Cancer Institute trial. J Clin Oncol 2007;25:2218–24.

89. Study of ramucirumab or IMC-18F1 with docetaxel or docetaxel alone as second-line therapy in participants with bladder, urethra, ureter, or renal pelvis carcinoma. Available at: http://clinicaltrials.gov/ct2/show/NCT01282463. Accessed July 17, 2014.

90. Pazopanib and vinflunine in urothelial cancer of the bladder. Available at: http://clinicaltrials.gov/ct2/show/NCT01265940. Accessed July 17, 2014.

91. Phase II pazopanib in combination with weekly paclitaxel in refractory urothelial cancer. Available at: http://clinicaltrials.gov/show/NCT01108055. Accessed July 17, 2014.

92. Cabozantinib for advanced urothelial cancer. Available at: http://clinicaltrials.gov/ct2/show/NCT01688999. Accessed July 17, 2014.

93. Docetaxel and lapatinib in metastatic transitional cell carcinoma in bladder. Available at: http://clinicaltrials.gov/show/NCT01382706. Accessed July 17, 2014.

94. A double blind randomised study of lapatinib and placebo in metastatic TCC of the urothelium (LaMB). Available at: http://clinicaltrials.gov/show/NCT00949455. Accessed July 17, 2014.

95. A Study of herceptin (trastuzumab) monotherapy in patients with metastatic urothelial cancer. Available at: http://clinicaltrials.gov/ct2/show/NCT02013765. Accessed July 17, 2014.

96. Phase 2 study of docetaxel þ/- OGX-427 in patients with relapsed or refractory metastatic bladder cancer. Available at: http://clinicaltrials.gov/ct2/show/ NCT01780545. Accessed July 17, 2014.

97. A phase I/II trial of AEZS-108 in urothelial cancer patients who failed platinum-chemotherapy. Available at: http://clinicaltrials.gov/ct2/show/NCT01234519. Accessed July 17, 2014.

98. TRC105 in adults with advanced/metastatic urothelial carcinoma. Available at: http://clinicaltrials.gov/ct2/show/NCT01328574. Accessed July 17, 2014.

99. BKM120 in metastatic transitional cell carcinoma of the urothelium. Available at: http://clinicaltrials.gov/ct2/show/NCT01551030. Accessed July 17, 2014.

100. F-03446962 in relapsed or refractory urothelial cancer. Available at: http:// clinicaltrials.gov/ct2/show/NCT01620970. Accessed July 17, 2014.

101. ASG-15ME is a study of escalating doses of AGS15E given as monotherapy in subjects with metastatic urothelial cancer. Available at: http://clinicaltrials.gov/ ct2/show/NCT01963052. Accessed July 17, 2014.

102. Sharpe AH, Wherry EJ, Ahmed R, et al. The function of programmed cell death 1 and its ligands in regulating autoimmunity and infection. Nat Immunol 2007;8: 239–45.

103. Boorjian SA, Sheinin Y, Crispen PL, et al. T-cell coregulatory molecule expression in urothelial cell carcinoma: clinicopathologic correlations and association with survival. Clin Cancer Res 2008;14:4800–8.

104. Xylinas E, Robinson BD, Kluth LA, et al. Association of T-cell co-regulatory protein expression with clinical outcomes following radical cystectomy for urothelial carcinoma of the bladder. Eur J Surg Oncol 2014;40:121–7.

105. Powles T, Vogelzang N, Gregg D. Inhibition of PD-L1 by MPDL3280A and clinical activity in pts with metastatic urothelial bladder cancer (UBC). J Clin Oncol 2014;32(Suppl):5s [abstract: 5011].

106. Jiang P, Lagenaur CF, Narayanan V. Integrin-associated protein is a ligand for the P84 neural adhesion molecule. J Biol Chem 1999;274:559–62.

107. Willingham SB, Volkmer JP, Gentles AJ, et al. The CD47-signal regulatory protein alpha (SIRPa) interaction is a therapeutic target for human solid tumors. Proc Natl Acad Sci U S A 2012;109:6662–7.

108. Duchesne GM, Bolger JJ, Griffiths GO, et al. A randomized trial of hypofractionated schedules of palliative radiotherapy in the management of bladder carcinoma: results of medical Research Council trial BA09. Int J Radiat Oncol Biol Phys 2000;47:379–88.

109. Siefker-Radtke AO, Walsh GL, Pisters LL, et al. Is there a role for surgery in the management of metastatic urothelial cancer? The M. D. Anderson experience. J Urol 2004;171:145–8.

Future Directions and Targeted Therapies in Bladder Cancer

Guru Sonpavde, MD[a], Benjamin S. Jones, MD[a],
Joaquim Bellmunt, MD, PhD[b], Toni K. Choueiri, MD[b],
Cora N. Sternberg, MD[c],*

KEYWORDS

- Urothelial carcinoma • Biologic agents • Therapeutic targets • Systemic therapy

KEY POINTS

- Current systemic therapy for metastatic urothelial carcinoma yields a median survival of 12 to 15 months in the first-line setting and only 6 to 8 months in the salvage setting.
- The Cancer Genome Atlas project has provided important insights regarding molecular tumor tissue alterations in bladder cancer.
- Emerging data provide promise for a potential role for programmed death 1 and programmed death ligand 1 pathway inhibitors, phosphatidylinositol 3 kinase/mammalian target of rapamycin pathway inhibitors, fibroblast growth factor receptor 3 inhibitors, antiangiogenic agents, epigenetic modulation, and stem cell drivers in selected patients.
- Novel clinical trial designs guided by predictive biomarkers based on preclinical data may accelerate therapeutic advances.

INTRODUCTION

Despite the high response rates seen in the first-line metastatic setting with cisplatin-based chemotherapy regimens for metastatic urothelial carcinoma (UC), the duration of response is brief and salvage systemic therapy with available agents (vinflunine, taxanes) is marginally active.[1–4] The limited efficacy of currently used first-line

Conflicts of interest: Research support from Onyx, Sanofi-Aventis; advisory board of GSK, Bayer, Merck, Genentech, Sanofi-Aventis (G. Sonpavde). None (B.S. Jones). Advisory board of Pierre Fabre, Sanofi-Aventis, GSK, Genentech, and Merck (J. Bellmunt). Institutional research support from Oncogenix, AstraZeneca, Amgen (T.K. Choueiri). Institutional research support from Oncogenix; GSK, Bayer, Novartis; honoraria, Bayer, Novartis (C.N. Sternberg).
[a] University of Alabama at Birmingham (UAB) Comprehensive Cancer Center, 1720 2nd Ave. S., Birmingham, AL 35294, USA; [b] Bladder Cancer Institute, Dana Farber Cancer Institute, Dana-Farber/Brigham and Women's Cancer Center, Boston, 450, Brookline Ave, MA 02215, USA; [c] Department of Medical Oncology, San Camillo Forlanini Hospital, Padiglioni Flajani, 1st Floor, Circonvallazione Gianicolense 87, Rome 00152, Italy
* Correspondence author.
E-mail address: cstern@mclink.it

Hematol Oncol Clin N Am 29 (2015) 361–376
http://dx.doi.org/10.1016/j.hoc.2014.10.008
0889-8588/15/$ – see front matter © 2015 Elsevier Inc. All rights reserved.

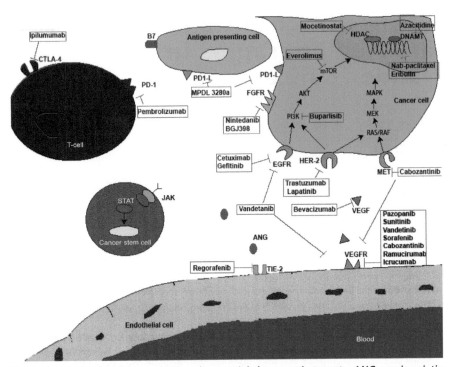

Fig. 1. Key molecular drivers of UC and potential therapeutic targets. ANG, angiopoietin; APC, antigen-presenting cell; DNMT, DNA methyltransferase; EGFR, epidermal growth factor receptor; FGFR, fibroblast growth factor receptor; HDAC, histone deacetylase; PD, programmed death; VEGF, vascular endothelial growth factor; VEGFR, VEGF receptor.

regimens and meager results with salvage chemotherapy translate to poor median survivals of only 12 to 15 months and 6 to 8 months, respectively. In addition, a large proportion of patients, especially elderly patients, do not receive chemotherapy or are ineligible for cisplatin-based combination chemotherapy because of poor performance status, renal dysfunction, and comorbidities, and show poor outcomes with carboplatin-based therapy.[5–8] The settings of perioperative systemic therapy, combined modality therapy with concurrent radiation, and bacillus Calmette-Guérin (BCG)–resistant non–muscle-invasive bladder cancer (NMIBC) also have suboptimal outcomes. Although no major advances have occurred for the systemic therapy for UC in more than 2 decades, better understanding of tumor biology has identified multiple potential therapeutic targets. This article discusses future directions and highlights emerging promising systemic agents for the treatment of UC.

POTENTIAL NOVEL THERAPEUTIC TARGETS

The Cancer Genome Atlas (TCGA) project recently provided multiple novel insights, although a single dominant tumor driver was not evident (**Fig. 1**).[9] Chromatin regulatory genes were more frequently mutated in muscle-invasive bladder cancer than in other common malignancies, suggesting a role for targeting epigenetic pathways. Most (76%) tumors harbored an inactivating mutation in 1 or more of the chromatin regulatory genes, and 41% had at least 2 such mutations. Recurrent mutations were observed in genes involved in cell-cycle regulation, chromatin regulation, and kinase signaling. RNA sequencing revealed 4 expression subtypes, including a papillarylike and basal-like/squamouslike subtype.[9] Activating FGFR3-TACC3 fusions and FGFR3 mutations were seen and potential therapeutic targets were noted in 69% of tumors, including targets in the phosphatidylinositol 3 kinase (PI3K)/AKT/mammalian target of rapamycin (mTOR), and mitogen-activated protein kinase (MAPK) pathway. Other studies of bladder cancer have also shown molecular subtypes and have suggested some actionable alterations, including those expressed in tumor initiating or stemlike cells (eg, Stat3, Gli1).[10–15] Stromal molecules, such as angiogenesis and T-lymphocyte checkpoints, may also represent broad therapeutic targets.

IMMUNOTHERAPY

Inhibitors of T-lymphocyte checkpoint receptors, especially programmed death (PD-1)/programmed death ligand 1 (PD-L1), are emerging as highly promising agents to induce durable remissions in multiple malignancies.[16,17] A phase II trial (n = 70) recently showed a high response rate coupled with potential response durability with MPDL3280a, a PD-L1 inhibiting monoclonal antibody (MAb), in the salvage setting.[18,19] Moreover, higher tumor expression of PD-L1 by immunohistochemistry (IHC) correlated with a robust response rate (2%), although a smaller proportion of patients with no PD-L1 expression also responded (4%). Responses occurred early and the duration of response appeared promising. The toxicity profile in the short term was reassuring with a low rate (3%–4%) of severe toxicities. Aggressive clinical investigation of MPDL3280a is ongoing in a large nonrandomized phase II trial in the salvage setting (NCT02108652), which also accrues to a smaller cohort of cisplatin-ineligible patients as first-line therapy. Furthermore, investigation of pembrolizumab, an MAb targeting PD-1, is planned as a phase III trial in the salvage context following promising results in a phase Ib trial (**Table 1**).[20] In this phase Ib trial, responses were seen in 24% of 33 pre-treated patients, and many responses were durable.

Ipilimumab, a cytotoxic T-lymphocyte (CTLA) 4–inhibiting monoclonal antibody modulated the immune state in a neoadjuvant trial, and an ongoing phase II trial is assessing the combination of ipilimumab and gemcitabine plus cisplatin (GC) chemotherapy as first-line therapy (NCT01524991).[21] ALT-801, a fusion molecule of interleukin (IL)-2 and a modified T-lymphocyte receptor designed to recognize a p53 epitope in the context of HLA-A*0201, is being evaluated.[22] At first, toxicities were manageable with outpatient administration and induction of an increase of serum interferon gamma, suggesting a favorable immune response. An ongoing phase I trial (NCT01326871) evaluates the combination of ALT-801 (intravenously) plus GC for patients progressing after prior GC for metastatic disease, and another trial (NCT01625260) evaluates ALT-801 plus gemcitabine (both intravenously) for BCG-resistant NMIBC.

FIBROBLAST GROWTH FACTOR RECEPTOR INHIBITORS

Dovitinib, a multitargeted tyrosine kinase inhibitor (TKI) that inhibits vascular endothelial growth factor (VEGF) and FGFRs, was evaluated as a single agent in a phase II second-line trial. Tumor tissue was evaluated for FGFR3 mutation and patients were stratified by mutational status. Of 44 patients, only 1 objective response was seen in a subject with wild-type FGFR3.[23] However, more potent and selective pan-FGFR inhibition by BGJ398 and JNJ-42756493 has preliminarily shown robust responses in UC harboring FGFR3 mutations, FGFR3/TACC3 translocation, or FGFR2 truncation.[24–26] Further clinical development of these agents and an Mab targeting FGFR3 are planned in randomized trials that will accrue a selected targeted population (see **Table 1**).

Table 1
Ongoing or planned randomized trials investigating new therapeutic targets in UC

Phase	Therapeutic Target	Control Arm	Experimental Arm	Trial Identifier
First-line for Cisplatin-eligible Advanced Disease				
III	VEGF	GC + placebo	GC + bevacizumab	NCT00942331, CALGB 90601
II	Tubulins	GC	GC + eribulin	NCT01126749
II	Heat shock protein 27	GC	GC + OGX-427	NCT01454089
First-line for Cisplatin-ineligible Advanced Disease				
II	VEGFR, EGFR	GCa	GCa + Vandetanib	NCT01191892
Second or Later Line for Advanced Disease				
III	PD-1	Vinflunine or paclitaxel	Pembrolizumab	Not available
II→III	Tubulins	Vinflunine	Cabazitaxel	2012-002826-55
II	VEGFR	Weekly paclitaxel	Pazopanib	73030316 (PLUTO)
II	Tubulins	Paclitaxel	Nab-paclitaxel	NCT02033993
II	Heat shock protein 27	Docetaxel	Docetaxel + OGX-427	NCT01780545
II	VEGFR1 or VEGFR2	Docetaxel	Docetaxel + ramucirumab Docetaxel + icrucumab	NCT01282463
II	FGFR3	Docetaxel	R3Mab	Not available
Switch Maintenance Therapy for Those with Stable Disease after First-line Chemotherapy				
II→III	Her2, EGFR	Placebo	Lapatinib	NCT00949455
Neoadjuvant Therapy				
II	VEGFR, FGFR	GC	GC + nintedanib	ISRCTN56349930
Adjuvant Therapy Following Radical Cystectomy				
II	Her2	No therapy	DN24-02 (APC-based vaccine)	NCT01353222

Abbreviations: APC, antigen-presenting cell; EGFR, epidermal growth factor receptor; FGFR, fibroblast growth factor receptor; GC, gemcitabine plus cisplatin; GCa, gemcitabine plus carboplatin; PD, programmed death; VEGF, vascular endothelial growth factor; VEGFR, VEGF receptor.

PHOSPHATIDYLINOSITOL 3 KINASE/AKT/MAMMALIAN TARGET OF RAPAMYCIN PATHWAY INHIBITORS

Mutations involving the PI3K/mTOR pathway are prevalent in a subset of patients and may represent potential therapeutic targets in UC.[27] Everolimus, an orally administered mTOR inhibitor, has been evaluated following prior platinum-based chemotherapy, alone in a phase II trial, and in combination with pazopanib in phase 1 clinical trial.[28–30] Despite poor overall activity and outcomes, a small subset of patients whose tumors harbored deletions in the *TSC1* (tuberous sclerosis complex 1) gene or activating mTOR mutations experienced exceptionally durable control of disease lasting for more than 1 to 2 years.[29] Everolimus is being evaluated in combination with gemcitabine plus weekly fractionated cisplatin in unselected patients with a baseline creatinine clearance greater than or equal to 40 mL/min in the first-line metastatic setting (NCT01182168). A nonrandomized study of unselected cisplatin-ineligible patients is assessing everolimus alone or with paclitaxel (NCT01215136). In addition, a selective oral PI3K TKI, buparlisib, is being evaluated in unselected patients initially and selected patients with tumors bearing PI3K mutations in the expansion cohort (NCT01551030).

AGENTS TARGETING EPIGENETIC PATHWAYS

A substantial amount of tumor tissue profiling (notably TCGA data) and preclinical data supports the aggressive evaluation of epigenetic modulators for UC.[9,31] Inhibition of histone deacetylase (HDAC) results in accumulation of acetylated histones and transcription factors leading to derepression of silenced tumor suppressor genes and antitumor activity. However, romidepsin and vorinostat showed marginal activity.[32] Nevertheless, more potent HDAC inhibitors are undergoing evaluation in patients with tumors harboring epigenetic alterations, such as mocetinostat, an oral second-generation HDAC inhibitor, for tumors bearing inactivating alterations in the histone acetyltransferase genes like EP300 or CREEBB. Azacitidine, a hypomethylating agent, showed significant activity in an autochthonous canine bladder cancer model.[33] Note that epigenetic modulation of tumor tissue may augment the activity of subsequent chemotherapy, as suggested in other malignancies.[34]

ANTIANGIOGENIC AGENTS
Bevacizumab

Data support targeting the tumor vasculature in general, and VEGF in particular, in UC.[35–38] In a phase II trial, bevacizumab, a humanized VEGF Mab, was evaluated in combination with GC as first-line chemotherapy.[39] The overall response rate (ORR) was 72%, including 19% with complete responses (CRs). The median progression-free survival (PFS) of 8.2 months and median overall survival (OS) of 19.1 months suggested a potential improvement compared with GC alone. Thromboembolic events occurred in 21% of patients, although the incidence diminished to 8% after the protocol was amended to administer a lower dose of gemcitabine (1000 mg/m^2). Bevacizumab has also been studied in a phase II trial in combination with gemcitabine plus carboplatin (GCa) in patients who were cisplatin-ineligible or deemed to be incurable by cisplatin because of visceral disease.[40] The ORR was 49%, including 6% CR and a median PFS and OS of 6.5 and 13.9 months, respectively. In addition, bevacizumab has been combined with GC and dose-dense MVAC (methotrexate, vinblastine, doxorubicin, cisplatin) preceding radical cystectomy in neoadjuvant nonrandomized trials.[41,42] However, the nonrandomized design renders them difficult to interpret. The phase III trial (see **Table 1**) comparing GC with either placebo or bevacizumab is expected to complete accrual in 2014, and will provide more definitive data. This important trial also allows maintenance bevacizumab or placebo in patients with at least stable disease following combination chemotherapy.

Sunitinib

Sunitinib, an oral small molecule, multitargeted receptor TKI with activity against VEGF receptor (VEGFR) and platelet-derived growth factor receptor (PDGFR) has been evaluated in multiple settings. As a single agent in the first-line setting in cisplatin-ineligible patients with Eastern Cooperative Oncology Group (ECOG) performance status (PS) 0 to 1 and calculated creatinine clearance less than 60 mL/min, sunitinib yielded an ORR of 8%, median time to progression of 4.8 months, and median OS of only 8.1 months.[43] Low IL-8 levels and tumor contrast enhancement greater than 40 Hounsfield units at baseline were associated with a better clinical outcome, suggesting their potential as biomarkers. When using sunitinib as second-line therapy, the

ORR, median PFS, and median OS were 5%, ~2.3 to 2.4 months, and ~6 to 7 months.[44] However, a placebo-controlled randomized phase II trial to evaluate a switch maintenance strategy of sunitinib after stability or response to first-line chemotherapy closed prematurely secondary to slow accrual and showed similar suboptimal median PFS (~2.8 months) and OS (~10.4 months) in both arms.[45] Substantial toxicities associated with sunitinib were noted in all of these trials. The efficacy of sunitinib in combination with GC was evaluated as preoperative therapy and as first-line therapy for metastatic disease in separate phase II trials, but toxicities forced premature closure of both trials.[46] In a phase II trial, sunitinib seemed to have clinical activity in patients with BCG-resistant NMIBC and increased immune activity.[47]

Pazopanib

Pazopanib, another TKI targeting VEGFR and PDGFR, has been evaluated as a single agent in the heavily pretreated platinum-refractory disease setting in which the ORR was 17%, but with a very low median PFS and OS of 2·6 months and 4·7 months.[48] However, a subset of patients seemed to garner durable benefits: 4 (10%) were progression free after a median follow-up of 19 months. Similar to the first-line sunitinib trial, high baseline IL-8 levels conferred poor outcomes, and early increases during treatment were also associated with poor outcomes. A second phase II single-agent study of pazopanib in the second-line setting was aborted because of futility.[49] Nevertheless, a randomized phase II trial is comparing second-line weekly paclitaxel versus pazopanib (see **Table 1**). A more recent nonrandomized phase II trial combined pazopanib with weekly paclitaxel as second-line therapy and suggested a potential improvement in outcomes with a high ORR and median OS of 10 months.[50] In contrast, another second-line trial combining vinflunine plus pazopanib showed prohibitive toxicities requiring substantial dose reduction of pazopanib to 200 mg once daily.[51] A frontline study of cisplatin-unfit patients treated with gemcitabine plus pazopanib (NCT01622660) is ongoing.

Vandetanib

Vandetanib, a VEGFR and epidermal growth factor receptor (EGFR) TKI, has been studied as salvage therapy after up to 3 prior lines of therapy. In this randomized phase II trial of docetaxel combined with placebo or vandetanib, there was no advantage in outcomes in term of PFS, OS, or responses.[52] A randomized phase II study to evaluate GCa with or without vandetanib for the first-line treatment of cisplatin-ineligible patients is recruiting (see **Table 1**).

Sorafenib

Sorafenib, a TKI targeting VEGFRs and PDGFRs, has shown virtually no activity as a single agent in the first-line and second-line settings.[53,54] A randomized phase II trial evaluating sorafenib combined with GC was closed prematurely because of slow accrual and showed no improvement in efficacy.[55] Sorafenib in combination with GCa showed excessive hematologic toxicities in a phase II trial and the efficacy was similar to that of GCa. However, sorafenib alone after the completion of GCa plus sorafenib seemed feasible and suggested a durable benefit.[56] A current phase I/II trial is evaluating the combination of sorafenib with vinflunine in the salvage setting (NCT01844947).

Cabozantinib

Cabozantinib is a TKI targeting VEGFR and MET, has shown promising bone metastasis–targeted activity in advanced prostate cancer and is currently under evaluation as salvage therapy for patients with metastatic UC (NCT01688999).[57,58] Preliminary responses have been observed and associated with low peripheral blood regulatory T cells (T_{regs}). Moreover, cabozantinib decreased T_{regs} and increased PD-1 expression in T_{regs}, suggesting a potential role for combination or sequencing with immunotherapy.

Other Antiangiogenic Agents

An ongoing 3-arm randomized phase II trial is evaluating docetaxel alone or combined with ramucirumab (VEGFR2 MAb) or icrucumab (VEGFR1 Mab) (see **Table 1**). Afliber-cept, a recombinant fusion protein that binds multiple VEGF isoforms and placental growth factor, showed poor activity as a single-agent salvage therapy.[59] TRC105, an antibody targeting CD105, a transforming growth factor beta (TGF-β) coreceptor expressed on the endothelium, is being studied in a phase II trial (NCT01328574). Acti-vin receptor–like kinase (ALK)-1, a TGF-β subclass receptor, is being targeted by PF-03446962 in the second-line setting (NCT01620970). Trebananib is an MAb that targets angiopoietin (Ang)-1 and Ang-2 and has shown promising activity in combina-tion with chemotherapy in a phase I trial.[60] Although the further development of treba-nanib in UC is not ongoing, a phase II trial of regorafenib, an oral TKI approved in colorectal carcinoma and gastrointestinal tumors with activity against VEGFRs, TIE2, PDGFR, and FGFR, is planned. CEP-11981, a TKI with similar spectrum of anti-angiogenic activity including TIE2, had significant preclinical activity.[61] The neoadju-vant setting is also being explored: nintedanib, a TKI targeting VEGFR and FGFR, is being investigated in a randomized phase II trial in combination with GC to evaluate pathologic complete response (pCR) as the primary end point (see **Table 1**). Lenalido-mide, an oral immune-modulating and antiangiogenic agent, seems to have antitumor activity in indolent UC preclinical models, and is being evaluated in combination with BCG for BCG-resistant NMIBC (NCT01373294).[62,63] The combination of lenalidomide and GC was terminated because of toxicities, but another ongoing phase I/II trial is combining lenalidomide with GCa (NCT01352962).

EPIDERMAL GROWTH FACTOR RECEPTOR AND HER-2 PATHWAY INHIBITORS
Epidermal Growth Factor Receptor Inhibitors

Both EGFR and Her2 are expressed, albeit not mutated, on most UC cells and corre-late with stage and outcomes.[64–66] The EGFR-targeting MAb, cetuximab, has been evaluated in UC in the first-line and second-line settings. However, no improvement in outcomes was seen with the addition of cetuximab to first-line GC in a randomized phase II trial in an unselected population.[67] In a phase II trial in the second-line setting, unselected patients were randomized to receive cetuximab with or without paclitaxel. Although poor activity was observed in the monotherapy arm, patients in the combi-nation arm showed an ORR of 25%, median PFS of 16.4 weeks, and median OS of 42 weeks.[68] Gefitinib, an EGFR TKI, showed poor activity in a phase II trial of unse-lected patients in the salvage setting and did not provide an incremental improvement in combination with GC in the first-line setting.[69,70]

Her2 Inhibitors

The HER2-directed monoclonal antibody, trastuzumab, was evaluated in combination with first-line gemcitabine, carboplatin, and paclitaxel for metastatic UC in a non-randomized phase II trial (n = 44) that defined Her2 expression by IHC, fluorescent in situ hybridization (FISH), and/or increased serum Her-2 levels. This regimen yielded an ORR of 70% and median OS of 14.1 months.[71] However, the addition of trastuzumab to GC in a randomized phase II trial accruing patients with Her2-expressing metastatic UC did not show an improvement in any efficacy end point.[72] Note that this trial screened 563 patients to identify only 75 eligible patients (13.3%) who had Her2 expression 3+ by IHC or 2+ by IHC plus FISH positive, and took ~5.5 years to recruit patients. There were no responses seen with salvage lapatinib, an EGFR, and Her2 TKI, in patients with UC in a randomized discontinuation study.[73] In a second-line trial of 34 evaluable patients with EGFR greater than or equal to 1+ and/or Her2 greater than or equal to 1+ by IHC treated with lapatinib, only 1 patient showed a partial response.[74] However, response plus stability correlated with EGFR 2+ or 3+ versus 0 or 1+ and HER-2 expression 2+ or 3+ versus 0 or 1+. A phase I trial combining GC plus lapatinib has completed accrual (NCT00623064). Interest remains in targeting Her-2. A randomized phase II trial that allows for transition to phase III is enrolling HER-2–amplified (IHC 2+ or 3+) UC and comparing lapatinib versus placebo in the maintenance setting following at least stable disease after first-line chemotherapy (see **Table 1**). Another strategy to target Her2 is the autologous antigen-presenting cell (APC) platform. APCs pulsed with the Her2 protein conjugated with granulocyte-macrophage colony-stimulating factor have been investigated in an open label randomized phase II trial in the adjuvant setting following radical cystectomy for patients with tumor Her2 greater than or equal to 1+ by IHC (see **Table 1**). Although efficacy results are awaited, preliminary results show safety of the product and biological activity with APC activation and upregulated T-cell cytokines.[75]

HEAT SHOCK PROTEIN INHIBITORS

Heat shock proteins (HSPs) are cytoprotective chaperones expressed in response to cellular stress and promote chemoresistance. Apatorsen is an antisense oligonucleotide directed at HSP27, which has been shown to sensitize the bladder to several cytotoxic chemotherapy drugs in a preclinical system.[76] This drug is actively being studied in randomized phase II trials in both the first-line metastatic setting in combination with GC (NCT01454089, accrual completed) and with docetaxel in the second-line setting (NCT01780545).

ANTIBODY-DRUG CONJUGATES

Antibody-drug conjugates (ADCs) are in the early stages of development for UC. The absence of a well-defined UC-specific membrane antigen may be a barrier, although one potential fairly specific antigen is SLITRK6. AGS15E, an ADC specific for SLITRK6, delivers monomethyl auristatin E, a tubulin toxin, and is being evaluated in a first-in-human phase I trial enrolling patients with advanced UC with progressive disease following prior systemic therapy (NCT01963052).

CYTOTOXIC AGENTS

Tubulin toxins have typically shown moderate activity and several are under investigation. In a phase II study of nanoparticle albumin-bound (nab) paclitaxel in the second-line setting, moderate activity was observed, with an ORR of 28% and median PFS and OS of 6.0 and 10.8 months, respectively.[77] A randomized phase II trial is comparing second-line paclitaxel versus nab-paclitaxel (see **Table 1**). Nab-paclitaxel was also evaluated in combination with GCa in the neoadjuvant setting, with 27% of subjects showing a pCR.[78] A phase II trial of this combination is underway in the first-line metastatic setting (NCT00995488). Cabazitaxel did not meet the minimum efficacy threshold to progress to the second stage of accrual in a phase II trial.[79] However, salvage therapy with cabazitaxel is currently being compared with vinflunine in Europe in a more selected population in the second-line phase II/III SECAVIN trial (see **Table 1**). Also, a neoadjuvant study (NCT01616875) is evaluating cabazitaxel. Eribulin, a halochondrin-B analogue and tubulin toxin, has shown modest activity as first-line or salvage therapy.[80,81] A first-line randomized phase II trial to investigate the impact of combining eribulin with GC has completed accrual (see **Table 1**). Pemetrexed, an anti-folate agent, has shown modest activity in a phase II trial (ORR, 28%) but little activity in another phase II trial.[82,83] To better understand the activity of pemetrexed as salvage therapy, a retrospective study was conducted (n = 135), which revealed marginal activity with ORR 8% and median PFS and OS of only 2.4 and 6.6 months, respectively.[84] Aurora kinase-A overexpression and spindle checkpoint dysregulation are prevalent in UC.[85] Alisertib, an oral selective small molecule inhibitor of Aurora kinase-A, is being studied as a single agent for relapsed UC in a phase II trial (NCT02109328).

INNOVATIVE CLINICAL TRIAL DESIGNS TO EXPEDITE DRUG DEVELOPMENT

The BCG-resistant NMIBC population and cystectomy-ineligible population receiving combined-modality systemic therapy plus radiotherapy constitutes large numbers of patients who may be eligible for trials and constitutes a relevant unmet medical need. Development of biologic agents as intravesical therapy for the BCG-resistant NMIBC population would be welcomed. The neoadjuvant paradigm remains underused for drug development. Although combinations of cisplatin-based neoadjuvant therapy and novel biologic agents may be studied in phase II trials to identify an improvement in pCR, patients proceeding to upfront cystectomy (eg, cisplatin-ineligible or chemotherapy-refusing patients) may be accrued on trials to compare the activity of multiple novel agents in a biomarker directed enrichment design to rapidly screen the most biologically active agents for further development. In this case, the improvement in pCR and biological activity need to translate to improved long-term outcomes.[86] However, reported trials evaluating neoadjuvant cisplatin-based chemotherapy have taken a long time to accrue and trials evaluating adjuvant cisplatin-based chemotherapy have been unable to complete accrual.[87–89] Nevertheless, both neoadjuvant and adjuvant therapy may be exploited for rational drug development and PFS at 2 years may be a useful intermediate end point, given its correlation with long-term survival.[90] Novel adaptive trial designs using predictive biomarker–informed therapy warrant strong consideration.

Clinical trials of locally advanced unresectable or metastatic disease have typically accrued slower than expected. The ongoing phase III CALGB 90601 trial comparing GC combined with either placebo or bevacizumab was amended to allow patients with a lower creatinine clearance of 50 to 60 mL/min in whom a template of gemcitabine plus weekly fractionated cisplatin is being used instead of the conventional GC, which uses 1 day of cisplatin per cycle. Because most patients are ineligible for cisplatin or chemotherapy, a new focus on such patients warrants serious consideration.[6,8] Future first-line trials should also account for recently reported new prognostic factors in addition to performance status and visceral metastasis (eg, hemoglobin, albumin, leukocytosis, and site of primary).[91,92] The use of PFS at 6 or 9 months as an intermediate end point may provide a signal of improved activity in the first-line setting.[93] The switch maintenance design using highly tolerable biologic agents warrants evaluation because patients generally progress after a brief treatment-free interval.

Second-line and salvage therapy trials have generally been designed as nonrandomized phase II trials using different eligibility criteria, rendering the results difficult to compare across trials. Guidelines have recently been proposed to use uniform eligibility criteria when enrolling patients in nonrandomized phase II trials of salvage systemic therapy.[94] In addition, prognostic factors (liver metastasis, hemoglobin level, performance status, time from prior chemotherapy) affect both activity and long-term outcomes; hence, a nomogram to compare expected versus observed outcomes using PFS at 6 months as a more optimal, universally applicable intermediate end point across cytotoxic and biologic agents may facilitate the interpretation of phase II salvage trials.[95–98] A more focused biomarker-enriched phase II design using a high threshold of activity of interest warrants consideration rather than phase III trials.

SUMMARY

Further progress in the treatment of UC will be determined by understanding the key molecular drivers and actionable therapeutic targets. Trials are currently underway or planned to validate the initial promise shown by PD-1 inhibitors, FGFR3 inhibitors, PI3K/mTOR inhibitors, and the potential activity of epigenetic modulation. In addition, aggressive accrual to trials requires multidisciplinary efforts with close collaboration between medical oncologists, urologists, radiation oncologists, basic/translational researchers, federal agencies, and industry.

REFERENCES

1. von der Maase H, Sengelov L, Roberts JT, et al. Long-term survival results of a randomized trial comparing gemcitabine plus cisplatin, with methotrexate, vinblastine, doxorubicin, plus cisplatin in patients with bladder cancer. J Clin Oncol 2005;23(21):4602–8.
2. Sonpavde G, Sternberg CN, Rosenberg JE, et al. Second-line systemic therapy and emerging drugs for metastatic transitional-cell carcinoma of the urothelium. Lancet Oncol 2010;11(9):861–70.
3. Bellmunt J, Theodore C, Demkov T, et al. Phase III trial of vinflunine plus best supportive care compared with best supportive care alone after a platinum-containing regimen in patients with advanced transitional cell carcinoma of the urothelial tract. J Clin Oncol 2009;27(27):4454–61.
4. Bellmunt J, von der Maase H, Mead GM, et al. Randomized phase III study comparing paclitaxel/cisplatin/gemcitabine and gemcitabine/cisplatin in patients with locally advanced or metastatic urothelial cancer without prior systemic therapy: EORTC Intergroup Study 30987. J Clin Oncol 2012;30(10):1107–13.
5. Galsky MD, Hahn NM, Rosenberg J, et al. Treatment of patients with metastatic urothelial cancer "unfit" for cisplatin-based chemotherapy. J Clin Oncol 2011; 29(17):2432–8.
6. Sonpavde G, Watson D, Tourtellott M, et al. Administration of cisplatin-based chemotherapy for advanced urothelial carcinoma in the community. Clin Genitourin Cancer 2012;10(1):1–5.
7. De Santis M, Bellmunt J, Mead G, et al. Randomized phase II/III trial assessing gemcitabine/carboplatin and methotrexate/carboplatin/vinblastine in patients with advanced urothelial cancer who are unfit for cisplatin-based chemotherapy: EORTC study 30986. J Clin Oncol 2012;30(2):191–9.
8. Sonpavde G, Galsky MD, Latini D, et al. Cisplatin-ineligible and chemotherapy-ineligible patients should be the focus of new drug development in patients with advanced bladder cancer. Clin Genitourin Cancer 2014;12(2):71–3.
9. Cancer Genome Atlas Research Network. Comprehensive molecular characterization of urothelial bladder carcinoma. Nature 2014;507(7492):315–22.

10. Damrauer JS, Hoadley KA, Chism DD, et al. Intrinsic subtypes of high-grade bladder cancer reflect the hallmarks of breast cancer biology. Proc Natl Acad Sci U S A 2014;111(8):3110–5.

11. Choi W, Porten S, Kim S, et al. Identification of distinct basal and luminal subtypes of muscle-invasive bladder cancer with different sensitivities to frontline chemotherapy. Cancer Cell 2014;25(2):152–65.

12. Sjodahl G, Lauss M, Lovgren K, et al. A molecular taxonomy for urothelial carcinoma. Clin Cancer Res 2012;18(12):3377–86.

13. Iyer G, Al-Ahmadie H, Schultz N, et al. Prevalence and co-occurrence of actionable genomic alterations in high-grade bladder cancer. J Clin Oncol 2013;31(25): 3133–40.

14. Volkmer JP, Sahoo D, Chin RK, et al. Three differentiation states risk-stratify bladder cancer into distinct subtypes. Proc Natl Acad Sci U S A 2012;109(6): 2078–83.

15. Chan KS, Espinosa I, Chao M, et al. Identification, molecular characterization, clinical prognosis, and therapeutic targeting of human bladder tumor-initiating cells. Proc Natl Acad Sci U S A 2009;106(33):14016–21.

16. Topalian SL, Hodi FS, Brahmer JR, et al. Safety, activity, and immune correlates of anti-PD-1 antibody in cancer. N Engl J Med 2012;366(26):2443–54.

17. Hamid O, Robert C, Daud A, et al. Safety and tumor responses with lambrolizumab (anti-PD-1) in melanoma. N Engl J Med 2013;369(2):134–44.

18. Powles T, Vogelzang N, Fine GD, et al. Inhibition of PD-L1 by MPDL3280A and clinical activity in patients with metastatic urothelial bladder cancer. J Clin Oncol 2014;32(5 Suppl) [abstract: 5011].

19. Bellmunt J, Petrylak DP, Powles T, et al. Inhibition of PD-L1 by MPDL3280A leads to clinical activity in pts with metastatic urothelial bladder cancer. ESMO congress 2014; abstract 8080.

20. Plimack ER, Gupta S, Bellmunt J, et al. A phase 1b study of pembrolizumab in patients with advanced urothelial tract cancer. ESMO Congress 2014; abstract LBA23.

21. Liakou CI, Kamat A, Tang DN, et al. CTLA-4 blockade increases IFNgamma-producing CD4+ICOShi cells to shift the ratio of effector to regulatory T cells in cancer patients. Proc Natl Acad Sci U S A 2008;105(39):14987–92.

22. Fishman MN, Thompson JA, Pennock GK, et al. Phase I trial of ALT-801, an interleukin-2/T-cell receptor fusion protein targeting p53 (aa264-272)/HLA-A*0201 complex, in patients with advanced malignancies. Clin Cancer Res 2011;17(24):7765–75.

23. Milowsky MI, Dittrich C, Martinez ID, et al. Final results of a multicenter, open-label phase II trial of dovitinib in patients with advanced urothelial carcinoma with either mutated or nonmutated FGFR3. J Clin Oncol 2013;31(Suppl 6) [abstract: 255].

24. Guagnano V, Kauffmann A, Wohrle S, et al. FGFR genetic alterations predict for sensitivity to NVP-BGJ398, a selective pan-FGFR inhibitor. Cancer Discov 2012;2(12):1118–33.

25. Sequist LV, Cassier P, Varga A, et al. Phase I study of BGJ398, a selective pan-FGFR inhibitor in genetically preselected advanced solid tumors. American Association for Cancer Research Annual Meeting 2014. San Diego, April 5–9, 2014; Abstract: CT326.

26. Bahleda R, Dienstmann R, Adamo B, et al. Phase 1 study of JNJ-42756493, a pan-fibroblast growth factor receptor (FGFR) inhibitor, in patients with advanced solid tumors. J Clin Oncol 2014;32(5 Suppl) [abstract: 2501].

27. Sjodahl G, Lauss M, Gudjonsson S, et al. A systematic study of gene mutations in urothelial carcinoma; inactivating mutations in TSC2 and PIK3R1. PLoS One 2011;6(4):e18583.

28. Wagle N, Grabiner BC, Van Allen EM, et al. Activating mTOR mutations in a patient with an extraordinary response on a phase I trial of everolimus and pazopanib. Cancer Discov 2014;4(5):546–53.

29. Iyer G, Hanrahan AJ, Milowsky MI, et al. Genome sequencing identifies a basis for everolimus sensitivity. Science 2012;338(6104):221.

30. Milowsky MI, Iyer G, Regazzi AM, et al. Phase II study of everolimus in metastatic urothelial cancer. BJU Int 2013;112(4):462–70.

31. Buckley MT, Yoon J, Yee H, et al. The histone deacetylase inhibitor belinostat (PXD101) suppresses bladder cancer cell growth in vitro and in vivo. J Transl Med 2007;5:49.

32. Cheung EM, Quinn DI, Tsao-Wei DD, et al. Phase II study of vorinostat (suberoylanilide hydroxamic acid, SAHA) in patients with advanced transitional cell urothelial cancer (TCC) after platinum-based therapy—California Cancer Consortium/University of Pittsburgh NCI/CTEP-sponsored trial. J Clin Oncol 2008;26(15 Suppl):16058.

33. Hahn NM, Bonney PL, Dhawan D, et al. Subcutaneous 5-azacitidine treatment of naturally occurring canine urothelial carcinoma: a novel epigenetic approach to human urothelial carcinoma drug development. J Urol 2012;187(1):302–9.

34. Clozel T, Yang S, Elstrom RL, et al. Mechanism-based epigenetic chemosensitization therapy of diffuse large B-cell lymphoma. Cancer Discov 2013;3(9):1002–19.

35. Miyake H, Hara I, Yamanaka K, et al. Elevation of serum levels of urokinase-type plasminogen activator and its receptor is associated with disease progression and prognosis in patients with prostate cancer. Prostate 1999;39(2):123–9.

36. Bernardini S, Fauconnet S, Chabannes E, et al. Serum levels of vascular endothelial growth factor as a prognostic factor in bladder cancer. J Urol 2001;166(4):1275–9.

37. Nakanishi R, Oka N, Nakatsuji H, et al. Effect of vascular endothelial growth factor and its receptor inhibitor on proliferation and invasion in bladder cancer. Urol Int 2009;83(1):98–106.

38. Bochner BH, Cote RJ, Weidner N, et al. Angiogenesis in bladder cancer: relationship between microvessel density and tumor prognosis. J Natl Cancer Inst 1995;87(21):1603–12.

39. Hahn NM, Stadler WM, Zon RT, et al. Phase II trial of cisplatin, gemcitabine, and bevacizumab as first-line therapy for metastatic urothelial carcinoma: Hoosier Oncology Group GU 04-75. J Clin Oncol 2011;29(12):1525–30.

40. Balar AV, Apolo AB, Ostrovnaya I, et al. Phase II study of gemcitabine, carboplatin, and bevacizumab in patients with advanced unresectable or metastatic urothelial cancer. J Clin Oncol 2013;31(6):724–30.

41. Chaudhary UB, Golshayan AR, Brisendine A, et al. Phase II trial of neoadjuvant cisplatin, gemcitabine, and bevacizumab followed by radical cystectomy (RC) in patients with muscle-invasive transitional cell carcinoma (TCC) of the bladder. J Clin Oncol 2011;29(Suppl 7) [abstract: 276].

42. Siefker-Radtke AO, Kamet AM, Corn PG, et al. Neoadjuvant chemotherapy with DD-MVAC and bevacizumab in high risk urothelial cancer: results from a phase II trial at the M. D. Anderson Cancer Center. J Clin Oncol 2012;30(Suppl 5) [abstract: 261].

43. Bellmunt J, Gonzalez-Larriba JL, Prior C, et al. Phase II study of sunitinib as first-line treatment of urothelial cancer patients ineligible to receive cisplatin-based chemotherapy: baseline interleukin-8 and tumor contrast enhancement as potential predictive factors of activity. Ann Oncol 2011;22(12):2646–53.
44. Gallagher DJ, Milowsky MI, Gerst SR, et al. Phase II study of sunitinib in patients with metastatic urothelial cancer. J Clin Oncol 2010;28(8):1373–9.
45. Grivas PD, Daignault S, Tagawa ST, et al. Double-blind, randomized, phase 2 trial of maintenance sunitinib versus placebo after response to chemotherapy in patients with advanced urothelial carcinoma. Cancer 2014;120(5):692–701.
46. Galsky MD, Hahn NM, Powles T, et al. Gemcitabine, cisplatin, and sunitinib for metastatic urothelial carcinoma and as preoperative therapy for muscle-invasive bladder cancer. Clin Genitourin Cancer 2013;11(2):175–81.
47. Garcia JA, Stephenson AJ, Ireland J, et al. Sunitinib in BCG-refractory non-muscle-invasive transitional cell carcinoma of the bladder. J Clin Oncol 2011;29(Suppl 7) [abstract: 262].
48. Necchi A, Mariani L, Zaffaroni N, et al. Pazopanib in advanced and platinum-resistant urothelial cancer: an open-label, single group, phase 2 trial. Lancet Oncol 2012;13(8):810–6.
49. Pili R, Qin R, Flynn PJ, et al. A phase II safety and efficacy study of the vascular endothelial growth factor receptor tyrosine kinase inhibitor pazopanib in patients with metastatic urothelial cancer. Clin Genitourin Cancer 2013;11(4):477–83.
50. Srinivas S, Narayanan S, Harshman LC, et al. Phase II trial of pazopanib and weekly paclitaxel in metastatic urothelial cancer. J Clin Oncol 2014;32(Suppl 4) [abstract: 299].
51. Gerullis H, Eimer C, Ecke TH, et al. Combined treatment with pazopanib and vinflunine in patients with advanced urothelial carcinoma refractory after first-line therapy. Anticancer Drugs 2013;24(4):422–5.
52. Choueiri TK, Ross RW, Jacobus S, et al. Double-blind, randomized trial of docetaxel plus vandetanib versus docetaxel plus placebo in platinum-pretreated metastatic urothelial cancer. J Clin Oncol 2012;30(5):507–12.
53. Sridhar SS, Winquist E, Eisen A, et al. A phase II trial of sorafenib in first-line metastatic urothelial cancer: a study of the PMH Phase II Consortium. Invest New Drugs 2011;29(5):1045–9.
54. Dreicer R, Li H, Stein M, et al. Phase 2 trial of sorafenib in patients with advanced urothelial cancer: a trial of the Eastern Cooperative Oncology Group. Cancer 2009;115(18):4090–5.
55. Krege S, Rexer H, vom Dorp F, et al. Prospective randomized double-blind multicentre phase II study comparing gemcitabine and cisplatin plus sorafenib chemotherapy with gemcitabine and cisplatin plus placebo in locally advanced and/or metastasized urothelial cancer: SUSE (AUO-AB 31/05). BJU Int 2014;113(3):429–36.
56. Mehnert JM, Mortazavi A, Stein MN, et al. A phase II trial of gemcitabine, carboplatin, and sorafenib in patients with transitional cell carcinoma: preliminary safety and outcome. J Clin Oncol 2011;29(Suppl 7) [abstract: 278].
57. Apolo AB, Parnus HL, Madan RA, et al. A phase II study of cabozantinib (XL184) in patients with advanced/metastatic urothelial carcinoma. J Clin Oncol 2013;31(Suppl) [abstract: 4577].
58. Apolo AB, Tomita Y, Lee MJ, et al. Effect of cabozantinib on immunosuppressive subsets in metastatic urothelial carcinoma. J Clin Oncol 2014;32(5 Suppl) [abstract: 4501].

59. Twardowski P, Stadler WM, Frankel P, et al. Phase II study of Aflibercept (VEGF-Trap) in patients with recurrent or metastatic urothelial cancer, a California Cancer Consortium Trial. Urology 2010;76(4):923–6.

60. Mita AC, Takimoto CH, Mita M, et al. Phase 1 study of AMG 386, a selective angiopoietin 1/2-neutralizing peptibody, in combination with chemotherapy in adults with advanced solid tumors. Clin Cancer Res 2010;16(11):3044–56.

61. Jian W, Levitt JM, Lerner SP, et al. The angiopoietin-tie2 pathway is a potential therapeutic target in urothelial carcinoma. Anticancer Res 2014;34(7):3377–82.

62. Jian W, Levitt JM, Lerner SP, et al. The preclinical activity of lenalidomide in indolent urothelial carcinoma. Anticancer Res 2014;34(7):3383–9.

63. Jinesh GG, Lee EK, Tran J, et al. Lenalidomide augments the efficacy of bacillus Calmette-Guerin (BCG) immunotherapy in vivo. Urol Oncol 2013;31(8): 1676–82.

64. Lonn U, Lonn S, Friberg S, et al. Prognostic value of amplification of c-erb-B2 in bladder carcinoma. Clin Cancer Res 1995;1(10):1189–94.

65. Sriplakich S, Jahnson S, Karlsson MG. Epidermal growth factor receptor expression: predictive value for the outcome after cystectomy for bladder cancer? BJU Int 1999;83(4):498–503.

66. Chaux A, Cohen JS, Schultz L, et al. High epidermal growth factor receptor immunohistochemical expression in urothelial carcinoma of the bladder is not associated with EGFR mutations in exons 19 and 21: a study using formalin-fixed, paraffin-embedded archival tissues. Hum Pathol 2012;43(10):1590–5.

67. Hussain M, Daignault S, Agarwal N, et al. A randomized phase 2 trial of gemcitabine/cisplatin with or without cetuximab in patients with advanced urothelial carcinoma. Cancer 2014;120(17):2684–93.

68. Wong YN, Litwin S, Vaughn D, et al. Phase II trial of cetuximab with or without paclitaxel in patients with advanced urothelial tract carcinoma. J Clin Oncol 2012;30(28):3545–51.

69. Petrylak DP, Tangen CM, Van Veldhuizen PJ Jr, et al. Results of the Southwest Oncology Group phase II evaluation (study S0031) of ZD1839 for advanced transitional cell carcinoma of the urothelium. BJU Int 2010;105(3):317–21.

70. Philips GK, Halabi S, Sanford BL, et al. A phase II trial of cisplatin (C), gemcitabine (G) and gefitinib for advanced urothelial tract carcinoma: results of Cancer and Leukemia Group B (CALGB) 90102. Ann Oncol 2009;20(6):1074–9.

71. Hussain MH, MacVicar GR, Petrylak DP, et al. Trastuzumab, paclitaxel, carboplatin, and gemcitabine in advanced human epidermal growth factor receptor-2/neu-positive urothelial carcinoma: results of a multicenter phase II National Cancer Institute trial. J Clin Oncol 2007;25(16):2218–24.

72. Oudard S, Culine S, Vieillefond A, et al. Multicenter randomized phase 2 trial of gemcitabine-platinum with or without trastuzumab (T) in advanced/metastatic urothelial carcinoma (A/MUC) with HER2 overexpression. ESMO Congress conference, Vienna, Austria, September 2012 [abstract: 1111].

73. Galsky MD, Von Hoff DD, Neubauer M, et al. Target-specific, histology-independent, randomized discontinuation study of lapatinib in patients with HER2-amplified solid tumors. Invest New Drugs 2012;30(2):695–701.

74. Wulfing C, Machiels JP, Richel DJ, et al. A single-arm, multicenter, open-label phase 2 study of lapatinib as the second-line treatment of patients with locally advanced or metastatic transitional cell carcinoma. Cancer 2009;115(13): 2881–90.

75. Bajorin DF, Gomella LG, Sharma P, et al. Preliminary product parameter and safety results from NeuACT, a phase 2 randomized, open-label trial of DN24-02

in patients with surgically resected HER2+ urothelial cancer at high risk for recurrence. J Clin Oncol 2014;32(5 Suppl) [abstract: 4541].

76. Kamada M, So A, Muramaki M, et al. Hsp27 knockdown using nucleotide-based therapies inhibit tumor growth and enhance chemotherapy in human bladder cancer cells. Mol Cancer Ther 2007;6(1):299–308.

77. Ko YJ, Canil CM, Mukherjee SD, et al. Nanoparticle albumin-bound paclitaxel for second-line treatment of metastatic urothelial carcinoma: a single group, multi-centre, phase 2 study. Lancet Oncol 2013;14(8):769–76.

78. Grivas PD, Hussain M, Hafez K, et al. A phase II trial of neoadjuvant nab-paclitaxel, carboplatin, and gemcitabine (ACaG) in patients with locally advanced carcinoma of the bladder. Urology 2013;82(1):111–7.

79. Hoffman-Censits JH, Vaughn DJ, Lin J, et al. A phase II study of cabazitaxel in patients with urothelial carcinoma who have disease progression following platinum-based chemotherapy. J Clin Oncol 2014;32(Suppl) [abstract: e15519].

80. Quinn DI, Aparicio A, Tsao-Wei DD, et al. Phase II study of eribulin (E7389) in patients (pts) with advanced urothelial cancer (UC)—Final report: a California Cancer Consortium-led NCI/CTEP-sponsored trial. J Clin Oncol 2010;28(15 Suppl) [abstract: 4539].

81. Quinn DI, Twardowski PW, Wei YE, et al. Phase II study of eribulin in platinum-treated, tubulin naive advanced urothelial cancer (UC) - A California Cancer Consortium trial (NCI/CTEP 7435). ECCO. Conference, Amsterdam, The Netherlands, September 2013, [abstract: 2704].

82. Galsky MD, Mironov S, Iasonos A, et al. Phase II trial of pemetrexed as second-line therapy in patients with metastatic urothelial carcinoma. Invest New Drugs 2007;25(3):265–70.

83. Sweeney CJ, Roth BJ, Kabbinavar FF, et al. Phase II study of pemetrexed for second-line treatment of transitional cell cancer of the urothelium. J Clin Oncol 2006;24(21):3451–7.

84. Benjamin DJ, Bamburg RM, Chaim J, et al. Efficacy of single-agent pemetrexed in platinum refractory metastatic urothelial cancer. J Clin Oncol 2014;32(Suppl 4) [abstract: 322].

85. Zhou N, Singh K, Mir MC, et al. The investigational Aurora kinase A inhibitor MLN8237 induces defects in cell viability and cell-cycle progression in malignant bladder cancer cells in vitro and in vivo. Clin Cancer Res 2013;19(7):1717–28.

86. Sonpavde G, Goldman BH, Speights VO, et al. Quality of pathologic response and surgery correlate with survival for patients with completely resected bladder cancer after neoadjuvant chemotherapy. Cancer 2009;115(18):4104–9.

87. Paz-Ares LG, Solsona E, Esteban E, et al. Randomized phase III trial comparing adjuvant paclitaxel/gemcitabine/cisplatin (PGC) to observation in patients with resected invasive bladder cancer: results of the Spanish Oncology Genitourinary Group (SOGUG) 99/01 study. J Clin Oncol 2010;28(18 Suppl), LBA 4518.

88. Grossman HB, Natale RB, Tangen CM, et al. Neoadjuvant chemotherapy plus cystectomy compared with cystectomy alone for locally advanced bladder cancer. N Engl J Med 2003;349(9):859–66.

89. Sternberg CN, Skoneczna IA, Kerst JM, et al. Final results of EORTC intergroup randomized phase III trial comparing immediate versus deferred chemotherapy after radical cystectomy in patients with pT3T4 and/or N+ M0 transitional cell carcinoma (TCC) of the bladder. J Clin Oncol 2014;32(5 Suppl) [abstract: 4500].

90. Sonpavde G, Khan MM, Lerner SP, et al. Disease-free survival at 2 or 3 years correlates with 5-year overall survival of patients undergoing radical cystectomy for muscle invasive bladder cancer. J Urol 2011;185(2):456–61.

91. Apolo AB, Ostrovnaya I, Halabi S, et al. Prognostic model for predicting survival of patients with metastatic urothelial cancer treated with cisplatin-based chemotherapy. J Natl Cancer Inst 2013;105(7):499–503.

92. Galsky MD, Moshier E, Krege S, et al. Nomogram for predicting survival in patients with unresectable and/or metastatic urothelial cancer who are treated with cisplatin-based chemotherapy. Cancer 2013;119(16):3012–9.

93. Galsky MD, Krege S, Lin CC, et al. Relationship between 6- and 9-month progression-free survival and overall survival in patients with metastatic urothelial cancer treated with first-line cisplatin-based chemotherapy. Cancer 2013; 119(16):3020–6.

94. Sonpavde G, Galsky MD, Bellmunt J. A new approach to second-line therapy for urothelial cancer? Lancet Oncol 2013;14(8):682–4.

95. Sonpavde G, Pond GR, Fougeray R, et al. Time from prior chemotherapy enhances prognostic risk grouping in the second-line setting of advanced urothelial carcinoma: a retrospective analysis of pooled, prospective phase 2 trials. Eur Urol 2013;63(4):717–23.

96. Bellmunt J, Choueiri TK, Fougeray R, et al. Prognostic factors in patients with advanced transitional cell carcinoma of the urothelial tract experiencing treatment failure with platinum-containing regimens. J Clin Oncol 2010;28(11):1850–5.

97. Pond GR, Agarwal N, Bellmunt J, et al. A nomogram including baseline prognostic factors to estimate the activity of second-line therapy for advanced urothelial carcinoma. BJU Int 2014;113(5b):E137–43.

98. Agarwal N, Bellmunt J, Maughan BL, et al. Six-month progression-free survival as the primary endpoint to evaluate the activity of new agents as second-line therapy for advanced urothelial carcinoma. Clin Genitourin Cancer 2014;12(2): 130–7.

Therapeutic Opportunities in the Intrinsic Subtypes of Muscle-Invasive Bladder Cancer

CrossMark

David J. McConkey, PhD[a],*, Woonyoung Choi, PhD[a],
Andrea Ochoa, BS[a], Arlene Siefker-Radtke, MD[b],
Bogdan Czerniak, MD, PhD[c], Colin P.N. Dinney, MD[d]

KEYWORDS

• Urothelial cancer • Basal and luminal • Neoadjuvant chemotherapy

KEY POINTS

• There seem to be strong associations between intrinsic muscle-invasive bladder cancer subtype membership and enrichment with clinically actionable genetic and epigenetic features.
• It seems that the intrinsic subtypes display differences in sensitivity to cisplatin-based combination chemotherapy.
• Because basal tumors are aggressive and chemosensitive, the overall impact of chemotherapy on disease-specific and overall survival should be carefully evaluated in patients with these tumors.
• Epigenetic mechanisms, including epithelial-to-mesenchymal transition and stromal fibroblast infiltration (plasticity), may impart resistance via mechanisms that are not captured in DNA mutation and copy number variation (CNV) analyses.
• Future trials with targeted agents should evaluate not only the presence of actionable DNA mutations, translocations, and CNVs, but also intrinsic subtype membership.
• Investigators should continue to exploit the neoadjuvant platform to accelerate the clinical development of targeted agents and to identify mechanisms of induced resistance.

M.D. Anderson has filed for patent protection for the subtype classifier.
[a] Departments of Urology and Cancer Biology, U.T. M.D. Anderson Cancer Center, 1515 Holcombe Boulevard, Houston, TX 77030, USA; [b] Department of Genitourinary Medical Oncology, U.T. M.D. Anderson Cancer Center, 1515 Holcombe Boulevard, Houston, TX 77030, USA; [c] Department of Pathology, U.T. M.D. Anderson Cancer Center, 1515 Holcombe Boulevard, Houston, TX 77030, USA; [d] Department of Urology, U.T. M.D. Anderson Cancer Center, Houston, TX 77030, USA
* Corresponding author. Department of Urology, U.T. M.D. Anderson Cancer Center, 1515 Holcombe Boulevard, Houston, TX 77030.
E-mail address: dmcconke@mdanderson.org

Hematol Oncol Clin N Am 29 (2015) 377–394
http://dx.doi.org/10.1016/j.hoc.2014.11.003
0889-8588/15/$ – see front matter © 2015 Elsevier Inc. All rights reserved.
hemonc.theclinics.com

INTRODUCTION

Muscle-invasive bladder cancers (MIBCs) are heterogeneous tumors with variable progression patterns and responses to frontline therapies.[1] Although approximately half of patients will be cured of their disease with definitive surgery with or without perioperative cisplatin-based chemotherapy, the others experience rapid progression and uniform mortality. There has been essentially no substantive progress in systemic therapy since the current cisplatin-based regimens were introduced more than 30 years ago. Many patients receive clear clinical benefit from chemotherapy, but no strategies have been developed to prospectively identify them; it has been estimated that their overall impact on disease-specific survival is only 5% to 15%.[2] The perception that perioperative chemotherapy provides only a modest benefit has resulted in its underutilization in patients with potentially lethal tumors, while at the same time our inability to prospectively identify chemoresistant tumors has resulted in the treatment of patients who received no clinical benefit. Finally, no biologically targeted agents have been approved to date, and no real clinical signal has emerged from the trials that have been performed with most of the traditional biological targets.[3]

There are many indications that a dramatic change in this dismal picture is about to occur. The first phase of The Cancer Genome Atlas' (TCGA's) bladder cancer project[4] and several parallel private efforts[5–8] have provided the first deep view of bladder cancer heterogeneity and have stimulated renewed enthusiasm for developing targeted agents in bladder cancer. Whole genome sequencing also provided the research community with its first targeted agent success story in the identification of *TSC1* and *NF2* mutations in a patient with bladder cancer whose tumor displayed a remarkable durable complete response to everolimus.[9] In addition, a community-wide effort to exploit the scientific opportunities afforded by the use of neoadjuvant therapy[10] has produced a very-high-profile clinical trial (the Southwest Oncology Group's CoXEN (coexpression extrapolation) trial)[11] that will allow for the prospective evaluation of multiple methods to predict sensitivity and resistance to chemotherapy, and a similar clinical trial that will assign patients to receive multiple targeted agents based on their tumor genomic profiles will open soon. Finally, exciting preliminary results from a phase I-II clinical trial of a blocking anti-PDL1 antibody suggest that immune checkpoint blockade is clinically active in a significant fraction of bladder cancers.[12] Together, these developments have prompted aggressive efforts to design and launch clinical trials that exploit our newly developed understanding of the biological properties of MIBCs stemming from these genomics efforts. However, past experience in other cancer types suggests that taking advantage of this information may not be entirely straightforward. Rather, it may be necessary to obtain a profound understanding of the biological mechanisms that explain *why* the alterations and particular patterns of gene expression are observed in certain tumors (and not others) and to determine exactly what they do for the cancer cells before the full potential of the genomics discoveries can be exploited.

It is now well established that cancer heterogeneity is controlled by both genetic and epigenetic mechanisms. One powerful strategy that has been used to visualize important epigenetic aspects of this heterogeneity is to use whole genome RNA expression profiling and unsupervised analyses to group tumors into intrinsic subtypes without considering their clinical properties (or sometimes even their tissues of origin).[13,14] This strategy has had a major impact on breast cancer, whereby knowledge of a tumor intrinsic subtype is used for clinical management.[15] Patients with luminal breast cancers are managed with surgery plus adjuvant endocrine therapy, whereas patients with basal-like or HER2-enriched tumors receive no benefit from endocrine therapy. Conversely, patients with basal-like or HER2-enriched tumors obtain substantial clinical benefit from perioperative chemotherapy, whereas most patients with luminal tumors do not.[16–18] These patterns of response and resistance are not obviously associated with tumor mutation profiles but rather seem to be more closely related to the tumors' cells of origin.[19] It is important that we consider and learn from this experience as the bladder cancer research community tries to fully exploit the emerging genomics information.

INTRINSIC SUBTYPES OF BREAST CANCER

Perou and colleagues[13] first observed the intrinsic molecular subtypes of breast cancer in a relatively small cohort of 65 tumors from 42 different patients. They used an in-house cDNA microarray that contained a total of 8102 different probes, filtered out the genes that displayed the greatest variations in expression across the dataset, and then used the filtered genes to perform an unbiased (unsupervised hierarchical clustering) analysis of the relationships among the gene expression patterns they observed in the tumors. They discovered that the tumors formed 4 distinct groups, and they recognized that 2 of them contained basal-like and luminal gene expression patterns that were similar to the ones found in cells at different stages of differentiation in the normal mammary epithelium.[19] They also appreciated that one subtype contained a signature characteristic of *ERBB2* (*HER2*) amplification.[13,14] The duplicated tumors within their discovery cohort consisted of samples taken before and 16 weeks after treatment with neoadjuvant chemotherapy as well as several matched primary tumor–lymph node metastasis pairs.[13] In almost all cases the clustering analyses revealed that these matched tumors were more similar to each other than they were to any of the other tumors in the dataset; in particular, the matched specimens always segregated to the same gene expression clusters.[13] Therefore, they suggested that the gene expression profiles that dictated subtype membership were intrinsic to the tumor (ie, stable) and did not depend on the site or timing of biopsy or even prior exposure to DNA-damaging chemotherapeutic agents. Since then, the breast cancer intrinsic subtypes have been consistently observed whenever cohorts of breast cancers are subjected to unsupervised hierarchical clustering.

The TCGA's breast cancer project afforded the opportunity to comprehensively characterize the genomic alterations associated with each intrinsic subtype.[20] Comparisons of tumor subtype membership as determined by unsupervised hierarchical clustering versus the use of an intrinsic subtype classifier (the PAM50)[15] revealed strong concordance between the two,[20] supporting the original conclusion that the intrinsic subtypes are associated with stable biological properties. Overall, the basal-like and HER2-enriched tumors exhibited the highest overall mutation rates consistent with greater genomic instability; but the luminal tumors contained a broader spectrum of different mutations.[20] Luminal tumors contained more activating mutations in *PIK3CA* and inactivating mutations in the differentiation-associated transcription factor *GATA3*, whereas the basal-like and HER2-enriched cancers had more p53 mutations, and the types of p53 mutations observed in the basal-like cancers were more damaging (nonsense and truncating).[20] One possible explanation for these differences in p53 mutation patterns could be that mutant p53 plays an oncogenic (gain-of-function) role in the luminal cancers,[21] whereas complete loss of function is more important in the basal and HER2-enriched tumors. Copy number variations (CNVs) also correlated with the tumor intrinsic subtypes, with the greatest frequencies observed in the basal-like and HER2-enriched tumors.[20]

The clinical characteristics of tumors within each breast cancer intrinsic subtype are also distinct.[14] Basal-like and HER2-enriched tumors are associated with shorter disease-specific and overall survival, particularly in the absence of neoadjuvant or adjuvant chemotherapy. However, most basal-like and HER2-enriched tumors respond to neoadjuvant chemotherapy[16–18]; patients whose tumors achieve a complete pathologic response have excellent outcomes. Patients with luminal A tumors have the longest disease-specific and overall survival, and most patients with luminal B tumors also have excellent clinical outcomes. These patients are treated with surgery and adjuvant hormonal therapy. Although luminal cancers are associated with excellent 5-year overall survival, they are also more often associated with late relapse, usually characterized by bone metastasis.[22] Together, the compiled genomic and clinical results support the original suggestions made by Perou and colleagues[13] that knowledge of a given tumor's intrinsic subtype carries important clinical information and that each subtype should be treated as a distinct disease entity.

INTRINSIC SUBTYPES OF BLADDER CANCER

One of the most important objectives in cancer research is to develop molecular classifiers that can inform prognostication and predict therapeutic efficacy. It might seem that the most straightforward way to do this would be to assemble cohorts of tumors from patients who experienced extreme clinical outcomes (ie, very short vs very long disease-specific survival or complete pathologic response vs progression with neoadjuvant or adjuvant chemotherapy), perform deep genomic profiling, and correlate the outcome with the genomic features observed. This strategy has been used successfully to develop prognostic classifiers, such as Genomic Health's Oncotype Dx platforms (Genomic Health, Inc, Redwood City, CA)[15] or GenomeDx's Decipher classifier (GenomeDx Biosciences Inc, Vancouver, BC, Canada and San Diego, CA).[23] Several academic groups have used this strategy to identify biomarker panels that correlate with clinical characteristics in bladder cancers, including recurrence, disease-specific survival, and/or metastasis; but the reproducibility of these signatures has been questioned.[24] From a biological perspective, the signatures do share general similarities across disease types (usually biomarkers associated with proliferation and tissue-specific differentiation). Indeed, high levels of Ki-67 and other cell cycle/proliferation biomarkers are consistently associated with poor prognosis in MIBC,[25] just as they are in breast or prostate cancers.[15] Past difficulties in reproducing specific signatures may be related to the use of different genomic platforms and tumor heterogeneity. Alternatively, it is possible that better classifiers could be developed by focusing on the gene expression differences associated with extreme clinical outcomes *within* a given intrinsic subtype.

A group at Lund University was the first to intentionally search for intrinsic subtypes in bladder cancers.[6,26] They performed whole genome mRNA expression profiling on a mixed cohort of more than 300 non-muscle invasive bladder cancers (NMIBCs) and MIBCs. They concluded that the tumors could be easily separated into 2 major subtypes, one that consisted almost entirely of grade 1 and 2 tumors (MS1) and another that contained mostly high-grade (G3) tumors (MS2).[26] Parallel analyses of mutations and focal genomic amplifications (FGAs) revealed that the MS1 tumors were enriched with activating mutations in *FGFR3* and *PIK3CA* and low levels of genomic instability, whereas MS2 tumors were enriched with mutations in *TP53*, amplification of *E2F3*, *RB* deletions, and large numbers of FGAs consistent with genomic instability.[26] In a subsequent study they used unsupervised hierarchical clustering to further define subtypes within the MS1 and MS2 tumors.[6] They concluded that the MS1 tumors could be subdivided into 2 subtypes and that the MS2 tumors formed up to 5 distinct subtypes. Importantly, they recognized that 2 of the MS2 subtypes (urobasal B and squamous cell carcinoma (SCC)-like) were enriched with high-molecular-weight basal cytokeratins, whereas 2 others (grouped together and termed *genomically unstable*) were enriched with low-molecular-weight luminal cytokeratins and uroplakins, which are urothelial terminal differentiation markers. Finally, one of the subtypes seemed to be infiltrated with stromal cells because it was enriched with extracellular matrix, immune cell, and fibroblast biomarkers; tumors in this infiltrated subtype also expressed low levels of genes involved in the late cell cycle.[6] They consistently observed these subtypes in multiple independent data sets and concluded that they corresponded to the intrinsic subtypes of bladder cancer.[6] Parallel work by another group used immunohistochemistry to show that MIBCs expressed basal and terminal differentiation-associated cytokeratins in a mutually exclusive fashion and concluded that cancers could be separated into subtypes resembling different states of differentiation within the normal urothelium.[27–29]

Parallel efforts by the authors' group and 2 others confirmed and extended these initial observations.[4,7,8] Using whole genome mRNA expression profiling and unsupervised analyses, the authors' group concluded that MIBCs could be grouped into 3 distinct subtypes characterized by differential expression of breast basal and luminal biomarkers.[7,30,31] In parallel, another group used a very similar approach on a large metadata set and concluded that the tumors formed 2 distinct basal and luminal clusters.[8] They also demonstrated that there was a subset of basal MIBCs that were very similar to the so-called claudin-low breast cancers.[8,32] Finally, using RNA sequencing (RNAseq) data from 128 MIBCs, the TCGA concluded that the tumors could be grouped into 4 mRNA expression-based subtypes and recognized that they were enriched with breast basal and luminal biomarkers.[4] Direct head-to-head comparisons of the 3 groups' calls in the TCGA data set revealed that the intrinsic subtypes identified by the 3 groups were extremely similar.[30,31] The differences in the number of clusters were explained by the fact that 2 of the groups subdivided the luminal tumors into 2 subsets, and the TCGA also subdivided the basal tumors into 2 subsets (**Fig. 1**). The significance of these divisions in the basal and luminal MIBCs is discussed later.

The authors also performed a head-to-head comparison of their subtype calls to the calls made by the group at the University of Lund.[6] Not unexpectedly, the results revealed strong similarities in the subtype calls made by the two groups (see **Fig. 1**). The Lund SCC-like tumors corresponded to the basal subtype; the Lund genomically unstable tumors corresponded to the luminal subtype; and the Lund infiltrated subtype corresponded to the MD Anderson p53-like subtype and the TCGA's cluster II tumors (see **Fig. 1**). Therefore, 4 independent groups using different cohorts of MIBCs discovered very similar subtypes; there can be very little doubt that they represent the intrinsic subtypes of MIBC.

Like their breast cancer counterparts, each of the intrinsic subtypes of bladder cancer possesses unique clinical characteristics. Patients with basal MIBCs tend to have more advanced stage and metastatic disease at presentation, whereas patients with luminal MIBCs tend to have better clinical outcomes.[7,8,33] Basal MIBCs are relatively more prevalent in women than in men[7,8] and are enriched with squamous histopathologic features.[4,6,7,34] On the other hand, luminal MIBCs were enriched with papillary histopathologic features,[4] and micropapillary MIBCs seem to be mostly luminal in origin (Choi W, Czerniak B, unpublished observations 2014). Finally, luminal MIBCs are enriched with activating *FGFR3* mutations,[7] which, as discussed earlier, are present in most low-grade NMIBCs. The presence of papillary features and *FGFR3* mutations suggests that luminal MIBCs may represent NMIBCs that have progressed to become muscle invasive. Recent lineage-tracing studies in a mouse model of bladder cancer support this idea.[35]

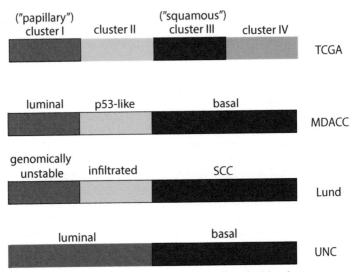

Fig. 1. Relationships between the intrinsic subtypes identified by the groups at the Lund University, MD Anderson Cancer Center (MDACC), the University of North Carolina (UNC), and the TCGA. Subtype calls made by the groups using the same tumor cohorts were compared. For the comparisons between the MDACC calls and those made by UNC or TCGA, the TCGA RNAseq dataset served as the reference. For the comparisons between the MDACC and Lund calls, the MDACC and Lund Illumina data sets were used. For the actual comparisons, see Choi and colleagues[30] and McConkey and colleagues.[74]

BIOLOGICAL PROPERTIES OF THE INTRINSIC SUBTYPES

Bioinformatic analyses of the gene expression signatures that characterized the MIBC subtypes revealed roles for transcription factors that had also been implicated in breast cancer.[7] The basal epithelial/stem cell transcription factors ΔNp63α and STAT3 were both identified as central regulators of basal MIBC gene expression, and ΔNp63 has also been implicated in basal breast cancers.[36–38] Basal expression of active STAT3 promoted carcinogen-induced tumorigenesis in a mouse model[39]; high-level expression of ΔNp63 in MIBCs was associated with poor clinical outcomes,[40,41] consistent with their central roles in basal MIBC biology. Aside from STAT3 and ΔNp63, basal cancers displayed gene expression features consistent with active NFκB, c-Myc, and hypoxia-induced factor (HIF) signaling. ΔNp63 knockdown resulted in downregulation of Myc[42] and the HIF signature (data not shown), indicating that both pathways are directly or indirectly connected to ΔNp63.

Luminal MIBCs were enriched with gene expression patterns that were similar to the ones found in luminal breast cancers, including active estrogen receptor (ER), TRIM24, FOXA1, and GATA3 signatures.[7,8] Luminal MIBCs also contained strong peroxisome proliferator activator receptor-gamma (PPARγ) signatures,[7] which are not recognized as an important feature of luminal breast cancers. (Perou and colleagues'[13] initial work actually identified PPARγ-associated biomarkers in basal-like cancers.) The TCGA's analyses of MIBCs demonstrated that *PPARG* is amplified in a fairly large fraction of tumors (16%),[4] and this *PPARG* amplification is enriched in the luminal subtypes (TCGA clusters I and II) (**Fig. 2**).

As introduced earlier, one group recognized that some basal MIBCs possess gene expression signatures that are similar to so-called claudin-low breast cancers.[8]

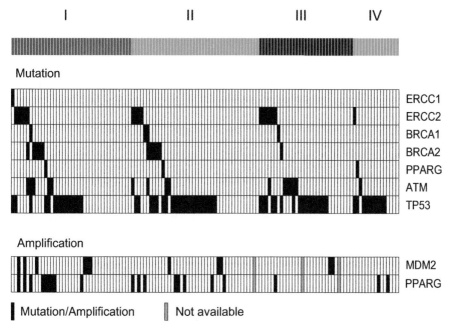

Fig. 2. Distribution of genomic alterations in DNA repair proteins and *PPARG* in the intrinsic subtypes in the TCGA cohort. Clusters I and II correspond to the luminal tumors, and clusters III and IV are basal. Note that *BRCA2* mutations and *PPARG* amplification are enriched in luminal cancers. Otherwise there are no clear associations with the subtypes; in particular, mutations in *TP53* display an even distribution.

Claudin-low breast cancers are characterized by expression of biomarkers associated with epithelial-to-mesenchymal transition (EMT),[16,32] a reversible physiologic process that has been implicated in tissue development, wound healing, cancer metastasis, and stemness.[43–45] ΔNp63 actually inhibits EMT by inducing expression of a micro-RNA (miR-205) that directly inhibits the critical EMT-inducing transcription factor, ZEB1.[46,47] Therefore, the observation that basal tumors were enriched with EMT biomarkers[7,8] was counterintuitive. The authors, therefore, explored the relationship between expression of ΔNp63 and EMT biomarkers in basal tumors within the TCGA's RNAseq cohort. The results revealed that the TCGA's cluster III corresponded to the basal tumors that possessed an epithelial molecular phenotype and expressed high levels of ΔNp63, E-cadherin, miR-205, and all 5 members of the miR-200 family, whereas the TCGA's cluster IV consisted of basal tumors that had undergone EMT (Ochoa A, Choi W, unpublished data). Furthermore, using a technique called gene set enrichment analysis, which evaluates the expression of gene expression signatures in mRNA expression profiling datasets, the authors confirmed that ΔNp63 was active in cluster III and ZEB1 was active in cluster IV (A. Ochoa, manuscript in preparation). Therefore, basal MIBCs can be subdivided into the TCGA's cluster III versus cluster IV based on whether or not they have undergone EMT. Epithelial-mesenchymal plasticity may be important for the propensity of basal tumors to produce metastases.[43]

As discussed earlier, the luminal MIBCs also seemed to segregate into at least 2 distinct subtypes, which the authors have called luminal and p53-like[7] and the TCGA termed cluster I and cluster II.[4] These luminal MIBC subtypes share similarities with the luminal subtypes of breast cancers.[30] Specifically, like luminal A breast cancers, the p53-like MIBCs express lower levels of cell cycle and proliferation biomarkers than do the tumors in any of the other subtypes.[6,7] Furthermore, the top 10 biomarkers that characterize the p53-like MIBCs are expressed by cancer-associated fibroblasts (CAFs)[6,7]; these same biomarkers are also enriched in luminal A breast cancers.[30] Therefore, CAF infiltration may be a major determinant of the biological properties that are unique to the p53-like MIBCs. Although the p53-like tumors contain a gene expression signature characteristic of active, wild-type p53, p53 mutation frequencies are identical to those observed in the other subtypes[7] (see **Fig. 2**), indicating that the p53-like signature is not driven by p53 itself.

EFFECTS OF CHEMOTHERAPY IN THE INTRINSIC SUBTYPES

Approximately 35% of patients receiving neoadjuvant cisplatin-based combination chemotherapy are downstaged to no residual muscle-invasive disease at cystectomy. These patients have excellent long-term survival, indicating that downstaging can serve as an excellent immediate surrogate for disease-specific survival. The same situation exists in breast cancer, which prompted the Food and Drug Administration to grant fast-track approval to agents that produce high pathologic complete response rates in the neoadjuvant setting.[48] Therefore, the neoadjuvant platform in bladder cancer provides the ideal setting to identify the molecular basis of chemosensitivity and resistance.[10] Tissue is readily available before and after therapy, providing the opportunity for deep molecular profiling. SWOG's open clinical trial of neoadjuvant gemcitabine/cisplatin versus dose-dense methotrexate-vinblastine-adriamycin-cisplatin (MVAC) (S1314) was designed specifically to test one candidate approach (CoXEN).[11]

As discussed earlier, previous studies demonstrated that the intrinsic subtypes of breast cancer display different sensitivities to neoadjuvant conventional chemotherapy. Response rates are highest in basal (80%) and HER2-enriched (65%) tumors, intermediate in luminal B tumors (about 20%), and lowest in luminal A tumors (0%–10%).[16–18] The authors, therefore, asked whether the intrinsic subtypes of MIBC also displayed differences in chemosensitivity in several independent cohorts of tumors from patients enrolled in clinical trials. The results revealed that the p53-like/luminal A MIBCs were largely chemoresistant.[7] About half of the basal and luminal (B) tumors were consistently downstaged to less than pT2, whereas only 10% to 15% of the p53-like tumors were downstaged, a fraction that is not different from what has been observed with surgery alone.

The authors also investigated whether differences in gene expression patterns could be observed in chemosensitive versus chemoresistant basal or luminal B tumors. The chemosensitive basal tumors in 2 of the cohorts were enriched with an immune signature characteristic of T and B lymphocyte infiltration.[7] The immune checkpoint biomarker CTLA4 was contained within this signature, indicating that the chemosensitive tumors might be enriched with anergic T-regulatory cells. Importantly, lymphocyte infiltration was also associated with chemosensitivity in breast cancer.[49] The significance of this immune infiltration remains unclear, but it is possible that chemotherapy reawakens these T anergic cells and that they directly contribute to tumor cell killing.

The authors also compared whole genome mRNA expression in the chemoresistant tumors before (transurethral resection of bladder tumor) and after (cystectomy) neoadjuvant chemotherapy with dose-dense MVAC.[7] Several of the tumors that had belonged to the luminal (B) subtype switched to the p53-like subtype after therapy, revealing significant plasticity between the luminal subtypes. In addition, all of the tumors were enriched with a wild-type p53 gene expression signature after therapy that included decreased expression of cell cycle and proliferation biomarkers. Although preclinical studies implicated wild-type p53 in chemotherapy-induced apoptosis, more recent studies have demonstrated that wild-type p53 and p53-ness can actually promote apoptosis resistance by inducing cell cycle arrest.[17,50] Therefore, therapy-induced p53-ness may contribute to chemoresistance in MIBC, interfering with the effects of regimens that are introduced after MVAC. It will be important to perform experiments in preclinical models to determine whether this chemotherapy-induced p53-ness decreases with time after withdrawal of chemotherapy and to develop new approaches to prevent it.

Preclinical and clinical studies concluded that inactivating mutations in homologous recombination or nucleotide excision repair (NER) genes, and in particular mutations in *BRCA1* or *BRCA2*, increase tumor cell sensitivity to cisplatin.[51,52] Therefore, it may be possible to prospectively identify chemosensitive MIBCs by screening pretreatment tumors for these mutations. A recent study tested this hypothesis using next-generation sequencing in a retrospective cohort of tumors from patients treated with neoadjuvant chemotherapy.[53] They concluded that inactivating mutations in the NER gene *ERCC2* were highly enriched in responders, and they performed functional studies in cell lines to confirm that these mutations did in fact cause increased cisplatin sensitivity. In addition, 2 chemosensitive tumors that did not contain inactivating ERCC2 mutations had inactivating mutations in *BRCA1* or *BRCA2*. Importantly, even though p53 plays a major role in DNA repair, inactivating *TP53* mutations were not associated with response.[53] However, it seems likely that inactivating mutations in other DNA repair genes produce similar downstream effects to those observed in tumors with *ERCC2* or *BRCA1/2* mutations, so a more comprehensive approach to detecting DNA repair defects may be necessary in order to prospectively capture 100% of chemosensitive tumors. Importantly, the chemosensitive tumors in this cohort also displayed increased CNVs.[53] Therefore, copy number-based assays to detect genomic instability may also be capable of estimating a tumor's potential to respond to neoadjuvant chemotherapy.

In light of these observations, the authors wondered whether there would be an inverse relationship between the presence of mutations in DNA repair genes and the p53-like intrinsic subtype. To explore this possibility, the authors examined the frequencies of major cisplatin sensitivity-associated DNA repair defects within the intrinsic subtypes in the TCGA data set. The results revealed that several of the cluster II tumors (which correspond to the p53-like subtype) contained in mutations *ERCC2*, *BRCA1*, and *BRCA2* (see **Fig. 2**). It will be important to determine whether tumors with these features are chemoresistant (as predicted by their gene expression profiles) or chemosensitive (as predicted by the mutations they contain). The authors are performing DNA sequencing in several of their neoadjuvant chemotherapy cohorts to directly address this question.

BIOLOGICAL TARGETS IN THE INTRINSIC SUBTYPES: RECEPTOR TYROSINE KINASES

One of the most important products of the recently completed first phase of the TCGA bladder cancer project was the identification of novel activating mutations, translocations, and copy number alterations in signal transduction pathways that can be targeted with clinically available inhibitors. For example, activating mutations in *PIK3CA* and *TSC1*, 2 central components of the PI3 kinase-AKT-mTOR pathway,[54] were observed in 20% and 8% of tumors, respectively; the pathway was predicted to be activated in more than 40% of tumors overall.[4] This finding has generated renewed enthusiasm for the creation of multi-arm (umbrella) clinical trials in bladder cancer whereby patients are enrolled to one or another arm of the trial based on the patterns of mutation observed in their tumors. Most of the MIBC targets are also present in other solid tumors; for example, *PIK3CA* mutations are also present in a large fraction of luminal breast cancers[20] and many other types of cancer. The fact that *PIK3CA* mutations are found in multiple types of cancer raises the possibility that trials could be designed to enroll patients across solid tumor types; the new National Cancer Institute Molecular Analysis for Therapy of Choice trial embodies this concept. Alternatively, trials could be designed to test the activity of a drug in patients whose tumors have specific genomic alterations that are predicted to cause sensitivity to the drug; such basket trials can be powered better to directly examine the relationship between the biomarker and drug activity than other trial designs can. Importantly, many of the actionable genomic alterations in bladder cancer are associated with the intrinsic subtypes, indicating that the alterations probably play important and distinct physiologic roles within each subtype during bladder cancer initiation and progression and that defining the molecular mechanisms underlying these biases could increase the predictive value of the genomic alterations to predict which patients will respond to these therapies.

Activating mutations in *FGFR3* are present in more than 70% of NMIBCs.[55] These mutations cause constitutive dimerization of the receptor, leading to constitutive mitogen-activated protein kinase activation.[55] In addition, recent work demonstrated that some FGFR3-dependent human bladder cancer cell lines contain activating *FGFR3* translocations that cause similar effects.[56] Preclinical studies demonstrated that these alterations cause FGFR3 dependency in human bladder cancer cell lines and xenografts.[56,57] The TCGA identified activating *FGFR3* mutations in 12% of MIBCs, and 3 out of 128 tumors contained *TACC3-FGFR3* translocations.[4] Some MIBCs also contained amplified *FGFR3*.[4] All of these *FGFR3* alterations were enriched in luminal MIBCs (**Fig. 3**), and parallel analyses of the mutations in the intrinsic subtypes from independent private data sets confirmed these results.[7] Based on the experience in preclinical models, it seems likely that these MIBCs will be sensitive to FGFR-targeted therapies.

Gene expression analyses revealed that HER2/ERBB2 and HER3/ERBB3 expression were enriched in luminal cancers.[4,7,8] Genomic alterations affecting *ERBB2* and *ERBB3* were also enriched in luminal MIBCs (see **Fig. 3**). Amplification of *HER2/ERBB2* was also observed in 7% of tumors, with high-level amplification (comparable with the levels in HER2-enriched breast cancers) present in two-thirds of them (6 out of 9).[4] Activating *ERBB2* mutations, localized to its cytoplasmic tyrosine kinase domain, were also observed in 7% of tumors.[4] Activating *ERBB2* mutations and amplification are highly prevalent in urothelial cancers with micropapillary histopathologic features (40%),[58,59] although the *ERBB2* mutations that accumulate in these cancers cluster in the extracellular rather than the tyrosine kinase domain. It seems likely these tumors will depend on ERBB2 for proliferation and/or survival, but this assumption is not yet supported by data from preclinical models. Activating mutations in *HER3/ERBB3* were observed in 11% of tumors, but no *ERBB3* amplification was observed.[4] Again, preclinical studies should be performed to determine whether *ERBB3* mutations can also be validated as a potential clinical targets.

On the other hand, many components of the epidermal growth factor receptor (EGFR) pathway were enriched at the mRNA level in basal MIBCs[6,7]; basal tumors were also enriched with *EGFR* amplification.[33] The TCGA project also reported amplification in 11% of tumors, and half of these (7 out of 14) exhibited high-level

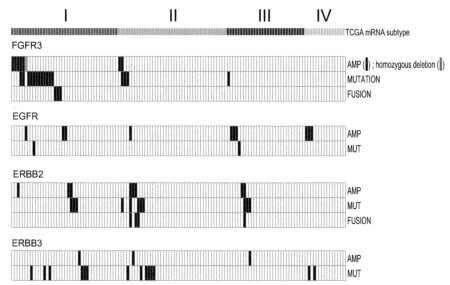

Fig. 3. Distribution of clinically actionable mutations in receptor tyrosine kinases in the intrinsic subtypes in the TCGA cohort. Clusters I and II correspond to the luminal tumors, and clusters III and IV are basal; cluster IV contains tumors that have undergone EMT. Note that *FGFR3*, *ERBB2*, and *ERBB3* alterations are more prevalent in luminal tumors, whereas epidermal growth factor receptor (*EGFR*) amplification is more common in basal tumors. AMP, amplification; MUT, mutation.

amplification (see **Fig. 3**).[4] Amplification of the *EGFR* was previously reported in small cell carcinomas of the bladder.[60] Studies in preclinical models suggest that basal tumors depend on EGFR signaling and are, therefore, sensitive to EGFR-targeted therapies.[33] However, molecular plasticity related to EMT could emerge as an important EGFR inhibitor resistance mechanism in basal tumors. In preclinical models of bladder cancer[61] and other solid tumors,[62] EMT is associated with resistance to EGFR inhibitors; as discussed earlier, basal bladder cancers are enriched with EMT biomarkers (particularly in the tumors represented by the TCGA's cluster IV).[7] Pharmacologic strategies exist that might prevent or reverse EMT and enhance EGFR inhibitor sensitivity within this subtype. Of particular interest are clinically available histone deacetylase inhibitors, which reverse EMT and promote EGFR inhibitor sensitivity preclinical models.[63]

It is important to remember that clinical trials have already been performed with drugs that target FGFR3, EGFR, and ERBB2; all of the trials were negative.[3] One explanation for this is that drug selection matters a lot; the first FGFR inhibitor trial used a drug that we now know has much lower potency than the best-in-class FGFR inhibitors have today. In addition, past trials were designed with expectations used in the setting of treating all patients with systemic chemotherapy and were underpowered to detect activity in the small group of patients with a potentially treatable signature. Rather than focusing on evaluating clinical activity in the 5% to 10% of patients with bladder cancer whose tumors clearly contained highly amplified EGFR or HER2, enrollment was based on a less precise determination of target levels (ie, with immunohistochemistry), so it can be argued that the potential value of all of these agents has not been determined.

OTHER CANDIDATE BIOLOGICAL TARGETS

One of the dominant features of luminal MIBC biology is PPARγ. As discussed earlier, luminal tumors are enriched with PPARγ gene expression signatures[7]; exposure to PPAR agonists promotes bladder cancer in rodent models.[64–66] In the TCGA cohort, *PPARG* was amplified in 17% of tumors[4]; this amplification was enriched in luminal tumors (see **Fig. 2**). In ongoing studies, the authors are defining its role in tumorigenesis and progression preclinical models. It is possible that PPARγ will emerge as a new therapeutic target.

Another attractive candidate subtype-associated target is ER. Luminal tumors were enriched for expression of ERβ (ESR2) and the ER coactivator FOXA1[4,7,8,33]; preclinical studies in human bladder cancer cell lines and mouse models have provided strong evidence for a role for the ER in bladder cancer initiation and progression, although on the surface the results seem somewhat contradictory. One group showed that the ER antagonist tamoxifen inhibited proliferation and induced apoptosis in human bladder cancer cells in vitro and blocked the growth of tumor xenografts and 4-hydroxybutyl(butyl)nitrosamine (BBN)-induced bladder cancers in vivo,[67–69] consistent with the idea that ER-induced gene expression promotes tumor growth. On the other hand, another group demonstrated that BBN-induced carcinogenesis was increased in mice lacking ERα.[70] The seemingly disparate results can be reconciled by the observation that mice lacking ERβ are protected from BBN-induced carcinogenesis,[71] indicating that ERα and ERβ play opposing roles in this mouse model. ERβ can promote gene expression in a tamoxifen-sensitive, ligand-independent fashion, which explains why tamoxifen can inhibit BBN-induced tumorigenesis. A chemo-preventative role for ligand-bound ERα would also explain why BBN-induced tumors are more common in male versus female mice and why bladder cancers are 2 to 3 times more common in men than in women. More difficult to understand is why ERα inhibits tumorigenesis in the BBN mouse model; the BBN tumors correspond to the basal intrinsic subtype, yet basal tumors are relatively more common in women than men. It is possible that the chemo-preventative effects of estrogen would be even stronger in a luminal cancer model.

Several other biological targets are enriched in basal MIBCs. The authors screened a panel of human bladder cancer cell lines for sensitivity to the mitotic kinesin inhibitor AZD4877 and correlated sensitivity with baseline gene expression profiles.[42] The results demonstrated that p63 was the top gene associated with response to the drug. Because AZD4877 inhibits the mitotic spindle checkpoint, the authors also screened the cell lines to determine their sensitivities to docetaxel, which induces apoptosis via similar mechanisms. The results confirmed that sensitivity correlated directly with p63 expression. Finally, the authors compared whole genome expression profiles in cells transduced with nontargeting or p63-specific siRNAs. One of the top downregulated genes in the latter was c-Myc, and knockdown of c-Myc also produced resistance to AZD4877 and docetaxel. Together, the results suggest that p63-induced Myc expression promotes sensitivity to antimitotic agents in bladder cancer cells. Therefore, basal bladder cancers, which are characterized by high-level ΔNp63 and Myc expression, could be especially sensitive to these agents.

HIF-1 is a transcription factor that is best known for its ability to induce expression of vascular endothelial growth factor. The authors' analyses of the gene expression patterns in the intrinsic subtypes of MIBC revealed that an HIF-1 signature was enriched in basal cancers.[7] Strikingly, p63 knockdown caused strong downregulation of this signature in human bladder cancer cell lines (Ochoa A, unpublished observation 2014), indicating that the HIF-1 signature is controlled by p63. High levels of vascular

389

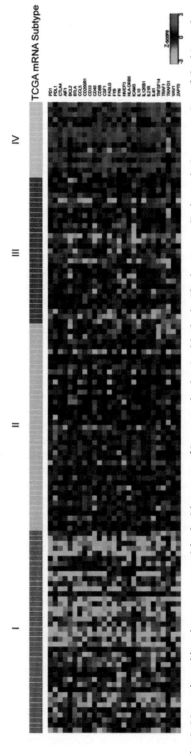

Fig. 4. Mesenchymal basal tumors are enriched with targets of immune checkpoint blockade. The heat map displays relative expression of the biomarkers contained within the immune signature reported in Choi and colleagues.[7] This signature contains the clinically actionable targets, CTLA4, PD-1, and PD-L1. Red, high relative expression; green, low relative expression.

endothelial growth factor (VEGF) correlated with poor outcomes in previous studies.[72,73] The authors recently performed intrinsic subtype assignments on tumors collected within the context of a phase II clinical trial of dose-dense MVAC plus bevacizumab (Avastin), a blocking antibody that is specific for the type-2 receptor for VEGF (VEGFR2). Patients with basal tumors experienced unusually good outcomes (Siefker-Radtke A, manuscript submitted), supporting the idea that HIF-1/VEGF signaling may be particularly important in basal tumors. A phase III clinical trial evaluating the efficacy of gemcitabine/cisplatin plus bevacizumab (NCT00942331) has nearly completed accrual. It will be interesting to determine whether patients with basal tumors obtained the most benefit from the combination.

Finally, as discussed earlier, a fraction of basal MIBCs is enriched with T and B lymphocyte and immune checkpoint biomarkers (CTLA4, PD-1, PD-L1).[7] In the recently completed phase I study of the blocking anti-PDL1 antibody MPDL3280A, 52% of patients with PD-L1–positive metastatic bladder cancers had objective Response evaluation criteria in solid tumors (RECIST) criteria responses, with complete responses observed in 7% of patients. The authors used the TCGA cohort to characterize expression of the immune signature they had linked to chemotherapy response (adding PD-1 and PD-L1) in their 4 intrinsic subtypes. The signature was highly enriched in the mesenchymal/claudin-low tumors represented by cluster IV (**Fig. 4**). The percentage of MIBCs contained within this mesenchymal subtype is very similar to the 7% of tumors that displayed complete responses in the completed phase I trial. It will be important to correlate the intrinsic subtypes with response to immune checkpoint inhibitors in future clinical trials.

SUMMARY AND FUTURE DIRECTIONS

There seem to be strong associations between intrinsic MIBC subtype membership and enrichment with clinically actionable genetic and epigenetic features. In addition, it seems that the intrinsic subtypes display differences in sensitivity to cisplatin-based combination chemotherapy. Because basal tumors are aggressive and chemosensitive, the overall impact of chemotherapy on disease-specific and overall survival should be carefully evaluated in patients with these tumors. Epigenetic mechanisms, including EMT and stromal fibroblast infiltration (plasticity), may impart resistance via mechanisms that are not captured in DNA mutation and CNV analyses. Therefore, future trials with targeted agents should evaluate not only the presence of actionable DNA mutations, translocations, and CNVs but also intrinsic subtype membership. In addition, investigators should continue to exploit the neoadjuvant platform to accelerate the clinical development of targeted agents and to identify mechanisms of induced resistance.

REFERENCES

1. Shah JB, McConkey DJ, Dinney CP. New strategies in muscle-invasive bladder cancer: on the road to personalized medicine. Clin Cancer Res 2011;17(9):2608–12.
2. Grossman HB. Neoadjuvant chemotherapy plus cystectomy compared with cystectomy alone for locally advanced bladder cancer. N Engl J Med 2003;349(9):859–66.
3. Sonpavde G. Second-line systemic therapy and emerging drugs for metastatic transitional-cell carcinoma of the urothelium. Lancet Oncol 2010;11(9):861–70.
4. Cancer Genome Atlas Research Network. Comprehensive molecular characterization of urothelial bladder carcinoma. Nature 2014;507(7492):315–22.

5. Iyer G. Prevalence and co-occurrence of actionable genomic alterations in high-grade bladder cancer. J Clin Oncol 2013;31(25):3133–40.
6. Sjodahl G. A molecular taxonomy for urothelial carcinoma. Clin Cancer Res 2012; 18(12):3377–86.
7. Choi W. Identification of distinct basal and luminal subtypes of muscle-invasive bladder cancer with different sensitivities to frontline chemotherapy. Cancer Cell 2014;25(2):152–65.
8. Damrauer JS. Intrinsic subtypes of high-grade bladder cancer reflect the hallmarks of breast cancer biology. Proc Natl Acad Sci U S A 2014;111(8):3110–5.
9. Iyer G. Genome sequencing identifies a basis for everolimus sensitivity. Science 2012;338(6104):221.
10. Dinney CP. Novel neoadjuvant paradigms for bladder cancer research: results from the National Cancer Center Institute Forum. Urol Oncol 2014;32(8):1108–15.
11. Lee JK. A strategy for predicting the chemosensitivity of human cancers and its application to drug discovery. Proc Natl Acad Sci U S A 2007;104(32):13086–91.
12. Powles T. Inhibition of PD-L1 by MPDL3280A and clinical activity in patients with metastatic urothelial bladder cancer (UBC). J Clin Oncol 2014;32(suppl):5s [abstract: 5011].
13. Perou CM. Molecular portraits of human breast tumours. Nature 2000;406(6797): 747–52.
14. Sorlie T. Gene expression patterns of breast carcinomas distinguish tumor subclasses with clinical implications. Proc Natl Acad Sci U S A 2001;98(19): 10869–74.
15. Prat A, Ellis MJ, Perou CM. Practical implications of gene-expression-based assays for breast oncologists. Nat Rev Clin Oncol 2012;9(1):48–57.
16. Prat A. Phenotypic and molecular characterization of the claudin-low intrinsic subtype of breast cancer. Breast Cancer Res 2010;12(5):R68.
17. Esserman LJ. Chemotherapy response and recurrence-free survival in neoadjuvant breast cancer depends on biomarker profiles: results from the I-SPY 1 TRIAL (CALGB 150007/150012; ACRIN 6657). Breast Cancer Res Treat 2012;132(3): 1049–62.
18. Esserman LJ. Pathologic complete response predicts recurrence-free survival more effectively by cancer subset: results from the I-SPY 1 TRIAL–CALGB 150007/150012, ACRIN 6657. J Clin Oncol 2012;30(26):3242–9.
19. Visvader JE. Keeping abreast of the mammary epithelial hierarchy and breast tumorigenesis. Genes Dev 2009;23(22):2563–77.
20. Cancer Genome Atlas Network. Comprehensive molecular portraits of human breast tumours. Nature 2012;490(7418):61–70.
21. Lozano G. The oncogenic roles of p53 mutants in mouse models. Curr Opin Genet Dev 2007;17(1):66–70.
22. Zhang XH. Latent bone metastasis in breast cancer tied to Src-dependent survival signals. Cancer Cell 2009;16(1):67–78.
23. Cooperberg MR. Combined value of validated clinical and genomic risk stratification tools for predicting prostate cancer mortality in a high-risk prostatectomy cohort. Eur Urol 2014. [Epub ahead of print].
24. Lauss M, Ringner M, Hoglund M. Prediction of stage, grade, and survival in bladder cancer using genome-wide expression data: a validation study. Clin Cancer Res 2010;16(17):4421–33.
25. Lotan Y. Prospective evaluation of a molecular marker panel for prediction of recurrence and cancer-specific survival after radical cystectomy. Eur Urol 2013;64(3):465–71.

26. Lindgren D. Combined gene expression and genomic profiling define two intrinsic molecular subtypes of urothelial carcinoma and gene signatures for molecular grading and outcome. Cancer Res 2010;70(9):3463–72.

27. Ho PL, Kurtova A, Chan KS. Normal and neoplastic urothelial stem cells: getting to the root of the problem. Nat Rev Urol 2012;9(10):583–94.

28. Chan KS. Identification, molecular characterization, clinical prognosis, and therapeutic targeting of human bladder tumor-initiating cells. Proc Natl Acad Sci U S A 2009;106(33):14016–21.

29. Volkmer JP. Three differentiation states risk-stratify bladder cancer into distinct subtypes. Proc Natl Acad Sci U S A 2012;109(6):2078–83.

30. Choi W. Intrinsic basal and luminal subtypes of muscle-invasive bladder cancer. Nat Rev Urol 2014;11:400–10.

31. McConkey DJ, Choi W, Dinney CP. New Insights into subtypes of invasive bladder cancer: considerations of the clinician. Eur Urol 2014;66:609–10.

32. Taube JH. Core epithelial-to-mesenchymal transition interactome gene-expression signature is associated with claudin-low and metaplastic breast cancer subtypes. Proc Natl Acad Sci U S A 2010;107(35):15449–54.

33. Rebouissou S. EGFR as a potential therapeutic target for a subset of muscle-invasive bladder cancers presenting a basal-like phenotype. Sci Transl Med 2014;6(244):244ra91.

34. Blaveri E. Bladder cancer outcome and subtype classification by gene expression. Clin Cancer Res 2005;11(11):4044–55.

35. Van Batavia J. Bladder cancers arise from distinct urothelial sub-populations. Nat Cell Biol 2014;16(10):982–91.

36. Carroll DK. p63 regulates an adhesion programme and cell survival in epithelial cells. Nat Cell Biol 2006;8(6):551–61.

37. Hoadley KA. Multiplatform analysis of 12 cancer types reveals molecular classification within and across tissues of origin. Cell 2014;158(4):929–44.

38. Cheung KJ, Gabrielson E, Werb Z, et al. Collective invasion in breast cancer requires a conserved basal epithelial program. Cell 2013;155(7):1639–51.

39. Ho PL, Lay EJ, Jian W, et al. Stat3 activation in urothelial stem cells leads to direct progression to invasive bladder cancer. Cancer Res 2012;72(13):3135–42.

40. Choi W. p63 expression defines a lethal subset of muscle-invasive bladder cancers. PLoS One 2012;7(1):e30206.

41. Karni-Schmidt O. Distinct expression profiles of p63 variants during urothelial development and bladder cancer progression. Am J Pathol 2011;178(3): 1350–60.

42. Marquis L. p63 expression correlates with sensitivity to the Eg5 inhibitor ZD4877 in bladder cancer cells. Cancer Biol Ther 2012;13(7):477–86.

43. Polyak K, Weinberg RA. Transitions between epithelial and mesenchymal states: acquisition of malignant and stem cell traits. Nat Rev Cancer 2009; 9(4):265–73.

44. Kalluri R, Weinberg RA. The basics of epithelial-mesenchymal transition. J Clin Invest 2009;119(6):1420–8.

45. Mani SA. The epithelial-mesenchymal transition generates cells with properties of stem cells. Cell 2008;133(4):704–15.

46. Tran MN. The p63 isoform DNp63a inhibits epithelial-mesenchymal transition in human bladder cancer cells: role of miR-205. J Biol Chem 2013;288:3275–88.

47. Gregory PA. The miR-200 family and miR-205 regulate epithelial to mesenchymal transition by targeting ZEB1 and SIP1. Nat Cell Biol 2008;10(5): 593–601.

48. Prowell TM, Pazdur R. Pathological complete response and accelerated drug approval in early breast cancer. N Engl J Med 2012;366(26):2438–41.
49. Denkert C. Tumor-associated lymphocytes as an independent predictor of response to neoadjuvant chemotherapy in breast cancer. J Clin Oncol 2010; 28(1):105–13.
50. Jackson JG. p53-mediated senescence impairs the apoptotic response to chemotherapy and clinical outcome in breast cancer. Cancer Cell 2012;21(6): 793–806.
51. Byrski T. Pathologic complete response to neoadjuvant cisplatin in BRCA1-positive breast cancer patients. Breast Cancer Res Treat 2014;147(2):401–5.
52. Narod SA. BRCA mutations in the management of breast cancer: the state of the art. Nat Rev Clin Oncol 2010;7(12):702–7.
53. Van Allen EM. Somatic ERCC2 mutations correlate with cisplatin sensitivity in muscle-invasive urothelial carcinoma. Cancer Discov 2014;4(10):1140–53.
54. Knowles MA, Platt FM, Ross RL, et al. Phosphatidylinositol 3-kinase (PI3K) pathway activation in bladder cancer. Cancer Metastasis Rev 2009;28(3–4): 305–16.
55. Knowles MA. Novel therapeutic targets in bladder cancer: mutation and expression of FGF receptors. Future Oncol 2008;4(1):71–83.
56. Williams SV, Hurst CD, Knowles MA. Oncogenic FGFR3 gene fusions in bladder cancer. Hum Mol Genet 2013;22(4):795–803.
57. Lamont FR. Small molecule FGF receptor inhibitors block FGFR-dependent urothelial carcinoma growth in vitro and in vivo. Br J Cancer 2011;104(1):75–82.
58. Ching CB. HER2 gene amplification occurs frequently in the micropapillary variant of urothelial carcinoma: analysis by dual-color in situ hybridization. Mod Pathol 2011;24(8):1111–9.
59. Ross JS. A high frequency of activating extracellular domain ERBB2 (HER2) mutation in micropapillary urothelial carcinoma. Clin Cancer Res 2014;20(1):68–75.
60. Wang X. Epidermal growth factor receptor protein expression and gene amplification in small cell carcinoma of the urinary bladder. Clin Cancer Res 2007;13(3): 953–7.
61. Black PC. Sensitivity to epidermal growth factor receptor inhibitor requires E-cadherin expression in urothelial carcinoma cells. Clin Cancer Res 2008;14(5): 1478–86.
62. Haddad Y, Choi W, McConkey DJ. Delta-crystallin enhancer binding factor 1 controls the epithelial to mesenchymal transition phenotype and resistance to the epidermal growth factor receptor inhibitor erlotinib in human head and neck squamous cell carcinoma lines. Clin Cancer Res 2009;15(2):532–42.
63. Witta SE. Restoring E-cadherin expression increases sensitivity to epidermal growth factor receptor inhibitors in lung cancer cell lines. Cancer Res 2006; 66(2):944–50.
64. Dominick MA. Urothelial carcinogenesis in the urinary bladder of male rats treated with muraglitazar, a PPAR alpha/gamma agonist: evidence for urolithiasis as the inciting event in the mode of action. Toxicol Pathol 2006;34(7):903–20.
65. Egerod FL, Brunner N, Svendsen JE, et al. PPARalpha and PPARgamma are co-expressed, functional and show positive interactions in the rat urinary bladder urothelium. J Appl Toxicol 2010;30(2):151–62.
66. Egerod FL. Biomarkers for early effects of carcinogenic dual-acting PPAR agonists in rat urinary bladder urothelium in vivo. Biomarkers 2005;10(4):295–309.
67. George SK. Chemoprevention of BBN-induced bladder carcinogenesis by the selective estrogen receptor modulator tamoxifen. Transl Oncol 2013;6(3):244–55.

68. Hoffman KL, Lerner SP, Smith CL. Raloxifene inhibits growth of RT4 urothelial carcinoma cells via estrogen receptor-dependent induction of apoptosis and inhibition of proliferation. Horm Cancer 2013;4(1):24–35.

69. Shen SS. Expression of estrogen receptors-alpha and -beta in bladder cancer cell lines and human bladder tumor tissue. Cancer 2006;106(12):2610–6.

70. Hsu I. Estrogen receptor alpha prevents bladder cancer via INPP4B inhibited akt pathway in vitro and in vivo. Oncotarget 2014;5(17):7917–35.

71. Hsu I. Suppression of ERbeta signaling via ERbeta knockout or antagonist protects against bladder cancer development. Carcinogenesis 2014;35(3):651–61.

72. Inoue K. The prognostic value of angiogenesis factor expression for predicting recurrence and metastasis of bladder cancer after neoadjuvant chemotherapy and radical cystectomy. Clin Cancer Res 2000;6(12):4866–73.

73. Slaton JW. Correlation of metastasis related gene expression and relapse-free survival in patients with locally advanced bladder cancer treated with cystectomy and chemotherapy. J Urol 2004;171(2 Pt 1):570–4.

74. McConkey D, Choi W, Dinney C. Reply to Mattias Aine, Fredrik Liedberg, Gottfrid Sjodahl, and Mattias Hoglund's letter to the editor re: David J. McConkey, Woonyoung Choi, Colin P.N. Dinney. New insights into subtypes of invasive bladder cancer: considerations of the clinician. Eur Urol 2014;66:609–10. Eur Urol 2014. [Epub ahead of print].

Index

Note: Page numbers of article titles are in **boldface** type.

Hematol Oncol Clin N Am 29 (2015) 395–407
http://dx.doi.org/10.1016/S0889-8588(15)00018-0
0889-8588/15/$ – see front matter © 2015 Elsevier Inc. All rights reserved.

Printed and bound by CPI Group (UK) Ltd, Croydon, CR0 4YY

07/10/2024

01040499-0006